T0334038

Child Welfare Systems and Migrant Children

International Policy Exchange Series

Published in collaboration with the
Center for International Policy Exchanges
University of Maryland

Series Editors
Douglas J. Besharov
Neil Gilbert

United in Diversity?
Comparing Social Models in Europe and America
Edited by Jens Alber and Neil Gilbert

The Korean State and Social Policy:
How South Korea Lifted Itself from Poverty and Dictatorship to Affluence
and Democracy
Stein Ringen, Huck-ju Kwon, Ilcheong Yi, Taekyoon Kim, and Jooha Lee

Child Protection Systems:
International Trends and Orientations
Edited by Neil Gilbert, Nigel Parton, and Marit Skivenes

The Age of Dualization:
The Changing Face of Inequality in Deindustrializing Societies
Edited by Patrick Emmenegger, Silja Häusermann, Bruno Palier, and
Martin Seeleib-Kaiser

Counting the Poor:
New Thinking About European Poverty Measures and Lessons for the United States
Edited by Douglas J. Besharov and Kenneth A. Couch

Social Policy and Citizenship:
The Changing Landscape
Edited by Adalbert Evers and Anne-Marie Guillemard

Chinese Policy in a Time of Transition
Edited by Douglas J. Besharov and Karen Baehler

Reconciling Work and Poverty Reduction:
How Successful Are European Welfare States?
Edited by Bea Cantillon and Frank Vandenbroucke

University Adaptation in Difficult Economic Times
Edited by Paola Mattei

Workfare Revisited:
Activation Reforms in Europe and America
Edited by Ivar Lødemel and Amílcar Moreira

Child Welfare Systems and Migrant Children:
A Cross Country Study of Policies and Practices
Edited by Marit Skivenes, Ravinder Barn, Katrin Križ, and Tarja Pösö

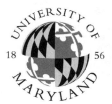

SCHOOL of
PUBLIC POLICY

CHILD WELFARE SYSTEMS AND MIGRANT CHILDREN

A Cross Country Study of Policies and Practices

Edited by

MARIT SKIVENES

RAVINDER BARN

KATRIN KRIŽ

TARJA PÖSÖ

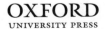

OXFORD
UNIVERSITY PRESS

OXFORD
UNIVERSITY PRESS

Oxford University Press is a department of the University of
Oxford. It furthers the University's objective of excellence in research,
scholarship, and education by publishing worldwide.

Oxford   New York
Auckland   Cape Town   Dar es Salaam   Hong Kong   Karachi
Kuala Lumpur   Madrid   Melbourne   Mexico City   Nairobi
New Delhi   Shanghai   Taipei   Toronto

With offices in
Argentina   Austria   Brazil   Chile   Czech Republic   France   Greece
Guatemala   Hungary   Italy   Japan   Poland   Portugal   Singapore
South Korea   Switzerland   Thailand   Turkey   Ukraine   Vietnam

Oxford is a registered trademark of Oxford University Press
in the UK and certain other countries.

Published in the United States of America by
Oxford University Press
198 Madison Avenue, New York, NY 10016

© Oxford University Press 2015

All rights reserved. No part of this publication may be reproduced, stored in
a retrieval system, or transmitted, in any form or by any means, without the prior
permission in writing of Oxford University Press, or as expressly permitted by law,
by license, or under terms agreed with the appropriate reproduction rights organization.
Inquiries concerning reproduction outside the scope of the above should be sent to the
Rights Department, Oxford University Press, at the address above.

You must not circulate this work in any other form
and you must impose this same condition on any acquirer.

Library of Congress Cataloging-in-Publication Data
Child welfare systems and migrant children : a cross country study of
policies and practice / edited by Marit Skivenes, Ravinder Barn, Katrin
Križ, Tarja Pösö.
   pages cm.— (International policy exchange series)
Includes bibliographical references and index.
ISBN 978-0-19-020529-4 (alk. paper)
1. Child welfare.   2. Immigrant children.   I. Skivenes, Marit.
HV713.C39537 2015
362.7′7912—dc23
2014022911

9 8 7 6 5 4 3 2 1
Printed in the United States of America
on acid-free paper

CONTENTS

ACKNOWLEDGMENTS

This project has received funding from the Norwegian Directorate for Children, Youth and Family Affairs covering expenditures for a meeting for the researchers in Bergen, Norway, in September 2012.

The research project "Norwegian Child Welfare Systems in a Comparative Perspective," funded by the Research Council of Norway (Program: FRISAM), has funded the work with the survey that was answered by almost 900 child welfare workers from nine countries. The editors wish to send a particular thanks to all child welfare workers who participated in our survey. We truly appreciate your important work. Hanne Stenberg shall have many thanks for her excellent work on organizing this complex survey process.

The editors are grateful for the hard work of the contributors to this book and for sharing their insights and interest on this important issue. Without them we would not have been able to turn this project into a book. Finally, we owe great thanks to Ida B. Juhasz for assisting us with the final rounds of the manuscript.

CONTRIBUTORS

RAVINDER BARN
School of Law
Centre for Criminology and Sociology
Royal Holloway
University of London
London, UK

ROBERTA TERESA DI ROSA
Department of Culture & Society
Area of Sociology
University of Palermo
Palermo, Italy

ILZE EARNER
School of Social Work
Hunter College
New York, NY

HANS GRIETENS
Centre for Special Needs Education &
    Youth Care
Faculty of Behavioral and Social Sciences
University of Groningen
Groningen, The Netherlands

ILAN KATZ
Social Policy Research Centre
University of New South Wales
Kensington, Australia

DEREK KIRTON
School of Social Policy
Sociology and Social Research
University of Kent
Kent, UK

KATRIN KRIŽ
Department of Sociology
Emmanuel College
Boston, MA

BRUCE LESLIE
Catholic Children's Aid Society of
Toronto and
Factor-Inwentash Faculty of
    Social Work
University of Toronto
Toronto, Canada

MERLE LINNO
Faculty of Social Sciences
   and Education
University of Tartu
Tartu, Estonia

SARAH MAITER
School of Social Work
Faculty of Liberal Arts and Professional
   Studies
York University
Toronto, Canada

ANTONIO LÓPEZ PELÁEZ
Department of Social Work
Faculty of Law
National Distance Education University
Madrid, Spain

TARJA PÖSÖ
School of Social Sciences and Humanities
University of Tampere
Tampere, Finland

CHRISTOPH REINPRECHT
Department of Sociology
University of Vienna
Vienna, Austria

SAGRARIO SEGADO SÁNCHEZ-CABEZUDO
Department of Social Work
Faculty of Law
National Distance Education University
Madrid, Spain

MARIT SKIVENES
Faculty of Health and Social Work
Bergen University College and
Department of Administration and
Organization Theory
University of Bergen
Bergen, Norway

JUDIT STRÖMPL
Faculty of Social Sciences and Education
University of Tartu
Tartu, Estonia

1

CHILD WELFARE SYSTEMS AND MIGRANT FAMILIES

AN INTRODUCTION

Ravinder Barn, Katrin Križ, Tarja Pösö, and Marit Skivenes

The aim of this book is to examine where, why, and how migrant children are represented in the child welfare systems[1] in 11 countries: Australia, Austria, Canada, England, Estonia, Finland, Italy, Norway, Spain, the Netherlands, and the United States. All of these countries have different histories and practices with migration, as well as various welfare state ideologies and child welfare system approaches. By comparing policies and practices in different types of child welfare systems and welfare states in terms of how they conceptualize and deal with migrant children and their families, we address an immensely important and pressing issue in modern societies. We understand "migrants" as people who move across national boundaries for whatever reason (out of free will or as refugees, displaced persons, etc.). In this book, we study the interactions between child welfare systems with migrants once they have arrived in a destination society of the global north—regardless of whether they intend to move on, return to their sending societies, or permanently settle in the new country as "immigrants."

Migrant children in the child welfare system are a critical issue, and they seem to face serious challenges that are evident across countries. Children may migrate with their parents, migrate alone, migrate as trafficking victims, or be left behind in the country of origin. Moreover, the contextual and temporal nature of migration has its own consequences for children in terms of health, education, social care, and crime. A range of factors including language and cultural barriers, uprootedness and instability, lack of access to basic services such as education and health, statelessness, discrimination, and social exclusion can all hamper the life chances of migrant children. And, of course, the vulnerability of children dramatically increases with irregular migration and the response of the receiving countries, whose laws may criminalize trafficked children or other migrant children and expose them to potential abuse during detention and deportation (UNICEF 2003, 2004; Touzenis, 2008). This book analyzes the child welfare systems' responses to the needs and rights of migrant children and families and is thus relevant for the wider field of health and social care professionals who meet and interact with migrant children and their families.

CONTEMPORARY CHILD WELFARE SYSTEMS

Societies differ in their ways of protecting children from abuse and neglect and providing for children's needs and interests. The recent cross-country analysis involving 10 high-income countries by Gilbert, Parton, and Skivenes (2011) highlights that a child-centric orientation is emerging within Western societies. The child-centric orientation regards children as individuals with particular rights and needs and complements the two traditional orientations: "family-service" and "child protection." Family service systems are concerned with service provisions to families; they are based on a therapeutic idea of rehabilitation and people's ability to revise and improve their lifestyle and behavior. The logic behind family service systems is that the child welfare system should provide services to prevent more serious harm and thus prevent out-of-home placements. The threshold for intervention is low. Child protection systems, on the other hand, are not built around service provision to prevent possible harm but around intervention when there is serious risk of harm for a child; therefore, the threshold for intervention is set to be high and the ambition is to provide services for a possible reunification. This book includes child welfare systems that represent all three orientations, with Finland, Norway, and the Netherlands as family service and child-centric child welfare systems; Austria, Spain, and Italy as family service–oriented systems; and Australia, England, Estonia, Canada, and the United States as child protection–oriented child welfare systems.

Child protection systems do not function in isolation but are related to the existing policy and legislation of each country. The systems are influenced by the general welfare of the countries and the welfare of families and children in particular. This is why we grouped the countries in this book by welfare state systems, based on the typology of welfare regimes by Esping-Andersen (1990) as further developed by Arts and Gelissen (2002). The Gilbert et al. (2011) study mentioned previously is based on the analysis of 10 wealthy Western countries that have traditions of social welfare that differ significantly from those of less economically developed countries, some of which have introduced only very limited and fragmentary forms of public services for children and families. When comparing the indicators of children's well-being, considerable differences among countries have been found. In a recent UNICEF study, inequality gaps for children were studied and children's well-being was measured along dimensions of material well-being, education, health, behaviors and risks, and housing. Table 1.1 shows the overall results, in which each country's overall rank is based on its average ranking for these five dimensions of child well-being (UNICEF, 2013: 2).

A light grey background indicates a place in the top third of the well-being score, mid-grey denotes the middle third, and dark grey represents the bottom third—the lower the score, the higher the children's well-being in that country. (UNICEF, 2013: 2).

Further, Table 1.2 shows poverty rates for children and the total population in the 11 countries analyzed in this book. According to the Organisation for Economic Co-operation and Development (OECD; 2011), 13% of all children (below age 18) lived in poverty across the 34 OECD countries in 2008. In the social democratic welfare states, child poverty rates were below 10%, whereas the conservative welfare states were around 15% to 18%, and the liberal welfare states varied from 12% to above 20% in the United States (OECD, 2011).[2]

We can see that the countries offering a wide provision of welfare services, such as the Nordic countries, tend to rank highly in these comparisons. Countries also regulate migration in different ways. In the literature on international migration research, it is common to distinguish between three policy

Table 1.1. Child well-being index

Country	Average rank (all five dimensions)	Material well-being (rank)	Health and safety (rank)	Education (rank)	Behaviors and risks (rank)	Housing and environment (rank)
Netherlands	2.4	1	5	1	1	4
Norway	4.6	3	7	6	4	3
Finland	5.4	2	3	4	12	6
United Kingdom	15.8	14	16	24	15	10
Canada	16.6	15	27	14	16	11
Austria	17	7	26	23	17	12
Spain	17.6	24	9	26	20	9
Italy	19.2	23	17	25	10	21
Estonia	20.8	19	22	13	26	24
United States	24.8	26	25	27	23	23

Note: Boldface indicates a place in the top one-third.
Source: UNICEF, 2013: 2.

Table 1.2. Poverty rates for children and the total population, 2008

Country	Total population (%)	Children (%)
Finland	8.0	5.4
Norway	7.8	5.5
Austria	7.9	7.9
Netherlands	7.4	9.7
Spain	14.0	17.7
Italy	11.4	15.3
United States	17.3	21.6
Canada	12.0	15.1
United Kingdom	11.0	12.5
Australia	14.6	14.0
Estonia	12.5	12.1
OECD 34-average	11.1	12.6

Source: OECD, 2011.

models concerning how states manage ethnic diversity (Sainsbury, 2006) and in particular how a country's rules and norms affect inclusion into and exclusion from social services (Castles and Miller, 2003). The three models are (a) the differential exclusionary model, (b) the assimilationist model, and (c) the multicultural model. In the differential exclusionary model, states treat migrants differently from the nonmigrant populations, for instance through social services and housing policies. States following the assimilation approach promote migrants' assimilation such as language learning and incorporating migrant children into the mainstream education system. In the multicultural model, the state supports ethnic community formation and provides services toward migrants' integration into the host society (Castles and Miller, 2003; Sainsbury, 2006). Typical of these models is their focus on adults. Therefore, our focus on migrant children and their needs and rights at the juncture of child protection and migration policies may cast new light on both the migration and welfare studies, as well as studies of child welfare policy.

CHILD WELFARE SYSTEMS AND MIGRANT CHILDREN

Countrywide child welfare systems are, by their very nature, based on national jurisdiction and policies. Such national legislation is, self-evidently, valid only in certain political and geographical areas. However, there are and have been child welfare activities that transcend the borders of nation states. For example, the United Nations Convention on the Rights of the Child has created a globally recognized norm structure for child welfare. Moreover, charity organizations, nongovernmental associations and international agencies such as UNICEF, among many others, have acted globally to promote the best interests of all children.

As migration has increased globally, national child welfare systems have become challenged in meeting the needs and concerns of migrating children and families. A key question has been raised by those working in the field of child welfare: how do and can public authorities meet the needs and rights of these children and families? In the welfare state literature, there is debate about the solidarity foundation for the social security net and how increased migration and heterogeneity may dissolve this foundation (cf., e.g., Mau and Burkhardt, 2009). Are we witnessing some of the same challenges in the child welfare systems and their approach to migrant children? Clearly a fundamental change in the welfare states meeting with migrants is that residency matters more and more. Some scholars conceptualize this as the denationalization of solidarity practices (Mau and Burkhardt, 2009), which shows how new population groups that are present in a nation are included in the welfare state on other premises than nationality.

People migrate from one country to another for several reasons. They may look for safety and refuge or employment and education; some may look for better living conditions or fulfilment of personal interests and family ties. Ecological disasters, military conflicts, and the uneven distribution of resources across the globe entice people to move to the extent that these changes are seen to be major challenges for social welfare and human rights globally. Existing studies suggest that people who migrate are younger than the population in general, and therefore the issue of families and children becomes a relevant migration concern. There are also such distinctive themes such as unaccompanied migrant children, transnational families, international adoptions, and child trafficking, which increase the complexity of migration issues of our time (Alba and Waters, 2011). The situation for an unaccompanied refugee child is different from the needs of a child whose family is moving to a new country because the parents were invited to work in a highly skilled job. Nevertheless, entering and living in a new country with its cultural norms and traditions may mean the newcomers encounter the kinds of problems that the child welfare systems are likely to deal with.

There are, for instance, challenges related to language proficiency, knowledge about cultural and social aspects, and knowledge about the public systems of the destination country (Barn, 2007; Chand, 2008; Dettlaff, 2008; Križ and Skivenes, 2009, 2010a, 2010b). Perhaps most significantly, the challenges may include collisions of ideas and beliefs about how to raise children, children's place in the family and society, and children's rights. Academic research evidence in this area from across the globe is growing and suggests the need to take into account the effects of immigration status, the impact of migration and acculturation, families' socioeconomic situation, and the need for comprehensive cultural assessments of children and families (Earner, 2005; Rome, 2010). However, overall we know little about how child welfare systems operate with newcomers who are children and families with a migrant background. Increasing the knowledge base about this important theme was the main rationale behind writing this book.

MIGRATION TRENDS AND PUBLIC POLICIES

The process of migration and its consequences for public service provision are an important concern among academics, practitioners, and policymakers. The impetus for this book arose from a recognition of the recent growth in migration, the resulting increase in racial and cultural heterogeneity in Western societies, and the question of how welfare states, especially child welfare service providers, deal with this heterogeneity when interacting with migrant children and their families. Although Western societies cannot claim to have been historically culturally homogenous, it is evident that in contemporary times the forces of globalization have led to greater movements of people resulting in vast changes in the social, cultural, economic, and political landscape.

While the economic processes of globalization are in evidence in regard to finance, communication, deregulation, and trade liberalization, we are also witnessing the impact of globalization on the relationships between people and cultures across international boundaries. Historically, while colonialism, slavery, and imperialism led to the transportation of Africans and South Asians to the Caribbean, the Americas, and Africa during the eighteenth and nineteenth centuries, we know that a desire among the colonizers to populate the newfound lands with white "stock" also resulted in the movement of white Europeans to Australia, Canada, New Zealand, and the Americas—thereby changing the racial and cultural demography of these spaces (Jupp, 2002).

Free mass migration—in which people migrate out of their own free will (and are not coerced to migrate as slaves or indentured servants)—is a phenomenon that is relatively recent (Williamson, 2006). In 2008, the United Nations (UN) estimated that the number of international migrants would reach 214 million (or 3.1% of the world population) by 2010; 16.3 million international migrants were refugees (UN, 2009). The proportion of migrants who were women was projected to be 49.0% by 2010. In terms of age, the median age of international migrants was 39 years in 2010, compared to the median age of 28 years in the total world population. Compared to the total world population, international migrants are overproportionally of working age and over age 65; young people are underrepresented among migrants (Henning, 2012). The regions of the global north are currently experiencing the major gains in in-migration (UN, 2009). In 2010, 59.7% of all international migrants lived in these regions, while 40.3% lived in the global south (Henning, 2012). Migration within the global south countries is as common as south–north migration (Henning, 2012). In terms of world regions, by 2010, the UN (2009) expected Europe to host 70 million migrants, Asia 61 million, North America 50 million, Africa 19 million, Latin America and the Caribbean 7 million, and Oceania 6 million international migrants (UN, 2009). Table 1.3 shows foreign-born populations in the 11 countries represented in this book.[3]

In contemporary times, whether as a consequence of economic inequalities, wars, or conflict, there have been movements of people across transnational borders in unprecedented numbers. World migration has dramatically increased especially since the 1960s (Williamson, 2006; Henning, 2012), even though the recent economic recession has decreased the movement of labor, particularly in the IT, construction, and manufacturing sectors (International Organization for Migration [IOM], 2012). The annual growth rate of migrants amounted to about 2.1% between 1965 and 1990. Today, it stands at 2.9% (IOM, 2012). Since World War II, there have been four significant trends in world migration: first, Latin America, formerly primarily a destination world region, has become a major sending region. Second, migration from Asia, Africa, and the Middle East has significantly increased. Third, the number of European emigrants has declined because of a growing migration within Europe. Fourth, since the 1980s, migration from Eastern Europe has increased (Williamson, 2006). Since the European enlargement in 2004, there has been an increase of migrant families and children from countries such as Albania, Bulgaria, Hungary, Latvia, and Poland. Labor migration within Europe has impacted more upon some countries than others. For example, three-quarters of the migrant population in Europe resides in a handful of countries—namely France, Germany, Italy, Spain and the United Kingdom (Council of Europe, 2011).

Table 1.3. Foreign-born population, by country

Country	Foreign-born as percentage of the total population (year of measurement)
Australia	26.8 (2010)
Austria	15.7 (2010)
Canada	19.9 (2010)
Estonia	16.3 (2010)
Finland	4.6 (2010)
Italy	8.0 (2009)
Netherlands	11.2 (2010)
Norway	11.6 (2010)
Spain	14.5 (2010)
United Kingdom	11.5 (2010)
United States	12.9 (2010)

Source: OECD, 2012.

The reasons why and conditions in which people migrate are numerous. They include a global trade and investment environment, particularly trade liberalization that favors the movement of labor and has resulted in a demand for labor in the global north, drawing on labor from the south. Migration cannot be understood without taking into account the economic disparities between the global south and north and recent demographic trends in the world population. Rapid population growth and economic hardship in the global south motivate people to migrate. At the same time, low fertility in the global north has resulted in smaller and aging populations, thus creating pull factors for migration toward the north. Transnational migrant networks between sending and destination societies have also played a key role in migration at the same time as modern transportation and communication technologies have fostered the international flow of people, information, skills, and remittances (IOM, 2012).

Migration to Western countries from non-OECD countries presents a challenge in a number of ways, from concerns about pressures on public services to a shared national identity and social cohesion. Such concerns are frequently located within racial and cultural demographic changes. Significantly, although Western nations need migrant labor, they continue to manifest ambivalence toward migrants from some parts of the globe, particularly those coming from non-OECD countries. In a study of European migration and policy trends, Boswell (2005: 5) reports that "anti-immigrant sentiment has manifested itself in public support for restrictive immigration and asylum policies, negative reporting on immigrants and asylum-seekers in the popular press, discrimination against resident ethnic minority groups, and racist or anti-immigrant harassment and violence."

Although some commonality is emerging with respect to citizenship, nationality, and language tests, there is tremendous variety in the ways in which nation-states seek to deal with immigration and its effects. Arguably, history and experience of immigration may be among the key factors in how governments and civil society take responsibility for the integration process (Haque, 2010). However, it cannot be assumed that length of exposure to migrants from a different culture is likely to result in what may be conceived as tolerance to diversity.

As migration is a problem-solving, as well as a problem-generating phenomenon (Soydan, 1998) and as social workers are, in many countries, the professionals meeting the social needs and social problems of migrant children and families, this book also examines the training of social workers and asks how the rights and needs of migrant children are included in the training of social workers. It is widely acknowledged that the term "social work" is increasingly difficult to pin down both within and across national boundaries (e.g., Williams, Soydan, and Johnson, 1998; Lyons, Manion, and Carlsen, 2006). The terms employed to refer to practitioners also vary (social workers, child welfare workers, care/case workers, social pedagogues, among many others) as do the educational programs. Within Europe, for example, some countries recognize only a university master's degree in social work while others accept a bachelor's degree from a university or polytechnic/university of applied sciences. The general trend is that an increasing number of these education programs are aiming at master's-level degrees (Matthies, 2011). Regardless of the differences in educational structures, there are global standards for education and training set by the International Federation of Social Workers (IFSW, 2012). The profession of social work is built on the core values of human rights and social justice. These values also characterize the frame for IFSW's approach to globalization. Notably, however, migration as a specific issue is not discussed in any detail in the resolution of globalization, educational standards, or the code of ethics. Cultural and ethnic diversity, within the frame of human rights and social justice, is highlighted in both educational standards and the code of ethics. Further, the IFSW underlines that the social work profession should recognize and act against the new inequalities resulting from social, economic, and ecological globalization (ISFW, 2012).

MIGRANT CHILDREN AND INTERNATIONAL LAW

Migration affects children in many and diverse ways and may expose them to violence and exploitation. Touzenis (2008: 13) notes that "there is no international or regional legislative framework dealing directly with child migrants." There are several international legal instruments that aim at protecting migrant children by creating legal obligations for those UN member states that ratify them. The United Nations Convention on the Rights of the Child, which has been ratified by all UN member states with the exception of the United States and Somalia, is intended to protect every child irrespective of their nationality, immigration status, or statelessness. Core principles include the child's best interests, participation, development, evolving capacities, and nondiscrimination (Touzikis, 2008). The principles that are particularly relevant for the protection of migrant children are "the right to a nationality, physical integrity, the highest attainable standard of health, education, and the right to be free from discrimination, exploitation, and abuse" (UNICEF, 2004: 55). The following articles are particularly pertinent for the protection of migrant children: Article 10 on family reunification; Article 36 on protection from all forms of exploitation; and Article 37 on protection from torture or other cruel, inhuman, or degrading treatment or punishment and from unlawful and arbitrary deprivation of liberty (UNICEF, 2004). Other protective international legal instruments, which have, however, not been ratified by all UN member states, include the Palermo Protocol, ILO Convention 182, the Optional Protocol on the Sale of Children, Child Prostitution and Child Pornography, and the Protocol to Prevent, Suppress and Punish Trafficking in Persons, Especially Women and Children that supplements the Convention against Transnational Organised Crime (UNICEF, 2003, 2004). While policymakers have focused on issues such as child trafficking, asylum-seeking, and refugee children, they have paid much less attention to how children are affected by immigration policies and how children left in sending societies are affected by adult migration (Touzenis, 2008).

CONTESTED AND VALUE-BASED CONCEPTS

The IOM underscores that there is "no universally accepted definition of migrant" (IOM, 2004: 40). Obviously an important reason for this is that concepts and terminology are disputed as they are embedded with normative and political values and interests. It is almost impossible to get it right, and within a cross-country study, the challenges and problems with concepts and cultural interpretations and practices are acutely present. We have chosen a set of definitions that is to be used within different countries and simultaneously provides direction and a framework for the comparative analysis this book sets out to undertake. The definition the IOM (2004: 40) provides of "migrant" emphasizes the free motivation behind the movement of migrating individuals:

> the term migrant is usually understood to cover all cases where the decision to migrate is taken freely by the individual concerned for reasons of "personal convenience" and without intervention of an external compelling factor. This term therefore applies to persons, and family members, moving to another country or region to better their material or social conditions and improve the prospect for themselves or their family.

"Migration," on the other hand, is defined as "any kind of movement of people, whatever its length, composition and causes; it includes migration of refugees, displaced persons, uprooted people, and economic migrants" (IMO 2004: 41). The IOM defines "immigration" as "the process by which non-nationals move into a country for the purpose of settlement" (IOM, 2004: 31). In this book, our focus is on the interactions between child welfare systems and migrants once they have arrived in a destination society of the global north, regardless of whether they intend to move on, return to their sending societies, or permanently settle there as "immigrants" (by the previously noted IOM definition). As terminology in the area of migration and immigration differs between countries, and to a varying degree is politically charged, each chapter brings forward how the child welfare literature and policies on migration or immigration in their respective country understand and use these terms.

The visibility of the migrant "others" who arrive with their own customs, values, traditions, and mores is often described by policymakers to be in direct conflict with the population of the receiving countries. It is this visibility expressed through clothes (e.g., headscarf, salwaar/kameez, sari), religion, language, food, and so on that marks these groups as "others"—the outsiders (Becker, 1963). The process of "otherisation," which marks out these individuals and groups as different, operates in essentialist terms to confer identities and ways of being to entire groups and communities whereby individual transgressions may be conceptualized as cultural and community problems. In other words, the entire group can come to be seen as problematic and associated with negativity through exposure in right-wing media and elsewhere through processes of politicking (e.g., with terms such "unwanted," "poor," "bogus," "drain on the economy," and "primitive") in highly dubious ways that challenge social cohesion and integration between groups and communities. Arguably, the continual reinforcement of such negative thinking widens the chasm whereby the settled and newly arrived immigrant groups bear the brunt of anti-immigrant sentiments.

Children may grow up in a hostile environment that looks at them only as members of a "migrant category" and overlooks their personality, interests, and agency. Children may develop strategies to cope with the hostility, change, or fight against it. The dilemmas and challenges in the processes of migration and discussions of how best to integrate the newly arrived children and their families are particularly relevant for the child welfare systems. Conflicts and tensions around child-rearing practices, the child's position in the family, children's rights, and generally the view on children's status and position are examples of issues that may be perceived very differently for a migrant and the society. Thus conflicts and tensions between newcomers and the host country about children's well-being are to be expected. The size of the gaps between migrant groups and host countries' values and standards is likely to have a huge impact on the roles and responsibilities a child welfare system has toward migrant children.

THE ORGANIZATION OF THE BOOK

Throughout this book we discuss how 11 countries' child welfare systems approach migrant children and families that are in need of child welfare intervention and help. Each individual chapter addresses the following five topics and questions:

(1) Law and policy: We outline what kind of platform the law and public policy creates for the well-being of migrant children and for child welfare systems working with migrant children who are at risk of neglect and abuse. To what degree are migrant children a focus of governmental policies? What critical issues do law and public policy

outline in terms of migrant children and their families? How do law and policy define problems and solutions?

(2) Organization: We examine the respective child welfare systems at the institutional and organizational levels, analyzing how different child welfare systems at the agency level interpret and develop politics, law, and policies into practice guidelines, procedures, manuals, and so on. We aim to analyze different domains in the child welfare system, including foster care, residential care, and child protection statistics. How are child welfare agencies organized to practice with migrant families? For instance, are there specific units working with migrant families?

(3) Training: We discuss the training and education that frontline child welfare workers practicing with migrant children and their families obtain. How are they trained in working with immigrant service users? Are they trained in culturally sensitive or antioppressive practice? What do training curricula look like?

(4) Representation of migrant children: We analyze to what extent migrant children are represented in the child welfare system and explore their characteristics: Are migrant children overrepresented or underrepresented compared to nonmigrant children? Who exactly are the migrant children represented in the child welfare system (ethnicity, country of origin, first- or second-generation status, etc.)? What are the types of risks and problems of the migrant children who have entered the child welfare system?

(5) Practice: We discuss what frontline practice with migrant families looks like in the respective countries. How do child welfare workers actually practice with migrants in different systems? This question is answered by an identical survey of child welfare workers in the countries represented in this book except Australia and the Netherlands. In each country, we used the same vignette, and in each country, we asked child welfare workers about their perceptions of the problem in the case vignettes and what they would do about the problem. Further, we asked workers about their experiences in interacting with service users with a migrant back ground. The survey methodology is discussed in the book's appendix.

For Canada, England, Finland, the Netherlands, Norway, and the United States, the book *Child Welfare Systems* (Gilbert et al., 2011) provides a comprehensive and detailed outline of their child welfare systems, but for the remaining countries there is a dearth of information in English on this matter and thus the chapters about these countries also present an outline of the basic features of their child welfare systems. The book contains 11 country chapters, followed by a concluding chapter and a methodological appendix. Following Gilbert et al.'s (2011) book on child protection systems and Arts and Gelissen's (2002) state-of-the-art article about welfare state typologies, combined with information from the country authors, we start with the four countries with a family service child welfare state that are considered social democratic welfare states: Finland, Norway, the Netherlands, and Austria. These countries are followed by family service child welfare systems within conservative (and Latin) welfare state countries—Spain and Italy. The third section comprises the countries with child protection–oriented child welfare systems that operate within liberal welfare states: the United States, Canada, England, Australia, and Estonia. In the conclusion, the editors summarize and discuss the most evident trends and challenges.

NOTES

1 We use the term "child welfare system" well aware that in many circumstances it is just as appropriate to use the term "child protection system." Empirically, we see that in comparative studies there can be difficulties differentiating between child welfare and child protection parts in a system that seeks to protect children (Hetherington et al., 1997; Gilbert, 1997; Gilbert, Parton, and Skivenes, 2011).
2 In this OECD report, the child poverty rate refers to "the share of all children living in households with an equivalised disposable income of less than 50% of the median for the population" (OECD, 2011: 1). The poverty rate for the total population is "the share of all individuals with an equivalised income of less than 50% of the median" (OECD, 2011: 1).
3 The term "foreign-born" applies to those individuals not born in the country to which they have migrated and does not denote ethnicity.

REFERENCES

Alba, R., & Waters, M. (2011). *The Next Generation: Immigrant Youth in a Comparative Perspective*. New York: New York University Press.

Arts, W., & Gelissen, J. (2002). Three worlds of welfare capitalism or more? A state-of-the-art-report. *Journal of European Social Policy*, 12(2), 137–158.

Barn, R. (2007). "Race," ethnicity and child welfare: A fine balancing act, critical commentary. *British Journal of Social Work*, 37(8), 1425–1434.

Becker H. (1963). *Outsiders: Studies in Sociology of Deviance*. New York: Free Press of Glencoe.

Boswell, C. (2005). *The Ethics of Refugee Policy*. Aldershot: Ashgate.

Castles, S., & Miller, M.J. (2003). *The Age of Migration: International Population Movements in the Modern World*. Basingstoke: Macmillan.

Chand, A. (2008). Every child matters? A critical review of child welfare reforms in the context of minority ethnic children and families. *Child Abuse Review*, 17(1), 6–22.

Council of Europe. (2011). Framework for Council of Europe Work on Migration Issues. Strasbourg: Council of Europe.

Dettlaff, A.J. (2008). Immigrant Latino children and families in child welfare: A framework for conducting a cultural assessment. *Journal of Public Child Welfare*, 2(4), 451–470.

Earner, I. (2005). Systemic issues in child welfare: Immigrant children and youth in the child welfare system. In G.P. Mallon & P. McCartt Hess (Eds.), *Child Welfare for the Twenty-First Century*, 655–664. New York: Columbia University Press.

Esping-Andersen, G. (1990). *The Three Worlds of Welfare Capitalism*. London: Polity Press.

Gilbert, N., ed. (1997). *Combatting Child Abuse: International Perspectives and Trends*. New York: Oxford University Press.

Gilbert, N., Parton, N., & Skivenes, M. (2011). *Child Protection Systems: International Trends and Orientations*. Oxford: Oxford University Press.

Haque, Z. (2010). *What Works with Integrating New Migrants? Lessons from International Best Practice*. London: Runnymede Trust.

Hetherington, R., Cooper, A., Smith, P., & Wilford, G. (1997). *Protecting Children: Messages from Europe*. Lyme Regis: Russell House.

Henning, S. (2012). Migration Levels and Trends: Global Assessment and Policy Implications. Retrieved August 18, 2012 from http://www.un.org/esa/population/meetings/tenthcoord2012/V.%20Sabine%20Henning%20-%20Migration%20trends.pdf.

International Federation of Social Workers (IFSW). (2012). Global Standards International Federation of Social Workers. Retrieved on October 14, 2012, from http://ifsw.org/policies/global-standards/.

International Organization for Migration (IOM). (2004). Glossary of Migration. Retrieved August 18, 2012, from http://publications.iom.int/bookstore/free/IML_1_EN.pdf.

———. (2012). About Migration. Retrieved August 18, 2012, from http://www.iom.int/jahia/Jahia/about-migration/lang/en.

Jupp, J. (2002). *From White Australia to Woomera*. Melbourne: Cambridge University Press.

Križ, K., & Skivenes, M. (2009). "Knowing our society" and "fighting against prejudices": How child welfare workers in Norway and England perceive the challenges of minority parents. *British Journal of Social Work*, 40(8), 2634–2651.

———. (2010a). Lost in translation: How child welfare workers in Norway and England experience language difficulties when working with minority ethnic families. *British Journal of Social Work*, 40, 1353–1367.

———. (2010b). "We have very different positions on some issues": How child welfare workers in Norway and England bridge cultural differences when communicating with ethnic minority families. *European Journal of Social Work*, 13(1), 3–18.

Lyons, K., Manion, K., & Carlsen, M. (2006). *International Perspectives on Social Work. Global Conditions and Local Practices*. Basingstoke: Palgrave Macmillan.

Matthies, A.-L. (2011). Social service professions towards cross-European standardisation of qualifications: Social work. *Social Work & Society*, 9(1), 89–107.

Mau, S., & Burkhardt, C. (2009). Migration and welfare state solidarity in Western Europe. *Journal of European Social Policy*, 19(3), 213–229.

Organisation for Economic Co-operation and Development (OECD). (2009). OECD Child Well-Being Module: Educational Deprivation. Retrieved on November 15, 2012, from http://www.oecd.org/els/familiesandchildren/48968185.pdf.

———. (2011). CO2.2: Child Poverty. Retrieved on November 16, 2012, from http://www.oecd.org/els/familiesandchildren/oecdfamilydatabase.htm#child_outcomes.

———. (2012). International Migration Outlook 2012: Country Notes. Retrieved on November 15, 2012, from http://www.oecd.org/migration/internationalmigrationpoliciesanddata/internationalmigrationoutlook-2012countrynotes.htm.

Rome, S.H. (2010). Promoting family integrity: The Child Citizen Protection Act and its implications for public child welfare. *Journal of Public Child Welfare*, 4(3), 245–262.

Sainsbury, D. (2006). Immigrants' social rights in comparative perspective: Welfare regimes, forms in immigration and immigration policy regimes, *Journal of European Social Policy*, 16(3), 229–244.

Soydan, H. (1998). Understanding migration. In C. Williams, H. Soydan, & M. Johnson (Eds.), *Social Work and Minorities: European Perspectives*, 20–35. New York: Routledge.

Touzenis, K. (2008). Human Rights of Migrant Children. Working Paper on International Migration Law 15. Retrieved August 18, 2012, fromvhttp://www.unicef.org/socialpolicy/index_48020.html.

UNICEF. (2013). Child Well-Being in Rich Countries: A Comparative Overview. Retrieved on December 17, 2013, from http://www.unicef-irc.org/publications/pdf/rc11_eng.pdf.

United Nations. (2009). Trends in International Migrant Stock: The 2008 Revision. Retrieved August 18, 2012, from http://www.un.org/esa/population/migration/UN_MigStock_2008.pdf.

United Nations Children's Fund. (2003). A Child-Right's Approach to International Migration: A UNICEF Perspective on Child Trafficking. Retrieved August 18, 2012, from http://www.un.org/esa/population/meetings/firstcoord2002/unicef.pdf.

———. (2004). A Child-Rights Approach on International Migration and Child Trafficking: A UNICEF Perspective. Retrieved August 18, 2012, from http://www.un.org/esa/population/meetings/thirdcoord2004/P06_UNICEF.pdf.

Williams, C., Soydan, H., & Johnson, M. (1998). *Social Work and Minorities: European Perspectives*. New York: Routledge.

Williamson, J.G. (2006). Global migration. *Finance and Development*, 43(3). Retrieved August 18, 2012, from http://www.imf.org/external/pubs/ft/fandd/2006/09/williams.htm.

PART I

FAMILY SERVICE–ORIENTED CHILD WELFARE SYSTEMS WITHIN SOCIAL DEMOCRATIC WELFARE STATES

2

HOW THE FINNISH CHILD PROTECTION SYSTEM MEETS THE NEEDS OF MIGRANT FAMILIES AND CHILDREN

Tarja Pösö

INTRODUCTION

In 2010, 4.6% of the people living in Finland were foreign-born. Ten years previously, in 2000, the number was 2.6% (Organisation for Economic Co-operation and Development [OECD], 2012). These figures indicate that Finland belongs to the OECD countries with the lowest levels of migration (Schierup, Hansen, and Castels, 2006). Consequently, Finland remains a homogeneous country in terms of people's national backgrounds. Finland's main indigenous ethnic, cultural, and language minorities have historically been very small, with the Swedish-speaking population comprising roughly 6% of the whole population, and the Roma and Saame people both less than approximately 1%. The country's homogeneity is also reflected in the fact that the social and economic differences between social classes have been relatively small.

Therefore, the notions of *unity* and *uniformity* have characterized Finnish society more so than those of diversity and differences (Raunio, Säävälä, Hammar-Suutari, and Pitkänen, 2011). However, the increase in migration, albeit small, means that the society is presently undergoing a change.

Considering the short history and low levels of migration to the country, migrant families and children constitute a new group in the welfare state system, challenging the system to react, adapt, and be reformulated (e.g., Brochmann and Hagelund, 2011). The challenges may differ fundamentally from those in countries with a long history of migration, and they may affect the Finnish ethos as a Nordic welfare state in a very particular way, as is demonstrated in this chapter.

This chapter describes and analyzes how the Finnish child welfare system responds to migrant families and children. Even though the message from the field suggests that social workers encounter new challenges when working with migrant families, the theme has not been studied to a great extent in the child welfare literature. The key text from the child welfare point of view is the study by Merja Anis (2008), which analyzes the encounters between migrant clients and child protection workers. This text emphasizes the cultural elements as the key aspect of child welfare with migrant families (e.g., Heikkilä-Daskalopoulos, 2008; Laakkonen, 2012). Other studies have examined migration from the point(s) of view of childhood, youth, and families (e.g., Keskinen, 2011; Honkatukia and Suurpää, 2007; Rastas, 2007), as well as social, educational, and health services and youth work (e.g., Clarke, 2004; Hammar-Suutari, 2009; Säävälä, 2011; Honkasalo, 2011).

The lack of specific research and statistics about migrant children in the child welfare system is demonstrated throughout this chapter. The results of a survey of 76 social workers working with migrant children and families in child protection are presented here in relevant contexts throughout the chapter (the details of the survey are discussed in the methodological appendix). The first part of the chapter provides an overview of the child protection system and migration and related legislation, organization, and practice, whereas the second part highlights and discusses the present challenges and dilemmas.

SETTING THE CONTEXT

The Finnish Child Protection System

When presenting the Finnish child welfare system in English, one always struggles with how to translate the concepts used, in particular the distinction between "child welfare" and "child protection" (Pösö, 2011). This is because Finnish society recognizes that its duties toward children are more encompassing than just protecting them from abuse, harm, and neglect. Therefore, all children and families with children are provided with a wide set of universal services and benefits as part of the Nordic welfare state model supporting child care (Eydal and Kröger, 2010). These services and benefits are often called "child welfare." Child and family-specific services for children and families experiencing some kind of risk, as defined by the Child Welfare Act, also exist. To draw a distinction between the universal child welfare services and the targeted statutory child welfare system, I use the term "child protection" to address the latter.

In Finland, the national Child Welfare Act regulates child protection. The latest Act was introduced in 2007 (417/2007). In line with the previous acts, it establishes the child's best interest as the leading principle but asks the authorities to enable children's participation in child protection issues. The task of providing services belongs to the 336 municipalities into which Finland, with its 5.4 million inhabitants, is currently divided. A mandatory reporting system combines all professionals and authorities working with children and young people with child protection. As the act provides only a general framework for the criteria for interventions and processes, the local authorities and social workers have a lot of discretion in how to implement the act with regard to the social and cultural context of the municipality. This means that child protection practices vary to some extent among the municipalities, child protection teams, and individual social workers.

In the previous cross-country analysis by Gilbert (1997) and Gilbert, Parton, and Skivenes (2011), it was shown that Finland belongs to the Nordic group of child welfare systems focusing on family services and recently even more so on child-focused services. The scope of child protection is wide, as it addresses both the circumstances in which children are being raised and that endanger or fail to safeguard their health or development, and the situations in which children's behavior itself endangers their health or development. The latter formulation calls upon the child protection authorities to act when the child is committing crimes or misuses alcohol and drugs, for example.

Consequently, there is a wide array of services provided by the local authorities. Most of the services are in-home services, voluntary by nature, which aim to support the child and the family in their own community. The emphasis on in-home services can be seen in the two case vignettes that we presented to 76 social workers as part of the survey research in this book, in which the majority of social workers estimated the risk level to be high or very high in both vignettes. Nevertheless, the main response was to provide in-home support services. Out-of-home placements are used only if in-home services turn out to be insufficient or inappropriate. The care orders leading to out-of-home placements may be voluntary or involuntary. The opinions of children ages 12 years and older are included in the formal decision-making process. Roughly a quarter of the care orders are given against the will of the child or his or her guardian (Heino, 2009).

The role of child protection has increased in Finland due to several factors. The latest act, especially, has expanded the tasks of the child protection authorities. However, even before the new act, starting from the mid-1990s, the number of children in the child protection system in terms of both in-home services and out-of-home placements has been greatly increasing. In 2011, 67 children per 1,000 children below the age of 18 were receiving in-home services, whereas 14 children per 1,000 children were placed out of their homes (Sotkanet, 2013). In 2011, 10,535 children were in care, whereas in 2000 the number was much lower (Lastensuojelu, 2011). The relative share of children between the ages of 16 and 17 has been increasing to a larger extent than that of younger children (Lastensuojelu, 2011). The increase in the number of children in the system is seen on the one hand as a reflection of the deterioration of universal public services and the increasing polarization of well-being among children and families and, on the other, of the expanding public governance of childhood and families (e.g., Heino, 2009; Hiilamo, 2009; Pösö, 2010; Harrikari, 2008).

As a consequence of the expansion of the tasks and service users in the system, there is currently a call for a fundamental restructuring of the child protection system and its relations with other service provision for children and families (Toimiva lastensuojelu, 2013). It is acknowledged that despite the welfare and service-orientated legislation, the children and families in need and at risk do not receive the services they require. There seem to be considerable problems in the quality of services, resources, and expertise provided by the local authorities. Most important, the emphasis on in-home services does not seem to reduce the need to place children out of their home. The formal emphasis on the participation of children does not seem to empower children and their parents to have their voice heard in child protection decision making (Toimiva lastensuojelu, 2013). There is, in other words, a considerable gap between the legislation and the practice of service provision in child protection.

Migration

According to Statistics Finland, "29,500 persons immigrated to Finland from foreign countries during 2011. The number is 3,100 higher than in the previous year and the highest during Finland's independence. Emigration from Finland also increased slightly and was 12,650 persons" (Official Statistic of Finland, 2012).

As was stated at the beginning of this chapter, 4.6% of people living in Finland were foreign-born in 2010 (OECD, 2012). The largest groups of migrants come from the ex-Soviet Union and Russia, Sweden, Estonia, Somalia, China, and Iraq (Väestöntutkimuslaitos, 2012). This definitional category of migrants is, however, rather limited as it ignores generational aspects (migrants of the first and second generation). If the category also includes the country of birth of one's parents, the number is almost 6%. This number is still considerably lower than in other Nordic countries (Ruotsalainen and Nieminen, 2012).

Although the most informative definition of migration is generally thought to be based on the country of a person's or his or her parents' birth, this definition is not systematically used in Finland. As a consequence, there is definitional variety and even confusion about how to address migration (Ruotsalainen and Nieminen, 2012). In national statistics, the categories of citizenship and language are used as well. In 2009, there were 155,700 people (2.9% of the total population) living in Finland who had non-Finnish citizenship. The largest groups were from Russia, Estonia, Sweden, Somalia, China, Thailand, and Iraq (Väestöntutkimuslaitos, 2012). Again, when looking at the people whose mother tongue is not Finnish or Swedish, we obtain the figure of 207,000 (3.7% of the Finnish population). In 2009, the largest groups of other mother tongues included Russian, Estonian, English, Somali, Arabic, Kurdish, and Chinese (Väestöntutkimuslaitos, 2012).

Looking at these statistics, we see that the majority of migration to Finland is from the neighboring countries of Estonia, Russia, and Sweden. Finland has had a long shared history with the latter two countries: Finland was a part of Sweden until the start of the nineteenth century and after that an autonomous part of Russia until the early twentieth century, thus many people may have had family roots of some kind in Finland already before the moment of migration. Linguistically, Swedish-speaking people moving from Sweden to Finland are not likely to experience any major language obstacles, as Swedish is a national language of Finland. In addition, the Estonian and Finnish languages are closely related, which facilitates communication. Most of the people also look alike.

The reasons for migrating to Finland are mainly family related. Based on a study carried out in 2005, it is estimated that 60% to 65% of all migrant people migrate due to family reasons. Fifteen percent of the migrants are refugees or asylum seekers, 10% are returning to Finland, and 5% to 10% migrate for occupational reasons (Väestöntutkimuslaitos, 2012). The OECD permit-based statistics show a similar tendency: 34.3% of the migration to Finland is family related, 39% is related to free movement, 17.4% is humanitarian, and 5.8% is work-related (OECD, 2012). In 2011, 3,088 asylum applications were filed and 3,576 asylum decisions were made. The largest groups among asylum seekers were from Iraq (738), Somalia (514), Afghanistan (289), and Russia (370). In the same year, asylum decisions were made about 132 unaccompanied minors, 59 of whom came from Somalia, 23 from Iraq, and 22 from Afghanistan. The number of unaccompanied asylum seekers has varied considerably during the past few years, showing, however, a more decreasing than increasing tendency (Väestöntutkimuslaitos, 2012).

This information is of an "official" nature; that is to say it is based on the national official statistics and statistics provided by state agencies and their record-keeping practices. It thus excludes information about undocumented migrants. It is estimated that every year Finnish authorities uncover a few thousand foreign nationals residing illegally in Finland ("Fight Against Illegal Immigration," 2012).

The people migrating tend to be younger than the population in general, and the great majority (80%) of the second migrant generation are 18 years of age or younger (Ruotsalainen and Nieminen, 2012; Martikainen and Tiilikainen, 2007). The family structures may differ from the Finnish family structures; for example, the number of family members tends to be higher in migrant families. However, it is noteworthy that the number of lone parents (20%) is at the same level as among the Finnish population in general (Martikainen and Tiilikainen, 2007: 27.) In other words, there is no single type of "migrant family."

Further, there is no single type of being a "migrant in Finland." The studies demonstrate, however, that first- and second-generation migrants are more likely to be unemployed than people in general. Young migrants tend to be less educated and less present in further education than their peers (Ruotsalainen and Nieminen, 2012.) It is estimated that a considerably high number of migrants in Finland belong to the most vulnerable groups in society in terms of poverty, health problems, and social exclusion. The risks are highest among migrant women with children (Malin, 2011; Ikäläinen, Martiskainen, and Törrönen, 2003). It is fairly common that migrant children and youth are addressed as the particular group at risk of social exclusion, and specific programs and policies are called for to tackle this risk. At the moment, migration and multiculturalism are highly debated and contested issues in local and national politics, and anti-migration views are expressed (e.g., Keskinen, Rastas, and Tuori, 2009). We also know that some migrant children face racism (Rastas, 2007).

LAW AND POLICY CONCERNING MIGRANT CHILDREN AND FAMILIES

In principle, migrant families and children are entitled to the same child protection services—as well as to other child welfare and health services and education—as anyone else in Finland. This is mainly for two reasons. First, the local authorities are obliged to provide welfare services, including child protection, to all people living in a municipal area. "Living in the municipal area" is the criterion used to allow people access to social services and is met when people have been registered in the municipal record-keeping system; to be registered, a migrant has to have permission to stay in the country, as defined by the Aliens Act (2004). The assumption is that everyone is registered and that registration is always updated if a person moves from one municipality (and address) to another. Emergency services should be provided to everyone in need, even to those staying in the municipality only temporarily or whose registration status is unclear. Second, the Finnish Constitution defines the principle of equality as one of the leading principles of the Finnish state:

> Everyone is equal before the law. No one shall, without an acceptable reason, be treated differently from other persons on the ground of sex, age, origin, language, religion, conviction, opinion, health, disability or other reason that concerns his or her person. Children shall be treated equally and as individuals and they shall be allowed to influence matters pertaining to themselves to a degree corresponding to their level of

development. Equality of the sexes is promoted in societal activity and working life, especially in the determination of pay and the other terms of employment, as provided in more detail by an Act. (Constitution of Finland, 1999)

The constitution emphasizes equality between the sexes, as well as children and adults especially; the notions of origin, language, and religion are important principles regarding migration. This principle applies to all legislation, and therefore the Child Welfare Act, among other acts, follows the same principle.

The right to services and the municipalities' obligation to provide services on an equal basis do not, however, cover all migrant groups and all situations, which is discussed later.

In 2010, a new act about the integration (resettlement[1]) of migrants (1386/2010) was introduced. The act targets all people who, as "foreigners," have received permission to stay in Finland. The target group of the act is wider than the previous act, which was aimed only at certain groups of migrants (e.g., refugees). In its own words, the new act aims to support the integration process of migrants and give migrants an opportunity to be active members of Finnish society. The municipalities have the duty to provide services for integration, with unemployed and job-seeking migrants forming special target groups. The services include individually tailored plans for integration, guidance to education and the labor market, as well as some financial support. The plan assigns obligations to municipalities (to provide the services in question), as well as to migrants (to follow the plan). The municipal employment agencies are the key actors for all migrants unless they are outside the labor market due to their age or other similar reasons.

According to the act, migrant families and children may be given plans of their own. Different from the previous act, the new act defines the position of minors within the frame of the Child Welfare Act and establishes that the principle of the child's best interest guides integration work. Special attention should be given to the participation of children in decision-making processes. The act also recognizes the migrant children's and young people's distinctive needs for integration and asks the municipalities to provide such services. Minors arriving and residing in Finland without a guardian should be given a guardian, and the municipalities are asked to provide group homes or other forms of residence for these children. Most interestingly, the act asks the municipal employment, traffic, and environment agencies to provide such units. The units, on the other hand, should follow the regulations set in the Child Welfare Act regarding staff, number of children, and living conditions, but they are not primarily child protection facilities. In other words, in terms of organization, the care of unaccompanied children is not the particular task of the child protection system.

On the level of national policy, the very first Government Integration Programme was approved by the Finnish government in June 2012. In his government website blog, the Minister for Employment and the Economy Lauri Ihalainen shares his views in English about the program and the challenges ahead and includes some thoughts about migrant children and youth:

> At present, Finnish society is in a phase where an increase in inequalities is a regrettable fact. This may have a particularly strong effect on immigrants, and at worst, lead to a vicious circle of marginalisation. Especially in the case of children and young people, feelings and experiences of marginalisation or discrimination can affect their whole life and hinder their growth into adulthood. In order to encourage positive attitudes, a lot of work must be done at day-care centres and schools, in leisure time activities and everywhere where children and young people can be found.
>
> For young people, it is crucial to find their own route to education, training and work. The Government Integration Programme includes two important initiatives: young immigrants will be provided with an opportunity to improve their study and language skills before entering upper secondary school, and the Ministry of Education and Culture will examine permanent solutions by 2015 to ensure that no young immigrant over the age of compulsory education is left without a comprehensive school leaving certificate.
>
> I believe that the most important factors behind strong integration are language skills, education, training and work. The importance of employment can never be overemphasised. (Ihalainen, 2012)

This long extract demonstrates well the present policy on migrants. Employment is seen as the key issue in integration and resettlement. Social exclusion is perceived as the main risk, and special attention should be given to children and young people to help them avoid social exclusion. For them, education and language skills are important. For adults, it is the responsibility of the employment authorities, and for children and young people, of the education authorities to act. In this general context, social work or the child protection system are not given any special responsibilities.

Some scholars (e.g., Keskinen, Vuori, and Hirsiaho, 2012; Raunio, Hammar-Suutari, and Säävälä, 2011) suggest that Finnish migration policy looks at migrants as (possible) labor force actors and focuses on related issues dealing mainly with adults. However, children become a focus as future members of the labor force—thus the educational interest. According to the minister's blog quoted previously, it is important to invest in (migrant) children and childhood to prevent them from being excluded from society. As the motivation is to avoid future risks and problems, migrant children and young people are thus viewed as constituting a potential risk to society. This is, inevitably, a narrow view of migrant children and youth.

CHILD PROTECTION FOR MIGRANT CHILDREN
AND FAMILIES—AN OVERVIEW

Organization of Services

In Finland, local authorities (municipalities) are responsible for providing child protection services. As mentioned previously, this means that child protection practices may vary among the municipalities due to the differences in the political climate, culture, history, and service structures in each municipality. Furthermore, as more than half of the migrants live in a small geographical area in the southern part of Finland, there are many municipalities that do not have—and have not had—any foreign-born inhabitants (Malin, 2011). According to the Child Welfare Act, only social workers working for the municipal social welfare agency have the legal authority to make decisions. Some social workers with child protection authority may, however, work in reception centers, emergency social services, and similar places.

The same mode of decentralized service provision is used in the "integration/resettlement services" for migrants: the key role and obligations belong to the municipalities. A clear distinction is drawn between integration, immigration, and child protection services. The integration/resettlement programme of the city of Tampere for 2010–2020, for example, states that child protection services do not belong to integration services but are provided, if ultimately necessary, outside integration services (Tampereen kaupungin kotouttamisohjelma, 2010–2012). Further, the care of unaccompanied minors and asylum-seeking families and children falls outside the purview of child protection services in organizational terms. Yet the duty to notify connects the authorities working in immigration or integration services with child protection authorities.

The low levels of migration and organizational arrangements are reflected in the survey data collected for the purposes of this book. Social workers who have experience working with migrant families and children were called to answer the survey. However, the ratio of migrant clients was very small among the respondents' case loads: 95% of them reported that one-third or less of their clients are migrants. Only one social worker had migrant clients constitute 60% of her clients. None of them worked solely with migrant children and families.

Professional Training and Practice

To act as a social worker with child protection authority, a five-year university degree (bachelor's and master's degree in social work) is required. This education combines both professional and research-based knowledge of social work. Ethics and legislation also play an important role in the curriculum, emphasizing human rights, as well as the rights of service-users and the duties of the public authorities. The education also includes language studies, and everyone holding an master's degree should demonstrate good language skills in one foreign language (which most often is English) in addition to Finnish and Swedish. Some universities—the University of Tampere, for example—encourage social work students to study the languages of their most likely client groups, such as Russian, but very few do so. However, in our survey data, 15% of respondents said that they spoke the same language as some of their migrant clients. This can be considered a surprisingly high figure, especially considering that only 5% of the social worker respondents were born outside of Finland and also considering their clients' reported countries of origin, with the major groups coming from Africa, Asia, and Eastern Europe.

Multiculturalism is a theme included in social work teaching programs. However, Finnish literature on social work and multiculturalism is very limited, and therefore most of the study literature comes from the United Kingdom or United States, countries with different histories and cultures of multiculturalism. Self-evidently, there are some discrepancies between the UK and US literature and the practice that Finnish social work students experience in their field placements during which they might never meet a migrant client. Other themes related to migration are touched on only in passing, if at all.

The fact that the right to social services is linked to one's residence tends to be the key message conveyed in many Finnish guidebooks and information about procedures. There is an Internet-based handbook of child welfare, edited by the National Institute for Health and Welfare, with a special section about migrants. The opening sentence underlines that everyone has equal rights to services; it does not mention any problems or tensions in this matter. Instead, multicultural practice, including especially the understanding of different cultures and related communication, is given major attention.

The cultural approach to migrant issues is the mainstream approach at the moment in training, as well as in practice. As important as it may be, it restricts the focus to social worker–client interactions or to the "migrant culture." There are proposals that the approach should be wider. Sari Laakkonen (2012), for example, calls for social workers to become advocates for the children of the Roma of Romania who beg on the streets. She claims that the present attitude to act only when Roma children are in immediate danger is not sufficient. Instead, social workers should look after the rights of these children from a wider rights perspective. This would mean, first, involvement in the public and political debates about the duties and rights of the European Union states and their citizens, and second, using their professional power to support the children even when they are not in immediate danger. This remains an obvious challenge for training and practice.

The challenges for training are visible in the survey data as well. Only one-quarter of the social workers had received some training to work with migrant clients, and two-thirds of them considered their skills poorer with migrant than nonmigrant clients. Two-thirds also considered work with migrants more demanding than with nonmigrants. There is an obvious gap between the skills and demands in these matters. The survey data does not, unfortunately, specify the thematic expectations for training.

Representation of Migrant Children and Young People

The national statistics of child protection do not list migrant children as such. The statistics are general in nature and recognize only the age, gender, and municipality of the children in the system and ignore a lot of important information about them. As research on this topic is almost nonexistent, *it is not possible to present any reliable figures* on the national level that would inform us about the representation of migrant families among the clients receiving different kinds of child protection services.

There are, however, hints of an overrepresentation of migrant children provided by studies focusing on some particular groups of clients. One study of this type focuses on youth residential institutions ("reform schools"). It shows that 8.6% of the young people in these institutions have a migrant (or minority) status (Kitinoja, 2005). In this study, the concept of "foreign-born" included— interestingly enough—all children who had at least one parent born outside Finland, as well as children belonging to the minority group of Roma. It was also noted that reliable information was not always available in the case files that were used as data, and thus the results are not highly reliable. However, the researcher draws the conclusion that migrant children are overrepresented in relation to their number in the population and that this is true for children from minority groups as well. Further, a study analyzing children who had been registered in the child protection system in 2006 in nine municipalities shows that 8% of the system's new clients live in "multicultural" families (Heino, 2007). The concept of "multicultural" included the citizenship status and language of the child and differs from the concept used in Kitinoja's study. Again, there were difficulties in finding out information about these matters as social workers do not automatically collect and store this information. These studies demonstrate vividly how unsettled and vague the notion of "migrant" is, as well as related knowledge production in child protection practice.

One of the few existing studies analyzing the needs of migrant families for child protection, based on interviews of professionals in social welfare and health care, suggests that the major "migrant issue" for child protection is experienced with teenagers (Heikkilä-Daskalopoulos, 2008). This is related to the conflicts between teenagers and their parents. These conflicts are rooted in the ways in which the different generations adapt to the Finnish way of life, allowing young people a wide degree of autonomy: the young people follow the Finnish norms of teenage life whereas the parents may follow a different norm structure. The study suggests that cultural negotiations with the help of family work are needed to bridge the gap between the different norms. On the other hand, issues related to violence were recognized as special "migrant and child protection" issues, including honor-related violence and corporal punishment, in which the Finnish social norms and ethics clash with those of some migrant families. Most interestingly, the problems presented were all of psychosocial nature, and such socioeconomic issues as poverty were excluded (Heikkilä-Daskalopoulos, 2008).

In fact, the issue of poverty is interrelated with child protection work with migrant families and children in a complex way. As part of the survey of Finnish social workers, a vignette about a 10-year-old girl, obviously mistreated by her parents and reported by a health nurse, was presented in two different ways: one included hard-working parents with long working hours (case 1) and the other unemployed parents living on income support (case 2). The Finnish social workers surveyed estimated that there was a considerable risk to the child in both cases. However, the risk was seen as less major in case 2, the child with unemployed and poor parents. Further, the social workers planned to provide services to help the girl to stay at home in the case of unemployed and poor parents (case 2) more often than in the case of hard-working parents (case 1). In the first case, almost half of the respondents (46%) thought of emergency placement as a child protection response whereas in the case of poor parents, this option was chosen by 37%.

Although the number of respondents is small (35 for case 1 and 41 for case 2), the differences in responses regarding families with different socioeconomic backgrounds can be seen to reflect a tendency to support parents in their parenting by first offering services to help the parents to change, especially if the poor parenting is linked to poverty. Poverty is a social problem, which has long been recognized by the Finnish child protection system, and social workers may feel comfortable in addressing poverty-related social problems. If poor parenting is not linked to poverty, the responses seem to be harsher. This may be a reflection of lower tolerance toward poor parenting by those without any economic hardship or else of a lack of professional tools and skills to work psychosocially with abuse in such conditions. The latter could even be interrelated with the lack of intercultural competencies in working with "different cultures" of a migrant family, and thus a harsher response was suggested.

PRESENT CHALLENGES AND DILEMMAS

In the following, some present challenges and dilemmas are discussed in relation to migrant children and families and the Finnish child protection system. Definitional and knowledge based issues are, self-evidently, among the first, followed by the notion of the normative nature of child protection and its boundaries and role in working with migrant children and families.

Definitional Challenges

"Since we do not have any refugees in our municipality, I will not participate in the survey" was the response that I heard when presenting the survey to a group of social workers attending a postqualifying course in child protection. I had just explained that the survey focuses on the issues that social workers encounter when working with migrant clients.

This response demonstrates the common practice among social workers to equate "migrants" with "refugees." This equation excludes the majority of migrant families and children and places the migrants into one specific category only. The category ignores the differences between refugees and asylum seekers, as well as other migrant groups, larger in size, and their differences regarding ethnic and cultural backgrounds, social situations, needs, and rights. Children adopted from abroad, for example, would not "naturally" be included in this category even though Finland is one of the European countries with considerably high rates of international adoption (Selman, 2012).

In fact, child protection research has not so far been helpful, on the one hand, in clarifying the concept of a migrant child/family and, on the other hand, in diversifying it. As has been shown here, migrant children have been defined with a variety of (unspecific) concepts in child protection research, and the national statistics do not provide any information at all about the migrant children in the system.

Fragmentary knowledge production in terms of research and statistics makes it difficult to build practice based on empirical knowledge. The over-/underrepresentation of migrant groups is not factually known, and therefore social policy cannot be formulated to meet the needs of the (possible) vulnerable groups or protect their rights. The vagueness of the use of the concept can lead to problematic, if not even misleading, conclusions and institutional responses. In child protection practice and research, sophisticated yet consistent definitions are needed to address "migrant children and families" as groups and individuals on which the empirical knowledge base, which is so urgently needed, can be built.

The Normative Nature of Child Protection and a Call for Diversity

Due to the holistic welfare-based approach to child protection, the criteria for services and interventions are formulated in a manner that leaves much for social workers and local authorities to define in actual practice. The responsibility of social workers is to adjust the needs and situations of a child they work with to what is generally seen as an appropriate childhood and family life (e.g., Pekkarinen, 2010; Kataja, 2012). Such a strong basis in social norms and their local interpretations have functioned well enough in a homogenous society in which family patterns and life courses are rather similar. However, these norm structures are contested by migrant clients.

Consequently, the system runs the risk that the different norms created by different religions, family patterns, customs, and traditions deviating from the traditional Finnish norms are seen as "problems." In her study of child protection workers meeting migrant families, Merja Anis (2008) found that migrant clients were seen as "different" from other families in need of child protection services. The perception of "difference" may lead to normative assumptions of "different" meaning troublesome and problematic (Anis, 2008; Keskinen, 2011). It is challenging to view norms in a fundamentally new, more diverse way and, consequently, reconsider the threshold for child protection services and their nature. Further, there is a need to communicate and elaborate the social norms and the role of the child protection system as a norm-keeper with migrant communities.

Studies in other fields of social welfare suggest that the role of the Finnish public welfare system as "a helping friend" is not recognized by people who have, for example, not trusted the public administration in their country of origin (e.g., Clarke, 2004). Trust is challenged in the child protection system, which functions in the field of private family relations, as well as cultural expectations and social norms about "appropriate" family life and childhood and deals with children and families in a bureaucratic manner, recording, for example, every visit and discussion. The idea of the child protection system being a "service system" might be viewed as very contested, as it may use some coercive power as well. This tension is especially complex in Finland because the child protection system includes both elements—providing services needed and wished for by the family and monitoring, intervening, and breaking the family relations even against the will of the family—and the same professionals can act in both of these two roles. It is therefore highly necessary that the norm structures employed by the child protection system and their relation to different migrant, ethnic, cultural, and religious positions are well known and explicitly explained to migrant children and families, as well as to the different professionals working with migrants.

The Role and Boundaries of the Child Protection System With Regard to Migrant Children

The Finnish child protection system focuses on children who are registered in a municipality and provides only emergency services to nonregistered children. This adversely affects some migrant children, especially undocumented children, as they do not have access to supportive services in the long term.

The rights of undocumented migrant children have been discussed in terms of their right to education and nonemergency health care (such as prenatal health care for pregnant women) but not in terms of child protection. The policy is somewhat unclear at the moment as, on the one hand, the recognition of children's rights asks the authorities to act regardless of the child's legal status, and, on the other hand, specific legislation sets restricting criteria for service provision (e.g., registration as a resident). Nevertheless, in the survey data gathered for this chapter, almost all Finnish social workers treated the case vignette about a newborn baby with parents living in obvious poverty as a child protection issue, regardless of the legal status of the migrant family. This suggests that practitioners tend to take a wide view of the role of the child protection system if there is a small baby and his or her parents needing attention. However, about half of the social workers did not know whether the child protection system should react if they met an undocumented child not attending school. If the child were documented, the child protection workers would be obliged to act in Finland. This suggests that the social workers hesitate more about their role and its legitimacy if the child's situation does not include an immediate risk of poor care. Yet, from the point of view of children's rights, the right to education should be considered as well.

The roles and boundaries are not set only by the legal status of migrants but also by the organizational division of duties. The care and upbringing of unaccompanied asylum-seeking children provide a good example: even though this group of children is a very vulnerable group in need of care, the task is not given to child protection practitioners but to immigration services and related expertise. The child is entitled to have a social worker to support him or her, but the process of examining the asylum application does not follow child protection ideology or children's rights. It is claimed that unaccompanied asylum seekers lose their right to be a child and have the attention that children in vulnerable positions normally get. Rather, they are treated as posing a risk to national security and are treated accordingly in specialized organizational arrangements (Pakolaisneuvonta, 2012).

Consequently, one could claim that the child protection system tends to approach migrant children as any children within the existing bureaucratic limits instead of trying to actively reach out to vulnerable groups of migrant children. The tensions that migrant young people experience in their families between different life-styles and values could also be a task for the outreach work of the child protection system. These tasks, as many others, have been left to other organisations, nongovernmental organizations in particular. Considering the philosophy of the present Child Welfare Act and the recognition of children's rights, one could assume that, in addition to the former issues, child protection could be active in working with children who are the object of human trafficking (e.g., "Child Trafficking in the Nordic Countries," 2011), those who "disappear" in transnational custody disputes, or those who are sentenced to return to their home country without any asylum in Finland. Child protection could possibly also deal with those children who are left in their home country when the parents migrate to Finland to work. The latter issue is relevant for women who, in increasing numbers, move to Finland to work as nurses and other care-workers to fill the need for care labor in an aging society and to financially support their families at home (Kröger and Zechner, 2009). This could be a child protection issue as well, although it is outside any (national) boundaries that the legislation draws at the moment.

CONCLUDING REMARKS

We have seen that Finland is a country with low but increasing levels of migration and that the child protection system is only gradually learning to address issues related to migration. Migrant children and families are entitled to full social and health services, education, and child protection on the basis of registration as any other resident in a Finnish municipality. The chapter has demonstrated that there is a need to rethink the criteria for child protection services, as well as the organizational duties of the child protection system and other agencies and their responses from the point of view of migrant communities, and especially from the point of view of very vulnerable migrant children. The full scale of migration should be recognized in service provision, and services should be provided accordingly. Moreover, the knowledge base should be strengthened to guide policy and practice so that it is sensitive to the voices of migrant children and families and the differences among them.

The recognition of migrants as users or possible users of child protection services challenges the overarching principles of sameness and universalism that have traditionally shaped the welfare responses in Finland (e.g., Keskinen, 2011). Further, it challenges the way the public child protection system expands its function and philosophy to meet the issues migration in a globalized world entails. It remains to be seen how the child protection responses will develop. There is, after all, a strong interest to include all children in (the aging) Finnish society, which may lead to sensitive and empowering child protection practice with and for migrant children in need and at risk. Unfortunately, other directions may be taken as well.

NOTE

1 The term *kotouttaminen*, the key term in this act, translates poorly into "integration," "inclusion," or "resettlement," which are, however, used in English texts. The translation lacks the tone of the original Finnish word *koti* (home), which forms the root of the term *kotouttaminen*.

REFERENCES

Aliens Act (301/2004). Helsinki: Ministry of Justice. Retrieved December 12, 2012, from www.finlex.fi.

Anis, M. (2008). *Sosiaalityö ja maahanmuuttajat* (Social Work and Migrants). Helsinki: Väestöliitto.

Brochmann, G., & Hagelund, A. (2011). Migrants in the Scandinavian welfare state. The emergence of a social policy problem. *Nordic Journal of Migration Research*, 1(1), 13–24.

Child Trafficking in the Nordic Countries: Rethinking Strategies and National Responses (2011). Florence: United Nations Children's Fund, UNICEF Innocenti Research Centre.

Child Welfare Act (417/2007). Helsinki: Ministry of Justice. Retrieved December 12, 2012, from www.finlex.fi.

Clarke, K. (2004). *Access and Belonging in the Age of Viral Epidemic: Constructing Migrants Living with HIV/AIDS in the Finnish Welfare State.* Tampere: University of Tampere.

Constitution of Finland (731/1999). Helsinki: Ministry of Justice. Retrieved December 12, 2012, from http://www.finlex.fi/fi/laki/kaannokset/1999/en19990731.

Eydal, G., & Kröger, T. (2010). Nordic family policies: Constructing contexts for social work with families. In H. Forsberg & T. Kröger (Eds.), *Social Work and Child Welfare Politics: Through Nordic Lenses*, 11–28. Bristol: Policy Press.

Fight Against Illegal Immigration. Helsinki: Ministry of the Interior. Retrieved December 13, 2012, from http://www.intermin.fi/en/migration/fight_against_illegal_immigration.

Gilbert, N., ed. (1997). *Combatting Child Abuse: International Perspectives and Trends.* New York: Oxford University Press.

Gilbert, N., Parton, N., & Skivenes, M., eds. (2011). *Child Protection Systems: International Trends and Orientations.* New York: Oxford University Press.

Hammar-Suutari, S. (2009). *Asiakkaana erilaisuus: Kulttuurien välisen viranomaistoiminnan etnografia* (Difference as a Client: An Ethnography on Intercultural Practice of Authorities). Joensuu: Karjalan tutkimuslaitos.

Harrikari, T. (2008). *Riskillä merkityt* (Marked with Risk). Helsinki: Nuorisotutkimusverkosto.

Heikkilä-Daskalopoulos, S. (2008). *Maahanmuuttajataustaiset lapset ja perheet palvelujärjestelmässä—asiantuntijoiden näkökulmia* (Children and Families of Migrant Background in the Service System—The Points of View of Experts) Helsinki: Lastensuojelun keskusliitto.

Heino, T. (2007). Keitä ovat uudet lastensuojelun asiakkaat? (Who Are the New Child Protection Clients?) Working Paper 30. Helsinki: Stakes.

———. (2009). Lastensuojelu—kehityskulkuja ja paikannuksia (Child protection—Tendencies and locations). In J. Lammi-Taskula, S. Karvonen, & S. Ahlström (Eds.), *Lapsiperheiden hyvinvointi 2009* (The Well-Being of Families with Children), 198–213. Helsinki: Terveyden ja hyvinvoinnin laitos.

Hiilamo, H. (2009). What could explain the dramatic rise in out-of-home placement in Finland in the 1990s and early 2000s? *Children and Youth Services Review*, 31, 177–184.

Honkasalo, V. (2011). *Tyttöjen kesken—Monikulttuurisuus ja sukupuolten tasa-arvo nuorisotyössä* (Among Girls Youth Work, Multiculturalism and Gender Equality). Helsinki: Nuorisotutkimusseura/Nuorisotutkimusverkosto.

Honkatukia, P., & Suurpää, L. (2007). *Nuorten miesten monikulttuurinen elämänkulku ja rikollisuus* (Young Men's Multicultural Life Course and Criminality). Research Report 232. Helsinki: Oikeuspoliittinen tutkimuslaitos.

Ihalainen, L. (2012). Lauri Ihalainen: At Home—In Finland. Ministry blog TEMatiikkaa. April 7. Retrieved October 15, 2012, from https://www.tem.fi/?106266_m=107172&l=en&s=4712.

Ikäläinen, S., Martiskainen, T., & Törrönen, M. (2003). Mangopuun juurelta kuusen katveeseen—asiakkaana maahanmuuttajaperhe (From under the Mango Tree to the Shelter of a Pine Tree—A Migrant Family as a Client). Helsinki: Lastensuojelun Keskusliitto.

Kataja, K. (2012). *Lapsuuden rajoilla. Normaalin ja poikkeavan määrittymnen huostaanottoasiakirjoissa* (On the Borders of Childhood: Defining Normality and Deviance in Care Order Records). Turku: Turun yliopisto.

Keskinen, S. (2011). Troublesome differences—Dealing with gendered violence, ethnicity, and "race" in the Finnish welfare state. *Journal of Scandinavian Studies in Criminology and Crime Prevention*, 12(2), 153–172.

Keskinen, S., Rastas, A., & Tuori, S., eds. (2009). *En ole rasisti, mutta... Maahanmuutosta, monikulttuurisuudesta ja kritiikistä* (I Am Not a Racist But...About Migration, Multiculturalism and Criticism). Tampere: Vastapaino.

Keskinen, S., Vuori, J., & Hirsiaho, A. (2012). *Monikulttuurisuuden sukupuoli. Kansalaisuus ja erot hyvinvointiyhteiskunnassa* (The Gender of Multiculturalism: Citizenship and Differences in a Welfare Society). Tampere: Tampere University Press.

Kitinoja, M. (2005). *Kujan päässä koulukoti* (At the End of the Road, a Reform School). Research Report 150. Helsinki: Stakes.

Kröger, T., & Zechner, M. (2009). Migration and care: Giving and needing care across national borders. *Finnish Journal of Ethnicity and Migration*, 4(2), 17–26.

Laakkonen, S. (2012). Sosiaalityöntekijän rooli sosiaalisten ongelmien esiin-nostajana—esimerkkinä kerjäläiskysymys (The role of social workers as the claims-makers of social problems—The issue of beggars as an example). In M. Strömberg-Jakka & T. Karttunen (Eds.), Sosiaalityön haasteet (Social Work Challenges), 54–71. Jyväskylä: PS-kustannus.

Lähteenmäki, M. (2013). Lapsi turvapaikanhakijana: Etnografisia näkökulmia vastaanottokeskuksen ja koulun arjesta (The Child as an Asylum Seeker: Ethnographic Perspectives on Reception Centres and Daily School Life). Studies in Educational Sciences 247. Helsinki: University of Helsinki.

Laki kotoutumisen edistämisestä (The Act about Supporting Integration) (1386/2010). Helsinki: Ministry of Justice. Retrieved December 12, 2012, from www.finlex.fi.

Lastensuojelu 2011 (Child Welfare 2011). (2011). Statistical Report 26/2012. Suomen virallinen tilasto, Sosiaaliturva 2012. Retrieved November 15, 2013, from http://www.stakes.fi/tilastot/tilastotiedotteet/2011/Tr29_11.pdf.

Malin. M. (2011). Maahanmuuttajien terveyteen ja hyvinvointiin vaikuttavat tekijät (Factors influencing on health and well-being of migrants). Yhteiskuntapolitiikka, 76(2), 201–213.

Martikainen, T., & Tiilikainen, M., eds. (2007). Maahanmuuttajanaiset: Koto utuminen, perhe ja työ (Migrant Women: Integration, Family and Work). Report D46. Helsinki: Väestöntutkimuslaitos.

Official Statistics of Finland (OSF). (2012). Migration. Helsinki: Statistics Finland. Retrieved December 2, 2012, from http://www.stat.fi/til/muutl/index_en.html.

Organisation for Economic Co-operation and Development (OECD) (2012). International Migration Outlook 2012. Country Notes: Finland. Paris: OECD. Retrieved December 2, 2012, from http://www.oecd.org/migration/internationalmigrationpoliciesanddata/internationalmigrationoutlook2012countrynotes.html.

Pakolaisneuvonta 2012: Yksintulleet turvapaikanhakijalapset (Regufee Advice 2012: Unaccompanied Child Asylum Seekers). (2012). Helsinki: Finnish Refugee Advice Centre. Retrieved December 14, 2012 from http://www.pakolaisneuvonta.fi/index_html?lid=136&lang=suo.

Pekkarinen, E. (2010). Stadilaispojat, rikokset ja lastensuojelu—viisi tapaustutkimusta kuudelta vuosikymmeneltä (Stadi-Boys, Crime and child Protection—Five Case Studies from Six Decades). Helsinki: Finnish Youth Research Society.

Pösö, T. (2010). Havaintoja suomalaisen lastensuojelun institutionaalisesta rajasta (Some remarks about the institutional boundaries of Finnish child welfare). Janus, 18(4), 324–336.

———. (2011). Combatting child abuse in Finland: From family to child-centered orientation. In N. Gilbert, N. Parton, & M. Skivenes (Eds.), Child Protection

Systems: International Trends and Orientations, 112–130. New York: Oxford University Press.

Rastas, A. (2007). *Rasismi lasten ja nuorten arjessa: Transnationaalit juuret ja monikulttuuristuva Suomi*. (Racism in the Everyday Life of Children and Young People: Transnational Roots and Multicultural Finland in the Making). Tampere: Tampere University Press and Nuorisotutkimusseura/ Nuorisotutkimusverkosto.

Raunio, M., Säävälä, M.,Hammar-Suutari, M., & Pitkänen, P. (2011). Monikulttuurisuus ja kulttuurien välisen vuorovaikutuksen areenat (Multiculturalism and the arenas for intercultural interaction). In P. Pitkänen (Ed.), *Kulttuurien kohtaamisia arjessa* (Cultural Encounters in Everyday Life), 17–50. Tampere: Vastapaino.

Raunio, M., Hammar-Suutari, S., & Säävälä, M. (2012). Kaupunkiseudut kulttuurien välisen vuorovaikutuksen ympäristöinä (Town regions as the contexts for intercultural interaction). In P. Pitkänen (Ed.), *Kultturien kohtaamisia arjessa* (Cultural Encounters in Everyday Life), 51–74. Tampere: Vastapaino.

Ruotsalainen, K., & Nieminen, J. (2012). Toisen polven maahanmuuttajia vielä vähän Suomessa (Second-generation migrants still only a few in Finland). *Tieto & Trendi*, 4–5. Retrieved March 14, 2013, from http://www.stat.fi/ artikkelit/2012/art_2012-07-04_003.html.

Säävälä, M. (2011). *Perheet muuttoliikkeessä: Perustietoa maahan muuttaneiden kohtaamiseen* (Families on the Move: Basic Information to Migrant Encounters). Katsauksia E41. Helsinki: Väestöliitto.

———. (2012). *Koti, koulu ja maahan muuttaneiden lapset: Oppilashuolto ja vanhemmat hyvinvointia turvaamassa* (Home, School and Migrated Children: School Care and Parents Supporting Welfare). Katsauksia E 43. Helsinki: Väestöliitto.

Schierup, C., Hansen, P., & Castels, S. (2006). *Migration, Citizenship, and the European Welfare State: A European Dilemma*. Oxford: Oxford University Press.

Selman, P. (2012). The global decline of intercountry adoption: What lies ahead? *Social Policy & Society*, 11(3), 381–397.

Tampereen kaupungin kotouttamisohjelma 2010–2020 (The Resettlement Programme of Tampere City for 2010–2020). (2012). Tampere: The City of Tampere. Retrieved August 21, 2012, from http://www.tampere.fi/hallinto-jatalous/organisaatio/konsernihallinto/maahanmuuttajatyo.html.

Toimiva lastensuojelu (Functioning Child Welfare). (2013). Raportteja ja muistioita 19. Helsinki: Sosiaali-ja terveysministeriö.

Väestöntutkimuslaitos. (2012). Helsinki: Family Federation of Finland. Retrieved December 5, 2012, from http://www.vaestoliitto.fi/tieto_ja_tutkimus/ vaestontutkimuslaitos/tilastoja-ja-linkkeja/tilastotietoa/maahanmuuttajat/.

3

HOW THE NORWEGIAN CHILD WELFARE SYSTEM APPROACHES MIGRANT CHILDREN

Marit Skivenes

INTRODUCTION

Children of the immigrant population and their families are a controversial topic in Norway. In particular, at the end of 2012, there were heated debates about the status of immigrant children in Norwegian society. Part of the back-story relates to a public uproar against immigration regulations that force children who have lived for extended periods in Norway to leave the country. Residents of many communities have demonstrated against the consequences of Norwegian immigration policies with public protests. The public debate heated up even further because of the documentary movie by the Norwegian filmmaker Margreth Olin titled *The Other* (*De Andre*) about unaccompanied minor asylum seekers, which was released in October 2012 and put additional pressure on the Norwegian government as preparations for the 2013 elections began. The Norwegian Parliament discussed the parliamentary report "Children on the Run" (Barn på flukt") during the autumn of 2012 but, like the government, was reluctant to take a stand on the issue. However, the courts had to take a stand, and, on December 21, 2012, the Norwegian Supreme Court— in a plenary ruling—decided that two children, 9 and 10 years of age, born in Norway to foreign-born parents could not remain in Norway. The court concluded that the children's rights under the Convention on the Rights of the Child were protected and that immigration regulations overrode the children's best interests. Neighbors, friends, and bishops protested that the ruling was inhumane, and many in the general public were stunned. Some were perhaps even more disappointed because they had gained hope from the ruling of the European Court of Human Rights on December 4, 2012, in which the court ruled for the siblings Abbas and Fozi Butt and against the Norwegian state on the matter of deportation.[1] The court stated that deportation was a breach of Article 8 of the European Convention on Human Rights and that the siblings should be granted permanent residence in Norway. The 11 years this case took, clearly is an intolerably long process for any child or young adult to be involved in. These recent cases involve children's rights and the principles of the best interests of immigrant children, up against states' rights to regulate who can enter a territory, reside there, and become a citizen. Regardless of the legal status of a child, in Norway the child welfare system has a responsibility for all children who are in particular need of assistance or are at risk of harm.

The aim of this chapter is to examine how the Norwegian child welfare system addresses issues involving immigrant children and their families that are considered to be at risk. Throughout the chapter the terms "immigrant" and "migrant" are used interchangeably. The immigrant population (or the newcomer population) is defined as (a) persons who are born abroad to foreign-born parents and (b) persons born in Norway to foreign-born parents. Norway is a country in northern Europe with a population of approximately 5 million and an immigrant population of approximately 600,000 (12.2%). Immigration to Norway is a fairly recent trend that began in the late 1960s and has steadily increased since that time. In 2000, 6.6% of the child population was composed of immigrants; in 2011, that figure had doubled to 12.7%. The five largest immigration groups in Norway comprise immigrants from Poland, Sweden, Pakistan, Iraq, and Somalia (Statistics Norway, 2011 [as of January 1, 2011]). The Norwegian state is obligated to ensure the rights of all children who are within the Norwegian jurisdiction, but the right to protection in Norway is secondary to the right to protection in the child's home country (St. Meld. 27, 2011–2012: 43). The Norwegian child welfare system has responsibility for *all* children who are at risk in Norway, including unaccompanied asylum-seeking children who are zero to 15 years old.[2]

The Norwegian child welfare system operates within a comprehensive welfare state that has a tight safety net with universal welfare services—the social democratic welfare state model (Esping-Andersen, 1990; Arts and Gelissen, 2002; Brochman, Hagelund, Borevi, Jønsson, and Petersen, 2010). The child welfare system has a child-centric orientation (Skivenes, 2011) and is characterized as a family-service system (Gilbert, Parton, and Skivenes, 2011). Within this system, the aim is to promote healthy childhoods and to prevent serious risk and harm (Skivenes, 2011). To achieve this goal, the state provides services to children and families at early stages of risk to prevent the development of situations that present serious risk of harm to children. Family-service systems provide services to families and are based on the therapeutic concept of rehabilitation and on people's ability to revise and improve their lifestyles and behavior. Thus the underlying goal is to provide services that prevent more serious harm and, therefore, prevent out-of-home placements. So the threshold for service provisions is low.

In the Norwegian context, issues relating to the immigrant population usually involve discussions about integration and inclusion of newcomers (Eide, Qureshi, Rugkåsa, and Vike, 2009). There are also discussions about how certain immigrant groups are not contributing to the community, are misusing the welfare system, and are not respecting Norwegian legislation and regulations, as well as about poverty, racism, and oppression of immigrant groups. In the child welfare system, we know that immigrant children are grossly overrepresented; in 2009, approximately 26.5 per 1,000 nonimmigrant children were in the child welfare system and 51.9 per 1,000 immigrant children were in the system. Why is that so?

This chapter examines the particular problems, challenges, and solutions that relate to migrant children and the child welfare system in Norway. It begins with an overview of the Norwegian context and system, followed by statistics and facts that are available to us in Norway. Thereafter, I offer an outline of descriptions of common problems found in the field, followed by an examination of legislation and policy perceptions. I then present the training program for child welfare workers and the results from a survey of 168 child welfare workers that includes questions about perceptions of, and experiences with, immigrant families. In the concluding section, I discuss how barriers for communication may be an important component in understanding some of the problems and challenges facing migrant children and families in the Norwegian child welfare system.

THE NORWEGIAN CONTEXT AND CHILD WELFARE SYSTEM[3]

Following the outline of Skivenes (2011), the Norwegian child welfare system is classified as a "family service—mandatory reporting" system similar to those in the other Scandinavian countries. The past 20 years have witnessed a steady increase in the responsibilities and services provided by the child welfare system. More children receive services, more children are placed out of their homes, and more workers are employed by the system. There has also been a juridification of the system, an emphasis on education and knowledge, and a steady stream of reforms. Today's system has high ambitions for children who might be at risk, and a child-centric policy is evident in the way that children are addressed as individuals who deserve respect and dignity as children and not only as future adults that can contribute to, and provide for, the welfare state.

In Norway, the child welfare system is an integral part of the welfare state. The Norwegian welfare state attempts to distribute services according to universal principles of human dignity and justice that guarantee all citizens "minimum standards of income, livelihood, housing accommodation, and education" (Eriksen and Loftager, 1996: 2). Children are included in these welfare arrangements as part of a family but also as individuals. They have rights to education, health services, and a decent childhood free from neglect and abuse. The Norwegian child welfare system is both protective and supportive in its approach to children at risk; it provides a wide range of welfare services and undertakes compulsory action when necessary.

Each of the 428 Norwegian municipalities is required by law to have a responsible child welfare administration. Because municipality sizes differ, agency sizes differs. For instance, Bergen, the second largest municipality in Norway, has a population of approximately 280,000 and a child welfare agency with 200 full-time positions (as of 2012). By contrast, the municipality of Tysnes, only an hour's drive from Bergen, has a population of 2,800 and only two full-time positions in its child welfare agency. The responsibility for children at risk is identical in these municipalities, and the services and quality of casework and decision making adhere to the same standards.

At the municipal level across Norway, there are 3,650 full-time positions (as of 2011)—3.6 positions per 1,000 children—and the number of child welfare workers has steadily increased since 1994. Approximately half of the child welfare workers hold a bachelor of arts degree in child welfare/protection work, and the rest have either a bachelor's degree in social work or a higher degree.

There are three main reasons for child service or interventions from the child welfare system.

1. At the lowest level, the child welfare system intervenes when a child due to conditions in the home or for other reasons is in particular need of assistance, as defined in the Child Welfare Act, Section 4-4 (1), by providing voluntary in-home services.

2. If the agency cannot help the child with in-home services, or if in-home services are inappropriate (if the child is maltreated or abused, for instance, as described in the Child Welfare Act, Section 4-12), out-of-home placement is sought.

3. If a youth is behaving destructively or violently (e.g., substance abuse), the child welfare agency can provide in-home services or an out-of-home placement under the Child Welfare Act, Sections 4-24 and 4-26.

Intervention may be voluntary or compulsory. Serious interventions, such as the use of force and out-of-home placements, must be decided by the county court. An overview of the rates of services and interventions are presented in Table 3.1.

Table 3.1. Norwegian national statistics on children and the child welfare system

	1994	2000	2005	2007	2008	2009	2010	2011
Referrals investigated, per 1,000 children	13.2	16.5	19.5	22.8	25.2	26.5	28.8	30.6
Children receiving services (all types), end of year, per 1,000 children	19.9	21.8	25.2	27.5	28.4	29.5	30.4	30.5
Children receiving in-home services, end of year, per 1,000 children	14.6	16.9	19.7	21.8	22.6	23.6	24.1	24.0
Children placed out of home (with and without care order), end of year, per 1,000 children	5.9	6.7	7.4	8.0	8.2	8.4	9.0	9.3
Children with a formal care order decision, end of year, per 1,000 children	5.3	4.8	5.5	5.7	5.8	6.0	6.3	6.5
Children placed out of home without a formal care order decision, end of year, per 1,000 children	0.6	1.9	1.9	2.3	2.4	2.5	2.8	2.8
Reunification cases decided by court, N = cases	*	*	*	174	191	208	203	214
Adoptions of children in the child welfare system, N = persons	*	*	*	*	*	30	29	40
Adoption cases decided by court,[a] N = cases	*	27	11	11	24	23	34	38
Workers in the child welfare system, 100% position, end of year, per 1,000 children	2.3	2.4	2.7	2.9	3.0	3.1	3.2	3.6
Young persons (18–22) receiving child welfare services, end of year, N = persons	*	1,722	2,348	2,472	2,570	2,922	3,459	3,899

(Continued)

Table 3.1. (Continued)

	1994	2000	2005	2007	2008	2009	2010	2011
New children in the system, N = children[b]	*	8,583	10,045	11,731	11,760	12,386	13,231	13,695
Child population, end of year, N = children	1,003,203	1,060,857	1,092,728	1,099,279	1,103,481	1,109,156	1,114,374	1,118,225
Immigrant child population, end of year	*	70,335	91,553	104,624	1,134,11	123,297	132,685	141,901
Unaccompanied asylum-seeking children	*	*	*	400	1,400	2,500	890	860

Sources: IMDi (2012a); Statistics Norway (2012); Skivenes (2011).

* Statistics not available/reliable.

ᵃ Outcome of decision is not known.

ᵇ This statistic may include several young adults (18 to 22 years old).

IMMIGRANT POPULATION AND THE CHILD WELFARE SYSTEM

The immigration population of 600,000 persons in Norway, as measured in January 2011, has roots in more than 175 countries. Approximately half of immigrants are originally from Asia (210,000), Africa (73,500), or Latin America (19,200; IMDi, 2012b). Most of the immigrant population consists of people born outside Norway (500,000; IMDi, 2012b). The population of children (zero to 17 years old) was approximately 1,118,225 as of January 1, 2012, and, of these, approximately 141,901 children were immigrants.

Approximately 860 unaccompanied minors sought asylum in 2011, and the majority of them came from (in descending order) Afghanistan, Somalia, Iraq, Sri Lanka, and Ethiopia. Approximately 68% of the unaccompanied asylum seekers were 16 years old or older, 14% were 15 years old, and 18% were 14 years old or younger. Only the latter group of children was the responsibility of the local child welfare agency, that is, those children 14 years old and younger. The goal of the child welfare agency is that unaccompanied children between the ages of 15 and 18 years shall become the responsibility of the child welfare agency, but this is delayed because the government anticipates that this will require more resources than local child welfare agencies have at present (cf. Ot.prp. nr. 28, 2007–2008; St. Meld. St. 27, 2011–2012). We do not have accurate numbers for unaccompanied minor asylum seekers in the child welfare system because there are differences between municipalities in their handling of the responsibility for the children who are 15 years old and over (Allertsen, Kalve, and Aalandsli, 2007). Some municipalities include these children and young persons in the child welfare system, while others do not. Table 3.2 presents a detailed overview of the statistics available about children in the child welfare system, distinguishing between children from the immigrant population (first and second generation) versus children outside the immigrant population. A clear finding is that the overrepresentation of immigrant children in the child welfare system is connected to the provision of in-home services. The rate of immigrant children placed out of home over the past 10 years has been lower than or equal to that of nonimmigrant children.

Table 3.2 sheds a somewhat positive light on the troubling issue of overrepresentation of immigrant children in the child welfare system because the overrepresentation relates to in-home services. It is, of course, a different matter to be overrepresented in receiving services than to be overrepresented in losing custody over a child as a result of neglect or abuse. It makes sense that families in the immigrant population are in need of more services because they are newcomers to a country, with looser connections to work and community and often with a smaller social network and fewer family members to rely on. However, the table does not show the number of voluntary out-of-home placements

Table 3.2. Facts and numbers for the immigrant and nonimmigrant child populations

	2009	2004	2002
Nonmigrant children in Norway	985,859	1,000,847	996,790
Migrant children in Norway	123,297	87,186	78921
Nonmigrant children in the child welfare system	26,143 (26.5/1,000)	22,848 (22.8/1,000)	21,284 (21.4/1,000)
Migrant children in the child welfare system	6,399 (51.9/1,000)	3,560 (40.8/1,000)	2,840 (36/1,000)
Nonmigrant children with in-home services	20,297 (20.6/1,000)	17,451 (17.4/1,000)	16,147 (16.2/1,000)
Migrant children with in-home services	5,655 (45.9/1,000)	3,168 (36.3/1,000)	2,529 (32/1,000)
Nonmigrant children with care orders	5,846 (5.9/1,000)	5,397 (5.4/1,000)	5,137 (5.2/1,000)
Migrant children with care orders	744 (6/1,000)	392 (4.5/1,000)	311 (3.9/1,000)

Sources: Kalve and Dyrhaug (2011); Statistics Norway (2011).

N = children, or n per 1,000 children.

(placement without a formal care order). Statistics Norway does not cover such information, and there is speculation (and worry) that voluntary placements may have an element of force in them and/or that it is easier to place a child "voluntarily" because there is a veil of parental authority over such a placement. Perhaps some workers find it more convenient to do voluntarily placements with immigrant families? We do not have much evidence or knowledge to substantiate these propositions, and there is an urgent need for more information about the nature and number of voluntarily placements.

Although the statistics may elicit comparatively good news about the matter of immigrant children versus nonimmigrant children in the child welfare system, several worrying aspects about the system should be examined. First, there are differences between immigrants born abroad and immigrant children born in Norway (first and second generation). Second, there are country differences—children from some countries are much more overrepresented in the child welfare system.

(1) As for differences between immigrant children and children with immigrant parents, 67.5 out of 1,000 immigrant children are in the child welfare system, while 41.4 per 1,000 children of immigrant parents are in the system. Further, examining the type of services that children receive, we find an important difference in the numbers for care orders; approximately 8.6 per 1,000 immigrant children are in care, versus 4.3 per 1,000 of the children with immigrant parents.

In the nonimmigrant child population, approximately 5.3 per 1,000 children are in care.

(2) The immigrant child population in the child welfare system contains children with backgrounds from over 175 countries, and there are disproportionate numbers of children from certain countries. Because accurate statistics about these matters do not exist, the following numbers are based on the zero- to 22-year-old age group and include approximately 2,934 young adults (cf. Kalve and Dyrhaug, 2011). At the end of 2009, the following countries were among the top seven most-represented countries: Afghanistan (163 per 1,000 children), Eritrea (96 per 1,000 children), Iraq (94 per 1,000 children), Russia (91 per 1,000 children), and Burma (Myanmar; 85 per 1,000 children). The list of countries of children in the child welfare system with immigrant parents is as follows (in descending order): Russia (85 per 1,000 children), Iran (77 per 1,000 children), Iraq and Afghanistan (both with 71 per 1,000 children), Morocco (62 per 1,000 children), Eritrea (62 per 1,000 children), and Vietnam (59 per 1,000 children). Table 3.3 presents an overview of this information. Kalve and Dyrhaug (2011) show that there are age differences between the group of immigrant children and immigrant children born in Norway. Of immigrant children, most are teenagers, and only one out of 10 is below the age of six. In the second-generation group, the opposite holds, with approximately three out of four children being below the age of 13 years, with many of preschool age (Kalve and Dyrhaug, 2011).

There is no comprehensive explanation for these country differences, but clearly the situation in the countries these families originate from are important to their abilities to establish themselves in a society such as Norway. A number

Table 3.3. Background country for immigrant population in the child welfare system

Immigrant children	Children with immigrant parents
67 per 1,000 zero to 22-year-olds (*n* = 5,146)	51 per 1,000 zero to 22-year-olds (*n* = 4,187)
Afghanistan 163/1,000	Russia 85/1,000
Eritrea 96/1,000	Iran 77/1,000
Iraq 94/1,000	Iraq 71/1,000
Russia 91/1,000	Afghanistan 71/1,000
Burma 85/1,000	Morocco 62/1,000
Iran 82/1,000	Eritrea 62/1,000
Somalia 80/1,000	Vietnam 59/1,000

Source: Kalve and Dyrhaug (2011). Numbers are from 2009 and include children and young adults who are zero to 22 years old.

of families have been through many hardships before entering Norway; these families will likely find it difficult and challenging to establish themselves and their children in Norway. Another important explanation for the high numbers for immigrant children in the child welfare system may be related to unaccompanied asylum-seeking children, which may explain the high numbers for Afghanistan, Iraq, and Somalia.

NORWEGIAN LAW AND POLICY IN THE CHILD WELFARE AREA AND MIGRANT CHILDREN

Children in the immigrant population who somehow are in a problematic situation that can activate the assistance of the child welfare system have not been high on the Norwegian political agenda. A systematic examination of major policy documents, legislation, and parliamentary reports during the past 12 years (2000–2012) reveals that neither have the child welfare system's role in regard to immigrant children, nor immigrant children themselves, been an issue that has been much discussed.[4] But, surely, with the recent court cases and the public criticism of the government's policies and lack thereof (cf. the introduction in this chapter), the issue has received independent and dynamic attention. The governments report to the Parliament ("Children on the Run") is a clear example of this. Further, in newer reports, the issue of immigrants and minorities are mentioned on a routine basis, in line with how gender and environment became concerns that should be considered, as is evident in the report "Better Protection of Children's Development" (NOU, 2012: 5).

Norway has a relatively short history with migrants and immigrants, and as early as 1975 the Norwegian government regulated migration to the country, stating that only persons with a certain status were admitted to the country; these included experts, those who sought family reunification, students, and refugee and asylum seekers (cf. Gullestad, 2002). For those who are admitted to the country, there is an explicit policy of inclusion, solidarity, and expectation that all should contribute according to abilities. For example, Rugkåsa (2009) shows how work is an integration strategy toward migrant women. The Stoltenberg's second government (2005–2013) states the following about its general ambition on the immigration field:

The Government will promote a tolerant, multicultural society and combat racism. Diversity enriches our society.

Rights, obligations and opportunities will be the same for all, regardless of ethnic background, gender, religion, sexual orientation or degree of functioning.

Gender equality is also a precondition for an inclusive society.

The government will combat discrimination, prejudice and racism in order to give everyone the same opportunities for social participation.

At the same time we will make it clear that all inhabitants are obliged to participate, comply with the law and support the fundamental democratic values of our society. (BLD, 2014)

In the government's action plans there are formulated concrete goals that directly target migrant children. Two of them directly involve the child welfare system and possibly the police, and that is the combat against genital mutilation and forced marriage. Both practices are banned and illegal in Norway, and the government uses different tools to fight these practices: information, a focus on changing attitudes, bringing forward knowledge, and advisors who communicate with the migrant population. Two other strategic measures the government uses are improved education and child care arrangements for migrant children, meant to reduce and combat poverty among immigrant children.

Regarding children in the immigrant population in Norway, three groups in particular have received attention in recent years and have created responses and measures from the government: children in families who have received a negative answer on their application of residence in Norway, unaccompanied minor asylum seekers, and migrant workers and their families.

First, children who are born in Norway or who have stayed in Norway for years but whose parents are denied permission to stay in Norway are part of the cases I mentioned in the introduction, and are creating an uproar in parts of the population. In 2012 the public debate was around 544 children who lived in a highly stressful and uncertain situation. Questions about amnesty were raised, but the government declined to give amnesty due to migration regulations and fear of promoting incentives for migrant families to come to Norway without proper cause (St. Meld. 27, 2011–2012: 47ff). The government is clear in its policy report to the Parliament in 2012 that it will not make any legislative changes, but the report presents some clarifications, for example, around the balancing of best interest and immigration control considerations. The starting point for the government is that the Convention on the Rights of the Child does not give a directive for solving immigration cases, with the implication that the best interest principle is not decisive. This is also the interpretation the Norwegian Supreme Court proposes (cf. Rt., 2009, s1261). However, the more serious the situation is for the child, the more it calls for emphasis on the child's interest (St. Meld. 27, 2011–2012: 46, cf. 50ff).

As for the child welfare system's responsibility for children living in these families waiting for an answer on their application or their appeal, they are not mandated *a particular* responsibility for these children. However, I wonder if the child welfare system should be given instruction to direct attention to these children because they are undoubtedly living in a difficult and uncertain situation. In particular, the situation is difficult when the family receives a rejection to an application or an appeal. An extreme example is a young woman and her one-year-old baby, who received a rejection on the asylum appeal; consequently she killed herself and the baby on January 16, 2012.[5]

The second group is the unaccompanied asylum seekers who are in Norway and who, according to Norwegian law and practice, are in need of help and assistance because they lack caregivers. The government is concerned for this group of children and has put in place several measures to improve their situation. However, it is also an explicit concern that children are sent from their home country in the hopes of being admitted residence in Norway. This is not in the children's best interest as the Norwegian government regards it, because there is a magnitude of dangers for vulnerable children traveling alone (St. Meld. 27, 2011–2012: 48). New legislation has been put into place to prevent and protect children who are victims of trafficking. The child welfare system has received a clear mandate to protect these children, with extended powers to keep children in a residential unit and to supervise children and those who want to reach them (Innst. 250 L, 2011–2012; cf. St. Meld. 27, 2011–2012: 47). The other measure put in place, in 2009, was to narrow the opportunities to be granted stays in Norway for children the age of 16 to 18 years who do not have a need for protection.

Third are the migrant workers and their children who come under the scrutiny of the child welfare system. In 2012 there were at least three high profile cases: a Polish family who lost custody of two boys due to neglect,[6] an Indian family who lost custody of their children of five months and three years old,[7] and another Indian family convicted of violence toward their 11-year-old boy.[8] The child welfare system was central in all three cases (although it was the court that decided about both care orders and violence). The migrants' home countries' governments and media have engaged themselves in the cases. The main tenant has been that the Norwegian child welfare system is oppressive and lacks cultural understanding. The child welfare system states that these cases are about the children's interest and the position children have in Norwegian society. Children's strong standing in all areas of the Norwegian society represents a new historical era that may be challenging for older generations of Norwegians and represents in a new cultural perspective—perhaps a very different approach to disciplining children and including them in family and society (cf. Križ and Skivenes, 2011).

Examining the child welfare systems approach to migrant children, the Norwegian Child Welfare Act of 1992 is guided by the "best interest" principle and instructs decision makers to take into regard the particular and individual needs and interests of the child concerned. Rarely does this law give additional recommendations for arguments and circumstances to consider. However, if a child is to be placed out of home, the legislator requests decision makers to consider ethnic, religious, cultural, and linguistic background. The paragraph reads like this:

> § 4-15. Selection of placement in a particular case.
> Within the framework set forth in § 4-14, the location chosen by the child's individuality and need for care and training in a stable environment. It should also be taken with due regard to the desirability of continuity in a child's upbringing and to the child's ethnic, religious, cultural and linguistic background. It shall also be given to how long it is likely that the position will last and whether it is possible and desirable that the child has visitation and other contact with the parents.

The wording chosen in this paragraph is quite similar to the English Children's Act of 1989, and there have not to my knowledge been discussions about making changes to this approach.

In sum, the policies and the legislation on vulnerable migrant children display a rather clear problem perception, that recently has made an attempt to draw a line between the principle of the child´s best interest and immigration regulations.

CULTURE CONFLICTS AND DISCRIMINATION

A pressing question is whether the numbers presented here show that the overrepresentation of immigrant children and families in the child welfare system is the result of oppression and/or racism. This topic elicits varying perceptions and explanations among Norwegian academics and from the general public. However, there is a recurring sentiment in the public discourse and in some academic discourse that the immigrant population is discriminated against. For example, the Norwegian sociologist Kaya (2010: 19) believes that Norwegian society is ethnocentric and oppressive: "In meetings between ethnic Norwegians and immigrants, it is the Norwegian cultural rules and norms that are applicable and seems totally dominant, while the migrant's own cultural rules are invalid." In Kaya´s opinion, there is also oppression and ethnocentrism in the practices conducted by social workers: "Bigotry and ethnocentrism dominate in most contexts. The first notion is that there is only one way to do things, i.e., one's own, and the other is perceived so that you are aware of the existence of more culturally specific ways of organizing businesses, but they think their own way is the best" (2010: 43).

Kaya does not substantiate these strong statements, and to my knowledge, there is no published research that supports them. The general opinion in the population (90%) is that immigrants are discriminated against (IMDi, 2012b). However, there is also in the population a "general agreement that immigrants with permanent residence in the country should have equal rights with the rest of the population" (IMDi, 2010b), and 90% of the population believes that all immigrants should have the same opportunity as Norwegians to employment (Statistics Norway, 2011).

Many findings show that immigrants believe that they are being discriminated against, and there are many observations of discrimination against migrants and minorities. For example, in the latest survey on "Integration in Norway," between 3% and 10% of the respondents say that they have experienced discrimination because of their ethnicity and/or cultural background (IMDi, 2012b). In a study of discrimination in the labor market, Rogstad (2006) identifies the subjective perception of discrimination to be between 14% and 18%. The study examined discrimination against newcomers in Norway with respect to the labor market and concludes that between 6% and 25% are discriminated against using a variety of methodological approaches (2006: 21). In a report from Statistics Norway, respondents from the 10 largest immigrant populations in Norway were asked in 2005 and 2006 about their experiences with discrimination in the labor market, education, housing, health, and other social areas. Approximately half of the respondents said that they had experienced discrimination once or more in one of these five areas. The author notes the following:

> The migrants most frequently report[ing] the experience of discrimination are Somalis and Iraqis. Both of these country groups are characterized by relatively short-lived, low education and low participation in the labor market. In other words, groups that are less included and are underrepresented in key areas of society. Their experience of discrimination can thus be marginalization. (Tronstad, 2009: 3)

Marginalization is a well-known problem for migrant families; in the period of 2005 to 2007, 12% of migrant children lived in poverty (Statistics Norway, 2011). Twenty-seven percent of children from Iraq, Afghanistan, and Somalia are in households that are economically poor. Other contextual factors are the lack of social network and difficulties finding employment. Clearly these stress factors influence a family's ability to raise their children the way they wish to and to use their resources effectively. Finally, it is important to be clear about the cultural differences and conflicts that may arise in a Norwegian society and to emphasize how these affect children's rights. In a book first published in 2002, *Rethinking Multiculturalism,* the Indian-English political theorist Parekh identifies and discusses the manner in which certain cultural practices create conflicts in Western societies (Parekh 2006: 273ff). Many of these practices concern children, and many violate Norwegian legislation and thus involve the child welfare system. Two clear examples of this are female circumcision and withholding children from education; these practices will not be part of a cultural dialog in Norwegian society (nor in other Western societies).

A lack of a cultural dialog on matters that create conflicts may be reason enough for migrants and others to express dismay and lack of trust in Norwegian society; this makes it critical to be aware of the possible pitfalls and the tyranny of being naïve with respect to minorities' experiences with oppression and discrimination. Two positive findings are encouraging: First, a recent survey shows that "between 60 and 80% of the population can envision giving various types of help to immigrant children, juveniles and adults to contribute to their integration in society" (IMDi, 2012b: 7). Second, in a recent court decision, the court of appeal (Gulating) examined a claim that child welfare agencies in Bergen municipality were discriminating an immigrant mother of African origin. The court expressed that it could not find any evidence to substantiate this claim (Jury Court, 2012).

TRAINING AND ORGANIZATIONAL STRUCTURES

In the Norwegian child welfare system, approximately 90% of the frontline child welfare force has a three-year bachelor of arts degree in social work (40%) or in child welfare work education (50%; NOU, 2009: 8, 93). The remaining 10% have some other type of education of three or more years or are unskilled. In the two largest municipalities in Norway, Oslo and Bergen, 89% of the sample of workers report having an education in social work at the bachelor's, master's, or doctoral level.

Training and education in working with immigrant groups/ethnic minorities is an area that is rather new in Norway. The government published an official report in 2009 (NOU, 2009: 8) concerning the general plans and development of competency in the child welfare system. An overt goal is to hire more workers with ethnic minority backgrounds; at present, the stipulation is that 3% to 5% of all the paid staff in the child welfare system (including foster homes and residential units) should come from the immigrant population or from a minority group (NOU, 2009: 8, 93). With respect to the child welfare system's approach to migrant families, the government states that child welfare workers must be culturally sensitive in combination with having specific knowledge about minority populations (NOU, 2009: 8, 37). However, there is also an explicit awareness that, although being culturally sensitive is a skill that is required in all child welfare work, it is important not to let the cultural focus overshadow matters such as poverty, lack of employment, and small social networks (NOU, 2009: 8, 37).

In September 2012, there were a handful of university colleges in Norway that offered courses of 15 to 30 ECTS, with a curriculum that focuses on culturally sensitive social work. As of December 2012, an overview of the number of child welfare workers who had attended these educational programs had not been provided. Among the survey sample from Bergen and Oslo, 37% of workers reported that they had received training to work specifically with immigrants. The educational programs on "Child Welfare from a Minority Perspective" funded by the Ministry of Children, Equality and Social Inclusion were evaluated in 2010. The conclusion was that they were of a high professional quality and had significant capacity for implementation (Thorshaug, Svendsen, and Berg, 2010).

Another way of working with specific aims is to focus on certain issues or functions; for example, the focus may be that child welfare agencies establish units to work with minority families. Norwegian legislation does not require a particular organizational form with respect to the interaction of child welfare agencies with migrant/immigrant families, and a request to the agencies involved in the survey shows that none of those who responded had established separate units for immigrant families (although several had undertaken responsibility for unaccompanied minors and had separate units for this). Further, none of the agencies had established guidelines specifically for working with immigrant families, whereas a few agencies had Internet sites available in English, Urdu, and Somali (Alna and Sagene in Oslo municipality).

PRACTICE—THE EXPERIENCES OF FRONTLINE WORKERS

We have responses from a sample of 168 child welfare workers working in Bergen and Oslo, the two largest cities in Norway.[9] All of these workers have experience working with migrant and immigrant families; at the time of the survey, their caseloads with immigrant children had an average of 50% and a mode of only 10%. Only 7% of the workers reported that they speak the language of one or more of their immigrant service users. Two out of three workers reported that they experienced more system barriers when working with immigrant families compared to nonimmigrant families.

When asked about irregular immigrant children, and whether they had responsibility for a child of school age that was not attending school, 84% confirmed that they did have such a responsibility. The remaining 16% of the workers either answered no (4%) or that they did not know (12%) in response to this question.

We created a vignette that we presented to the workers about a marginalized migrant family with a newborn baby (see appendix for full description of the vignette). We return to the results from this vignette later, but the responses from the sample of Norwegian child welfare workers show the close connections between the child welfare system and the welfare state system. The majority of workers (82%) responded that they would let the baby stay with the parents and provide services. Presented with a list of different solutions and services, we observed that workers would link the parents with the general welfare service system (93%) and provide them with other services available in Norway (89%). In response to whether the workers would find the family a place with amenities and running water, fewer than one out of three (29%) said they would; 46% said that was not an option in the Norwegian system. Helping parents find employment was clearly a service that child welfare workers could not assist with (66% answered "no" or "not an option in our system" to this statement).

In the questionnaire, we also included a possible value-charged statement that read: "I would encourage the parents to return to their home country." Only 13% said they would do this, and 46% answered no to this question.

To explore how child welfare workers understand their mandate and how the borders between immigration and child welfare are drawn, we asked workers to consider three statements, each followed by fixed-answer categories. The results are presented in Table 3.4 and show that most workers are certain they have the authority to act in these types of cases, but they are less certain that the interests of the child trump immigration issues. A majority of the workers are clear about the responsibility of the child welfare agency and that they shall act although immigration issues may be pending.

We also wondered whether child welfare workers in Norway would discriminate or show bias toward parents who are working versus parents who are recipients of welfare services, even though Norway is a country with a strong work ethic and in which public debates sometimes revolve around the opinion that immigrants are parasitic on the welfare state's generous and universal services. Testing for this variable in a vignette, we see that the result is that the sample group did not discriminate between parents who are working versus parents who are unemployed and living on child welfare benefits. There are no noteworthy differences in the risk assessments and their suggested decisions. I find it interesting that such a fact does not matter for worker assessments and choice in the case. For example, the recent "Integration Barometer 2012" indicates that a majority (71%) of the Norwegian population considers an immigrant's ability to support oneself and one's family through work an important criteria for successful integration (IMDi, 2012b: 8).

Table 3.4. Role and responsibility of the child welfare agency (*n* = 138)

	True	Not true	I don't know
"This is a case in which the child welfare agency would have the authority to act"	88%	3%	6%
"This is a case in which the interest of the newborn child would trump immigration issues."	48%	13%	28%
"This is a case in which immigration issues must be sorted out before we could do any child welfare work."	6%	74%	7%

When I presented this result to workers in a child welfare agency in Bergen municipality, they did not seem to be surprised by the similarity in the assessments. They thought this reflected their child focus, an interpretation that resonates with other research findings (Križ and Skivenes, 2010; Skivenes, 2011). Additionally, this might be a finding that is correlated with the violence aspect of the case, as violence against children is clearly illegal and a crime in Norway. There have been several high-profile media cases in which migrant families have used physical discipline and violence against their children and have been brought to court as a result; in such cases, the child welfare system has become involved to supervise the family and protect the children.

Recurrent issues in the Norwegian child welfare system and in public debates are the question of competency and whether child welfare workers have the right and necessary qualifications to work with service users from another ethnic, cultural, and religious background than the "typical" Norwegian majority. In the literature, there is no a universal recipe with which to work with newcomers and migrant children; cultural competency or cultural sensitivity in the approach seems to be common. Perhaps the clearest disagreement is about the amount of specific knowledge a worker should have about a country, minority group, ethnicity, religion, and so on of a service user. One position is that a worker should have such insights; the converse position is that a sensitive and respectful approach is sufficient (and the only feasible approach; Quershi, 2009).

Previous research has found that workers in Norway and England find it challenging to work with immigrant families because of language problems, cultural gaps, and miscommunication (Križ and Skivenes, 2010, 2012, cf. Holm-Hansen, Haaland, and Myrvold, 2007). We therefore asked the Norwegian sample ($n = 168$) whether they experience their work with immigrant families to be more, equally, or less challenging than working with nonimmigrant families and whether they believe that they are more, equally, or less competent in working with immigrant families versus nonimmigrant families. Approximately half of the sample (51%) expressed the belief that they are more or equally competent in working with immigrant families, and 65% of the sample stated that they experience their work with immigrant families to be more challenging than working with nonimmigrant families.

CONCLUSION

This chapter has shown how the Norwegian child welfare system approaches migrant children and their families and draws a picture of a system that, on many dimensions, is universal in its meeting with children at risk. In particular, the findings from the survey identify a unison perception among workers that migrant children are their responsibility. The government's policies and the platform that outline the Norwegian state's handling of migrant children are controversial within the general public, and there are critical voices that demand stronger political action and standpoint in the cases of migrant children. As it is now, it seems that many decisions that could have been handled by the politicians are now left to the court to decide. In a historical perspective, the Norwegian state was early to establish strict rules for immigration and settlement in 1975, and it has continued to do so. Even though children are a new issue on this political map, and bear with it difficult cases that challenge the Norwegian focus on child-centrism, the government has kept a firm focus on balancing best-interest considerations against immigration regulations. I think that is a conclusion to be drawn from the government report on migrant children, "On the Run," published in 2012.

Interestingly, the overrepresentation of migrant children in the child welfare system is an issue of providing in-home services. This indicates that the overrepresentation is less worrying because it is expected that migrant children are in need of more help, and it is in line with the general ideas of the welfare state and the ambitions of reducing poverty among immigrant children and their families. The cultural conflicts that have been identified in Western societies, and that often involve children, are also evident for the Norwegian child welfare system, and at both the policy and the practice level there are developed strategies to handle it together with a culturally sensitive practice. What continues to be problematic is the actual interaction with migrant children and their families. It is clear that frontline work demands more resources and time to communicate and create a common understanding between families and the child welfare system, and language barriers are continuously hindering fruitful collaboration.

Finally, the case of migrant children makes it evident how the rights of the child may collide with the rights and the actions of the parents, for example when parents' migration history and actions have huge consequences for their children. The case of *Norway v. Butt* (2012) and cases of irregular children are examples of this. In some of the cases that have been reviewed by the court, parents are then an appendage to their children's rights and can, for example, be grated admission to Norway based on the child's best-interest consideration. The possible side effect of this, and a fear the Norwegian state explicitly considers, is that children are used as means to gain access to Norway. As it is today, the answer to this problem, as the Norwegian state regards it, is to keep a clear focus on immigration regulations and, when necessary, include considerations of best interests for the child. I think we need an explicit political standpoint on the balancing point between these two considerations.

ACKNOWLEDGMENTS

Many thanks to Hanne Stenberg for her help providing statistics for the immigrant child population and for facilitating the practical work of the online survey. I am also grateful to Berit Crosby for collecting e-mail addresses from the child welfare agencies and examining official documents. Dr. Marianne Rugkåsa has given important comments on the chapter. Employees in the Bergenhus child welfare agency have kindly commented on the findings from the survey. Thanks also to the other editors and fellow authors in this book for their interest and comments during my writing process, and, finally, as always, my deepest gratitude to the child welfare workers for participating in the survey and, most of all, for the important work they do.

NOTES

1 Case of *Butt v. Norway* (Application no. 47017/09).
2 The ambition is that the child welfare system shall have responsibility for all asylum-seeking children but, because of resource limitations, the government has implemented this process in two steps. As of September 2012, the child welfare system is responsible for children zero to 14 years of age, and the immigration authorities has responsibility thereafter.
3 A comprehensive overview of the Norwegian child welfare system can be found in Skivenes (2011).
4 The following documents are examined: Endringer i barnevernloven—nye bestemmelser om midlertidig plassering av barn utsatt for menneskehandel 2012; Handlingsplaner mot tvangsekteskap og kjønnslemlestelse 2012; Handlingsplan for å fremme likestilling og hindre etnisk diskriminering 2009; Handlingsplan mot tvangsekteskap 2007; Handlingsplan mot seksuelle og fysiske overgrep mot barn 2005; Handlingsplan mot tvangsekteskap 2001; Handlingsplan mot kjønnslemlestelse 2000; NOU 2012:5; NOU 2011:20; NOU 2011:14; NOU 2011:7; NOU 2009:21; NOU 2009:14; NOU 2009:9; NOU 2009:8; NOU 2008:9; NOU 2006:9; NOU 2005:9; Ot.prp. Nr. 69 2008–2009; Prop. 132L. 2011–2012; Prop. 50L. 2011–2012; Prop. 43L. 2011–2012; Prop. 7L. 2009–2010; St. Meld. 27 2011–1012; St. Meld. 40 2001–2002; St. Meld. 39 2001–2002; St. Meld. 43 2000––2001; St. Meld. 17 1999–2000; St. Meld. 39 1995–1996; Tiltaksprogram—Fornyet innsats mot tvangsekteskap 2002.
5 Bergens Tidende: http://www.bt.no/nyheter/Om-ein-time-set-ho-fyr-pa-seg-sjolv-2821432.html.
6 District court decision of December 14, 2012. 12-031176MED-STAV.
7 http://www.aftenbladet.no/nyheter/lokalt/stavanger/Barnevernet-har-tvangsplassert-indiske-barn-2909674.html

8   District court decision of December 3, 2012, cf. Aftenposten, 4. Desember 2012.
9   The details and methodology for this cross-country survey are provided in
     the appendix.

REFERENCES

Allertsen, Linda M., Kalve, Trygve, & Aalandsli, Vebjørn. (2007). *Enslige min-dreårige asylsøkere i barnevernet* (Unaccompanied Asylum Seekers in the Child Welfare System). Oslo: Statistisk sentralbyrå.

Arts, Wil, & Gelissen, John (2002). Three worlds of welfare capitalism or more? A state-of-the-art-report. *Journal of European Social Policy*, 12(2), 137–158.

BLD. (2014). Intergration and Diversity, Barne-, Likestillings- og Inkluderingsdepartementet, 29.08.14. Available at: http://www.regjeringen.no/templates/Tema.aspx.html?idkeep=true&id=1138_712429&epslanguage=en-GB.

Brochmann, Grete, Hagelund, Anniken, Borevi, Karen, Vad Jønsson, Heidi, & Petersen, Klaus. (2010). *Velferdens grenser: innvandringspolitikk og velferds-stat i Skandinavia 1945–2010* (The Limits of Welfare: Integration Politics and the Welfare State in Scandinavia 1945-2010). Oslo: Universitetsforlaget.

Eide, Ketil, Qureshi, Naushad A., Rugkåsa, Marianne, & Vike, Halvard. (2010). *Over profesjonelle barrierer* (Beyond Professional Barriers). Oslo: Gyldendal Akademisk.

Eriksen, Erik Oddvar, & Loftager, Jørn, eds. (1996). *The Rationality of the Welfare State*. Oslo: Scandinavian University Press.

Esping-Andersen, Gøsta. (1990). *The Three Worlds of Welfare Capitalism*. Cambridge: Polity Press.

Gilbert, Neil, Parton, Nigel, & Skivenes, Marit, eds. (2011). *Child Protection Systems: International Trends and Emerging Orientations*. New York: Oxford University Press.

Gullestad, Marianne. (2002). *Det norske sett med nye øyne: Kritisk analyse av norsk innvandringsdebatt* (The Norwegian Seen from a New Position: Critical Analysis of Norwegian Immigrant Discourse). Oslo: Universitetsforlaget.

Holm-Hansen, Jørn, Haaland, Thomas, & Myrvold, Trine. (2010). *Flerkulturelt barnevern* (Multicultural Child Welfare). NIBR Report 10. Oslo: Norsk insti-tutt for by- og regionforskning.

Directorate of Integration and Diversity (IMDi). (2012a). Fakta om asylsøkere og flyktninger (Facts about Asylum Seekers and Refugees). Oslo: Integrerings- og mangfoldsdirektoratet. Retrieved August 1, 2013, from: http://www.imdi.no/no/iFAKTA/Fakta-om-asylsokere-og-flyktninger.

———. (2012b). Integreringsbarometeret 2012 (Integration Barometer 2012). Oslo: Integrerings- og mangfoldsdirektoratet. Retrieved August 1, 2013, from http://www.imdi.no/no/Nyheter/2012/Integreringsbarometeret-2012/.

Innst. 250 L. (2011–2012). Instilling til familie- og kulturkomiteen om endringer i barnevernloven (Proposal to the Committee for Family and Culture about Changes in the Child Welfare Act). *Familie- og kulturkomiteen.* Retrieved August 1, 2013-13 from http://www.stortinget.no/no/Saker-og-publikasjoner/Publikasjoner/Innstillinger/Stortinget/2011-2012/inns-201112-250/.

Jury Court. (2012). Gulating Court of Appeal. Decision. 12-096303ASD-GULA/AVD1.

Kalve, Trygve, & Dyrhaug, Tone. (2011). Barn og unge med innvandrerbakgrunn i barnevernet 2009 (Children and Youth with Immigrant Origin in the Child Welfare System 2009). SSB Report 39/2011. Oslo: Statistics Norway.

Kaya, Mehmed. (2010). Innledning (Introduction). In Mehmed Kaya, Halvor Fauske, & Asle Høgmo (Eds.), *Integrasjon og mangfold: Utfordringer for sosialarbeideren* (Integration and Diversity: Challenges for the Social Worker), 13–16. Oslo: Cappelen.

Križ, Katrin, & Skivenes, Marit. (2010). Lost in translation: How child welfare workers in Norway and England experience language differences when working with minority ethnic families. *British Journal of Social Work*, 40(5), 1353–1367.

———. (2011). How child welfare workers view their work with racial and ethnic minority families: The United States in contrast to England and Norway. *Children and Youth Services Review*, 33(10), 1866–1874.

———. (2012). Challenges for marginalized minority parents in different welfare systems: Child welfare workers' perspectives. *International Social Work*, doi: 10.1177/0020872812456052.

Norwegian Child Welfare Act. (1992). Oslo: Ministry of Children, Equality and Social Inclusion.

NOU 2009:8. (2009). Kompetanseutvikling i barnevernet (Development of Competency in the Child Welfare Services). Oslo: Barne-, likestillings- og inkluderingsdepartementet. Retrieved August 1, 2013, from http://www.regjeringen.no/templates/GenerellSide.aspx?id=579153&epslanguage=no

NOU 2012:5. (2012). Bedre beskyttelse av barns utvikling (Improved Protection of Child Development). Oslo: Barne-, likestillings- og inkluderingsdepartementet. Retrieved August 1, 2013, from http://www.regjeringen.no/nb/dep/bld/dok/nouer/2012/nou-2012-5.html?id=671400

Ot.prp. nr. 28. (2007–2008). Om lov om endringer i lov 17.juli 1992 nr. 100 om barneverntjenester mv. (About Law about Changes in Law 17th July 1992 Child Welfare Act). Oslo: Barne-, likestilling- og inkluderingsdepartementet. Retrieved August 1, 2013, from http://www.regjeringen.no/nb/dep/bld/dok/regpubl/otprp/2007-2008/Otprp-nr-28-2007-2008-.html?id=496950.

Parekh, Bhikhu. (2006). *Rethinking Multiculturalism: Cultural Diversity and Political Theory.* Cambridge: Harvard University Press.

Quershi, Naushad A. (2009). Kultursensitivitet i profesjonell yrkesutøvelse (Cultural sensitive professional practice). In Ketil Eide, Naushad A. Qureshi, Marianne Rugkåsa, & Halvard Vike (Eds.), *Over profesjonelle barrierer* (Beyond Professional Barriers), 206–228. Oslo: Gyldendal Akademisk.

Rogstad, J. (2006). Usaklige hindringer for ikke-vestlige minoriteter på arbeidsmarkedet i Norge. Oslo: ISF.

Rugkåsa, Marianne. (2009). Etniske minoritetskvinners inntreden i arbeidslivet og konsekvenser for barn og familieliv (Ethnic minority women's involvement in work life and its consequences for children and family). In Ketil Eide, Naushad A. Qureshi, Marianne Rugkåsa, & Halvard Vike (Eds.), *Over profesjonelle barrierer* (Beyond Professional Barriers), 129–148. Oslo: Gyldendal Akademisk.

Rt. (2009). Norwegian Supreme court decision. Rt-2009-1261

Skivenes, Marit. (2011). Norway—Toward a child centric perspective. In Neil Gilbert, Nigel Parton, & Marit Skivenes (Eds.), *Child Protection Systems: International Trends and Emerging Orientations*, 154–179. New York: Oxford University Press.

Statistics Norway. (2011). Innvandrere blir værende i fattigdom (Immigrants Remain in Poverty). SSB Report, 28–33. Oslo: Statistics Norway. Retrieved August 1, 2013, from http://www.ssb.no/ssp/utg/201101/04/.

———. (2012). Enslige mindreårige flyktninger i arbeid og utdanning. SSB Report 13/2012. Oslo: Statistics Norway.

St. Meld. 27. (2011–2012). Barn på flukt (Children on the Run). Oslo: Justis- og Beredskapsdepartementet.Retrieved August 1, 2013, from http://www.regjeringen.no/nb/dep/jd/dok/regpubl/stmeld/2011-2012/meld-st-27-2011-2012. html?id=684767.

Thorshaug, Kristin, Svendsen, Stina, & Berg, Berit. (2010). *Barnevern i et minoritetsperspektiv* (Child Welfare in a Minority Perspective). NTNU Report. Trondheim: Norwegian University of Science and Technology.

Tronstad, Kristin Rose. (2009). Opplevd diskriminering blant innvandrere med bakgrunn fra ti ulike land (Perceived Discrimination amongst Immigrants with Origin from Ten Different Countries). SSB Report 2009/47. Oslo: Statistics Norway.

4

IMMIGRANT CHILDREN AND FAMILIES IN THE CHILD WELFARE SYSTEM

THE NETHERLANDS

Hans Grietens

INTRODUCTION

This chapter contains four parts. In the first part, we give a state of the art on the migration of children and families to the Netherlands, including a discussion of migration trends, demographics, and research evidence on the well-being and risks in children and families. In the second part, we provide a general overview of the Dutch child welfare system. We outline the structure and organization of the system and give recent figures. Next, we present some of the major problems the Dutch child welfare system is currently facing, as well as some forthcoming changes. We discuss the recent shift toward evidence-based working in child welfare and its implications. The third part is on immigrant children and families in the child welfare system. We discuss the access of immigrants to child welfare services, summarize Dutch research on child welfare professionals' experiences with helping immigrant clients and immigrant clients' perceptions of help received, and review evidence-based interventions and good practices. Finally, we give some concluding remarks on how access to preventive and lower end services for immigrant children and families may be improved.

IMMIGRANT CHILDREN AND FAMILIES IN THE NETHERLANDS

Immigration Trends since the Second World War

The colonial history of the Netherlands means the country has a long tradition of being a host country for immigrants. Being a safe, rich, and affluent society, it attracted and still attracts people from abroad. As in other countries in Western Europe, there have been consecutive waves of immigration since the Second World War (Eldering, 2012). A distinction needs to be made between economical and political immigrants, although the line between both groups is often thin, and they may not be considered categories.

The first wave of economical immigrants is observed in the 1950s. Men from Mediterranean countries (in particular Italy and Spain) moved to the Netherlands to work in industry, for instance as coal miners in the south of the country. Their goal was to stay only for a few years, earn money, and return to their family in the home country. A majority of them returned. A second wave took place in the 1960s. From the mid-1960s on, increasing numbers of economic immigrants from North Africa (mainly from Morocco) and Turkey moved to the Netherlands to work in industry. Here a different process developed. Although these immigrants had planned to stay temporarily and return to their family shortly, the economical instability in their homeland made this very difficult. Many of them decided to stay in the Netherlands and let their wives and children migrate in order to reunify. A third wave of economical immigrants was seen in the 1990s. The fall of the iron curtain and the collapse of the Soviet Union initiated great moves of economic immigrants from Central and Eastern Europe. In addition, the globalization of the world caused people from all continents (in particular, Africa, Southeast Asia, and South America) to move to the Netherlands. Finally, since the beginning of the 1970s, the Netherlands has had economic immigrants from the former colonies and overseas (Indonesia, the Dutch Antilles, Suriname).

Openness, democracy, and political stability have made the Netherlands a safe haven for political immigrants, war refugees, and asylum seekers. In the mid-1970s, there was a stream of war refugees from Vietnam, followed in the 1980s by people fleeing from the dictatorial regimes in Iran and Central and South America. In the past three decades, civil wars in Europe (former Yugoslavia), Asia (Chechnya, Iran, Iraq, Afghanistan), and Africa (Somalia) has led to an increasing number of refugees and asylum seekers, adults, as well as minors, individuals, as well as families.

Immigrant Populations in the Netherlands: Some Figures[1]

The Netherlands are a small but densely populated country. In November 2013, the country had 16,848,317 inhabitants. The majority of them (about 4 out of

10) live in the cities of Amsterdam, Rotterdam, and The Hague, which are situated in the western part of the country in the provinces of North Holland and South Holland.

Since 1999, Statistics Netherlands (www.cbs.nl) defines an immigrant (*allochtoon*) as a person with at least one parent born in a country other than the Netherlands. A distinction is made between Western and non-Western immigrants. Western includes people coming from Europe (except Turkey), North America, Oceania, Japan, and Indonesia (including the Dutch East Indies). Non-Western countries include Turkey and all countries in Africa and Asia, except Japan and Indonesia, which both are considered industrialized countries. The reason for the distinction between Western and non-Western immigrants is the difference in socioeconomic position and culture between countries. The socioeconomic position and culture of Western countries is considered to be relatively similar to that of the Netherlands. Further, a distinction is made between first- and second-generation immigrants. First-generation immigrants are born outside the Netherlands with at least one parent who is also born outside the Netherlands. Second-generation immigrants are born in the Netherlands and have at least one parent who is born outside the Netherlands. People born outside the Netherlands with both parents born in the Netherlands are not considered for statistical purposes as immigrants.

According to this definition, in November 2013, the Netherlands counted 3,543,081 immigrants (21.0% of the total population). More than half of them (55.5%) were of non-Western origin, with Turkey (395,302), Morocco (368,838), Surinam (347,631), and the Dutch Antilles/Aruba (145,499) being most represented. The number of non-Western first-generation immigrants is larger than that of non-Western second-generation immigrants, whereas the reverse is true for Western immigrants. More than 3 out of 10 (30.7%) of the children and young people between zero and 20 were immigrants, with the number of non-Western immigrants being more than twice as high as that of Western immigrants. The percentage of immigrant people (*allochtonen*) in the general population has increased in the past decade from 17.5% in 2000 to 21.0% in 2013 and is expected to increase further in the coming years (CBS Statline, 2013). Immigrants are unequally spread across the country. About two out of three immigrants live in the western part of the country where the three largest cities are situated. About 30% of the immigrants live in the eastern and the southern part of the country (about 15% each), and only 5% live in the northern part. The distribution of immigrants across regions differs from that of nonimmigrants in that the highest concentrations of immigrants are to be found in the larger cities and the western part of the country and far less in the northern part (e.g., about 10% of the Dutch citizens versus about 5% of the migrants live in the northern provinces of Drenthe, Groningen, and Friesland).

Due to the lack of a clear definition and a uniform registration system, it is impossible to give the exact number of refugees in the Netherlands. The

Dutch Council for Refugees, a private supportive organisation for refugees, estimates the total number between 200,000 and 250,000 (www.vluchtelin-genwerk.nl). This figure includes individuals and families living in illegality. Official figures from Dutch Statistics (CBS Statline, 2013) are lower (about 75,000). According to the Dutch Council for Refugees, the number of parents and children living in illegal circumstances is growing in the Netherlands, because it has become more difficult to obtain political asylum during the past decade. This is also demonstrated by the declining figures of requests for asylum (first and following). In 1993, there were 35,399 requests, com-pared to 13,170 in 2012. Another reason for this decline may be the end of the war in former Yugoslavia in the late 1990s. About half of the requests for asylum are approved, and there is little variation in this rate across time. Nowadays, most approvals go to refugees from Somalia, Iraq, Afghanistan, and the Democratic Republic of Congo. Finally, the (official) number of unac-companied young minors has also been declining (1,562 in 1996 vs. 484 in 2011; www.pharos.nl).

Well-Being and Risks in Immigrant Children and Families

Most immigrant children and families, both Western and non-Western, are doing well. They gradually integrate into the Dutch society by learning the lan-guage and participating in work, school, and community life. However, as a group, immigrant children and families are more vulnerable as compared to nonimmigrant citizens. They run higher risks for developing (mental) health, psychosocial, and socioeconomic problems (e.g., Eldering, 2012). A summary of the Dutch research learns that immigrant non-Western families (e.g., Moroccan and Antillean families) are more often single-parent families and have larger numbers of children, lower socioeconomic status, and lower parental educa-tional levels (particularly in first-generation immigrants) as compared to non-immigrant families. Further, higher risks for teenage pregnancy (particularly in Dutch Antillean immigrants) and higher levels of parental stress have been reported in immigrant families (www.nji.nl).

There is little difference between the psychological well-being of Dutch and immigrant young people, and, among the latter, the number of people with a high education level is increasing. It remains difficult, however, for young immi-grants to find a job. In general, rates of problem behavior between Dutch and immigrant children and adolescents do not differ significantly. Interestingly, some differences between immigrant groups were found in epidemiological studies. Turkish parents, for instance, reported more emotional problems in their children than Moroccan or Dutch parents. Turkish children themselves also reported higher levels of emotional problems than Moroccan or Dutch children. Reports on Moroccan children strongly differed, according to the type of informant, with children reporting lower levels of emotional and behav-ioral problems than teachers and parents (Stevens, Bengi-Arslan, Verhulst,

Vollebergh, and Crijnen, 2003; Stevens, Pels, Vollebergh, and Crijnen, 2004). Further, immigrant girls are overrepresented in statistics on youth prostitution (MOVisie, 2009b; www.nji.nl). The ratio of Moroccan versus Dutch girls in prostitution is about 10 to 1; the ratio of Surinam/Turkish versus Dutch girls is about 3 to 1. Finally, immigrant boys and girls are overrepresented in official crime statistics. In particular, Moroccan and Antillean/Aruban boys are highly overrepresented. Rates on crime by young people, based on self-reports, do not show differences however (www.nji.nl).

Confirming international research (see, e.g., De Haene, Grietens, and Verschueren, 2007; Fazel and Stein, 2003; Groark, Sclare, and Raval, 2011; Hodes, 2010; McCarthy and Marks, 2010), Dutch studies showed that refugee children and children from asylum-seeking families have elevated rates of mental health problems and needs. In particular, these children suffer from internalizing problems, including depression, anxiety, and posttraumatic stress (Wiegersma, Stellinga-Boelen, and Reijneveld, 2011; Zijlstra, 2012).

THE CHILD WELFARE SYSTEM IN THE NETHERLANDS

Structure and Organization
According to Esping-Andersen's (1990) typology of welfare states, the Netherlands can be characterized as a social democratic/corporatist state. The country has an extensive child welfare system, which aims to help vulnerable children and families and includes preventive/supportive, as well as child protection/juvenile justice services. Child welfare falls under the Ministry of Public Health, Welfare and Sports, as do mental health care, youth health care, and care for people with disabilities. The organization is based on the Youth Care Act of 2005 (*Wet op de Jeugdzorg*), with provinces and communities as the main responsible authorities (van der Linden, Ten Siethoff, and Zeijlstra-Rijpstra, 2005). In general, the Dutch child welfare system can be typified as a family support system, looking for an appropriate balance between child welfare and child protection (Knijn and van Nijnatten, 2011).

Services can be grouped into three levels, depending on the target group on which they focus and the intensity of the care they provide:

- Level 0: community-based services. These have a preventive function and focus on regular developmental and parenting processes in all children between zero and 18 years old and their families; they are directly accessible to all children and their carers (e.g., schools, child care services, youth welfare work, youth organizations).
- Level 1: nonspecialized services. These function to screen problems related to the development and parenting of children at an early stage,

to offer early intervention, to refer if necessary, and to coordinate referral. These services should be easily and directly accessible to children and carers, and two types of services that play a major role at this level are the Centres for Youth and Family (*Centra Jeugd en Gezin*) and the Care and Advisory Teams (*Zorg- en Adviesteams*).

- Level 2: specialized services. These services offer intensive care and are accessible only on indication; the indication is provided by the Youth Care Agencies (*Bureau Jeugdzorg*). Care is given by the service providers, and coordination and follow-up are done by both the service providers and the Youth Care Agencies; the indication can lead to different types of care, provided by the following services:
  - Specialized youth care services (e.g., intensive family support, out-of-home placement in residential or family foster care);
  - Services making decisions about child protection and probation measures (Youth Care Agencies and national services);
  - Juvenile justice services and *Jeugdzorg Plus* services (services for minors with severe behavioral disorders);
  - Youth mental health care services;
  - Youth care services for children and young people with mild mental disabilities;
  - Special education for children and young people with behavioral disorders.

The first three Level 2 services are "true" child welfare services, organized at the level of provinces; the latter three are services that are part of other care systems (mental health care, care for people with disabilities, education). This shows that the child welfare system is not a completely separate system, disconnected from the other systems.

At all levels, efficient communication between carers, professionals, and other people involved is needed in order to make the system function well. Of particular interest is the role of the Centres for Youth and Family. These centers have a low threshold and must be easily accessible to parents, teachers, and professionals who have concerns about the upbringing of a child.

Within the second level, the Youth Care Agencies (*Bureau Jeugdzorg*) play a key role. The professionals working in these offices make up the indication. Their decision process ends up in a referral of children and families to the best fitting service. The offices make up indications for clients entering the care system voluntarily, but they are also make up indications following the imposition of a care order by the court (child protection measures, probation measures). In addition to the offices, which operate at the provincial level, there are services that work at a national level. These services implement child protection and probation measures for specific target groups, for instance children and youth with intellectual disabilities.

Different disciplines are involved in child welfare practice. The main disciplines involved are social work and social pedagogy. Social work is taught in (professional) bachelor degree programs. Social workers have direct contact with children and families, for instance through home visits, follow-up of family placements, and so forth. Social pedagogy is taught both in (professional) bachelor and master degree programs. Social pedagogues with a bachelor's degree have direct contact with children and used to be employed as group care workers. Social pedagogues with a master's degree are employed as staff members, for instance in family support services, foster care services, or children's homes. They monitor care plans and trajectories, supervise teams, and maintain supportive contacts with the children's families (Grietens, 2014).

The Dutch Child Welfare System: Some Figures

Each specialized service (Level 2) keeps records of children and families entering care and of their care trajectories. These figures are the basis of province reports and nationwide reports on youth care. A recent report was based on cases registered in 2009 (Jeugdzorg Nederland, 2010). That year, more than 300,000 children and young people (zero to 17 years) received some form of help within the child welfare system. This is approximately 9.5% of the total population. The number of minors who are being helped by services of the child welfare system has been increasing since 2002, particularly in the specialized youth care services and the mental health care services. The number of child protection measures has been increasing as well, while a slow decrease of probation measures has been noted.

However, this rate must be considered as the maximum rate of minors having a file in the child welfare system, and it probably is an overestimation of the actual rate (www.nji.nl). This has to do with the fact that some children are counted twice, for instance when a referral is made from one type of service to the other. Further, the figures do not include young people continuing youth care after 18. The exact number of children and families having contact with child welfare services is difficult to calculate. In Table 4.1, we present the estimated figures for each of the specialized services.

By the end of 2010, 27.1 per 1,000 children in the Netherlands had contact with child welfare services, not including children living in crisis situations receiving in-home or out-of-home services[2] and children with severe conduct disorders receiving help in *Jeugdzorg Plus* services.[3] The majority of children were receiving help while remaining in home (17.8 per 1,000). The number of children in out-of-home services was 9.3 per 1,000. More than half of these children (51.6%) were living in foster families, while 48.4% were living in residential settings (Jeugdzorg Nederland, 2011). No countrywide figures about the percentage of immigrant children having contact with the child welfare system are available, and neither are figures about the distribution of out-of-home placed immigrant children across living arrangements. Local statistics

Table 4.1. Estimated number and percentage of children (zero to 17 years) across the different types of specialized services (Level 2) in the child welfare system, 2009

Service	Number of clients	Percentage of youth
Specialized youth care services	75,323	2.1
Child protection and probation measures	74,153	2.1
Mental health care services	142,323	4.0
Services for children with disabilities	10,493	0.3
Special education services	27,698	0.8
Juvenile justice and *Jeugdzorg Plus*	3,819	0.1

Source: Jeugdzorg Nederland.

(www.nji.nl) show that in large cities and more densely populated areas, immigrant children tend to have more contact with the child welfare system and are high-resource-using. Compared to nonimmigrant children, they have more contacts with *Jeugdzorg Plus* services, for instance.

Current Problems and Planned Changes

Although the last reform of the child welfare system took place less than a decade ago, when the Youth Care Act (*Wet op de Jeugdzorg*) was implemented (van der Linden, Ten-Siethoff, and Zeijlstra-Rijpstra, 2005), it has become clear that some of the problems the system has been facing for many years still are not solved (www.nji.nl). Moreover, new problems have arisen. For these reasons, further reforms of the system are planned.

One issue is the rather one-sided focus on problems in youth. Screening, early identification of problems, and referral to specialized services are core activities of the services in Level 0 and 1 (see Structure and Organization). Too little attention is given to actions strengthening children and families; building up, restoring, and maintaining social networks; and primary prevention. In other words, child welfare has become too reactive and too synonymous with "help in case of problems related to the growing up and upbringing of children and youth." Focusing on preventive actions would give the system a more positive image in the public opinion. Further, it may decrease the high rates of children entering care. The one-sided focus on problems and the hyperreactivity of the system may be explained by some scandals of fatal child abuse and neglect in the late 1990s. Well known is the case of Savannah, a three-year-old girl who died after having been severely neglected and maltreated by her mother and stepfather (Knijn and van Nijnatten, 2011). The child welfare system was involved in this case but reacted too slowly and indolently. Legal action was taken against some professionals (Baartman, 2005).

A second issue is the strong fragmentation of services. The system is complex, and although it is linked to other systems like education, mental health care, and care for people with disabilities, these links are not really strong.

Further, services are organized at different levels. The Centres for Youth and Family, for instance, are organized by the local communities. But the specialized services (e.g., services for intense family support, family foster care services) are organized at the provincial level. And some other services (e.g., child protection and probation services) operate nationwide. Finally, the Youth Care Agencies are fully separated from the specialized services to which they refer clients. The fragmentation of authorities and responsibilities implies that many professionals are involved in a case. Consequently, it increases the risk of miscommunication between professionals, slowing down the care process.

Third, it turns out that many children are shifting through the system, going from one service to the other. Due to the complexity of the system, the shift of clients often is not visible. Reasons for the shift are the different entrances to the system, the lack of efficient communication between professionals, and the lack of a national registration system.

Fourth, the high numbers of children entering care (specialized services) shows there is a high "consumption" of care. The way the system is structured and organized stimulates this consumption. There is a broad range of rather easily accessible services for parents, teachers, and carers who have questions regarding the upbringing and (psychosocial) development of children. Clients have a passive role in the care process and develop a "shopping" attitude.

Policymakers concluded that the child welfare system has become unmanageable. Further, the system is too expensive. Costs are too high and are not balancing out effectiveness. A reform is necessary in order to tackle the aforementioned problems and to bring costs and effectiveness in balance. The reform will imply that the child welfare system will be further decentralized. More autonomy and responsibility will be given to the communities, and communities will be invited to collaborate in organizing the child welfare system in their region. This transition is planned to start in 2015 (www.nji.nl). Preparatory analyses made by academics and other experts (e.g., Meijs, Roza, van Baren, and Hoogervorst, 2012; van Yperen and Stams, 2010) learn that policy plans should stress (a) the "civil society" idea and the improvement of the living environment for all children and young people, including those from other cultures and (b) the need for an integrative and stepped care system, with a continuum of services going from preventive family support initiatives to intensive parent training programs and substitute care.

A Shift Toward Evidence-Based Working

Since the beginning of the 1990s, Dutch policymakers have increasingly been insisting on offering evidence-based help to clients in the child welfare system. This demand is not unique to the Netherlands. In many Western countries, a shift toward more evidence-based working in child welfare can be observed (Grietens, 2013). In the Netherlands, this has led to a boom of new initiatives in practice to increase the effectiveness of care and a growing number of studies on the evidence of these interventions. The Dutch Youth Institute (www.nji.nl), an agency bridging the gap between the field of practice and the academic world, has formulated clear-cut criteria of what evidence-based interventions are and has installed a committee that evaluates if an intervention can be considered evidence based (Veerman and van Yperen, 2007). Practitioners and researchers can apply to the institute for an intervention to be evaluated. Only interventions that have been proven effective by means of randomized control studies are recognized as efficacious. Interventions that do not meet this criterion can be evaluated as empirically efficient (but not tested by means of randomized control trial), theoretically efficient, or promising. The institute has developed a database of effective interventions in child welfare. The database is growing continuously, but until now only few interventions have the highest standard of efficiency. In Evidence-Based Interventions and Good Practices, we give a state of the art of the evidence base of interventions focusing on immigrant children and families.

In addition to the shift toward evidence-based working, the specialized youth care services are requested by the authorities to describe their activities in terms of performance. Ten indexes of performance are formulated, for instance goal achievement, client satisfaction reports, reduction of problems, and prevention of recidivism. Together, these indexes cover the core aims of child welfare: providing adequate help to clients, increasing the autonomy of clients, restoring children's safety, and protecting society from young people's criminal behavior. Each year services must report to the (provincial) authorities about their performance. The indexes are measured by means of standardized instruments (http://prestatieindicatoren.jeugdzorgnederland.nl)

IMMIGRANT CHILDREN AND FAMILIES IN THE CHILD WELFARE SYSTEM

Access

The Youth Care Act (*Wet op de Jeugdzorg*) states that all children living in the Netherlands have the right to care, irrespective of their cultural and socioeconomic background. So, in principle, all immigrant children and families have access to the services of the child welfare system. However, many services at Levels 0 and 1 report that immigrant children and families are underrepresented in their files, and empirical studies confirm that immigrants have less easily access to child welfare services (Broeze, 2011; van der Gaag and Speet, 2010). At least two reasons for the underrepresentation can be given. First, immigrants are not sufficiently familiar with the Dutch care system. This may be particularly true for first-generation migrants and refugees. The Centres for Youth and Family, for instance, are unfamiliar to many immigrants, as are the Youth Care Agencies. Second, services may expend too little effort on reaching immigrant children and families.

As a consequence, a number of immigrants enter the care system when problems have been escalating. A recent analysis of the indications made by the Youth Care Agency in Utrecht (one of the five largest cities in the country) showed that problems of immigrant children and youth were more complex, as compared to those of nonimmigrant children and youth. Problems of relational and interpersonal violence (e.g., domestic violence, child abuse) were highly prevalent. For this reason, specialized care was needed, and intrusive measures had to be taken to safeguard children (e.g., out-of-home placement; van der Gaag and Speet, 2010). Another finding of this study was that fewer immigrant than nonimmigrant children and youth were entering the care system on a voluntary basis. In other words: larger proportions of immigrant children and youth were entering care, following the imposition of a care order by the court.

Figures of immigrant children and youth in services at the end of the continuum of care illustrate this. Some groups of immigrants are overrepresented in these services. More than half of the children in juvenile justice services (57% in 2007), for instance, are immigrants, with Moroccan youth being the largest group (www.nji.nl). Similarly, high numbers of children placed in out-of-home in residential settings have a non-Dutch background (Kromhout, 2002). Stigmatization by police and judicial authorities and media and high visibility of youth from ethnic minorities in streets and public places may be another reason for the overrepresentation of immigrants in juvenile justice services, whereas the lack of foster families from ethnic minorities may be an alternative explanation of the high number of immigrant children and youth in residential care settings. In the mental health services, children and youth from ethnic minorities are also highly represented. Numbers have been increasing since the beginning of this century. In some parts of the country (e.g., Amsterdam), 30% to 40% of the clients have a non-Dutch origin, including refugee children and unaccompanied young minors. Consequently, the interculturalization of the mental health care services has become a major theme for professionals and policymakers (Beunderman, Savenije, Mattheijer, and Willems, 2004; Trienekens, 2008).

Experiences of Professionals and Immigrant Care Users

Although most bachelor and master programs (e.g., social work, social pedagogy) offer at least one compulsory course on intercultural aspects (e.g., communication) of child and family welfare, little is known about how child welfare professionals perceive their intercultural competence. Bellaart and Azrar (2002) and Oude Breuil (2005) reported that professionals working in Youth Care Agencies (*Bureaus Jeugdzorg*) perceived difficulties in communicating with immigrant children and parents and in reaching them. Jap-A-Joe and Jap-A-Joe (2012) interviewed a small sample of 17 family guardians (*gezinsvoogden*) who were caring for Surinam families in one countrywide service for clients with intellectual disabilities. Half of them perceived the quality of the contacts with clients as satisfying. According to the unsatisfied guardians, parents were inflexible and had a noncooperative attitude. It may be that the professionals overestimated the quality of the contacts with their clients, as only 30% of the parents reported the contacts with guardians were satisfying. Surinam parents had difficulties trusting the guardians and found their expectations were not met. They found that professionals did not sufficiently respect their cultural identity and took for granted that they were fully assimilated to the Dutch culture, as they officially were Dutch citizens.

These findings on child welfare professionals' views of their intercultural competencies correspond well with what is reported by professionals in other fields, for instance preventive parenting support (Pels, Distelbrink, and Postma, 2009) and mental health care (Beunderman et al., 2004). In several places in the Netherlands, efforts are undertaken to increase the intercultural competence of child welfare professionals. An example is the recent formulation of four specific competencies related to child welfare work with immigrant children and families by van de Haterd, Poll, Felten, Vos, and Bellaart (2010): mapping cultural frameworks, dealing with barriers in intercultural communication, building up trustful relationships with immigrant clients, and collaborating with professionals and partners from different ethnic groups. Every professional in the field has to acquire these skills by training and supervised reflected practice. First steps are undertaken to implement these competencies in training programs and curricula.

Studies on immigrant clients' perceptions of the help they receive confirm the lack of truly intercultural communication and the risk of serious mismatches between clients and professionals in child welfare (see, e.g., Kalthoff, 2009; van de Haterd et al., 2010). Notwithstanding their acculturation process, immigrant families want to keep their cultural identity, appreciate the professionals' interest for their culture (e.g., eating habits, decoration of the house), and feel discriminated when their cultural identity is ignored (Eldering, 2012). A parental behavior that may be subject of misunderstanding and severe conflict between immigrant families and professionals is corporal punishment of children. Slapping a child has been forbidden by law in the Netherlands since 2007 (www.kinderrechten.nl). Consequently, a "pedagogical" slap, a common practice in childrearing in non-Western cultures, may be considered by many professionals as child abuse and a sign to take child protection measures (Pels et al., 2009).

Jurrius, Bauer, Rutjes, and Stams (2011) developed a database of Dutch self-report studies on clients' satisfaction with child welfare services. The number of studies is growing, and self-reports are collected from clients—parents and children—in ambulatory, as well as out-of-home care (foster families, foster homes, residential settings). But the authors conclude that there is a lack of data on the satisfaction of clients from non-Western origin. It is not clear why this group is underrepresented in the database. Language problems may be a reason, in particular in first-generation migrants. Another reason may be a high non-response of immigrants in surveys, due to a lack of trust in the child welfare system and fear that reports will be misinterpreted or used against them.

Evidence-Based Interventions and Good Practices

Has the shift toward evidence-based working in child welfare led to the development of interventions targeting the specific problems (e.g., problems related to migration, stress, acculturation, war trauma) and needs of immigrant children and families? One would expect this, given the growing numbers of immigrant children and families in the population and their notable presence in the specialized services of the child welfare system.

However, in the database of effective interventions kept up by the Dutch Youth Institute (www.nji.nl) we found only 28 interventions targeting immigrant children and families. This is but a small proportion (<20%) of the 180 interventions comprising this database.[4] Moreover, only two interventions have been developed exclusively for immigrants: *Marokkaanse buurtvaders* (Moroccan neighborhood fathers) and *Hulpmix* (Helpmix). The former is a community-based intervention aimed at reducing problem behavior in Moroccan children and youth and restoring safety in risky neighborhoods. Immigrant fathers with high authority in the neighborhood play a key role in this intervention. The latter is an online intervention for non-Western immigrant youth. Youth are invited to bring up at an early stage questions regarding identity formation, relationships, sexuality, and future perspectives so they can be referred to appropriate services and an escalation of problems can be prevented. The other 26 interventions were developed for the general population of children and families but take into account cultural diversity or include culturally sensitive elements. They can be grouped into four categories: family support interventions, interventions focusing on the development of children and the reduction of educational delays, interventions promoting health (including healthy sexual behavior) and socioemotional development, and interventions reducing or preventing problem behavior.

Until now, none of the interventions have been proven to be empirically efficient. All have reached the level of "theoretically efficient."[5]

Ince and van den Berg (2009) reviewed 162 interventions for children and youth on the promotion of development and the prevention of psychosocial and educational problems. The results of their study are highly comparable to what we find in the database of the Dutch Youth Institute. Only 14 interventions were targeting exclusively for immigrant children and families. Forty-four interventions were culturally sensitive and could be used with immigrants. None of the interventions could be labelled "empirically efficient" and only one as "theoretically efficient."

In addition to these interventions, numerous local initiatives and participatory projects have been developed during the past ten years. The Verwey-Jonker

Institute (see http://www.nji.nl/eCache/DEF/1/32/051.html) has made a short list of initiatives and projects representing good practices. The list includes specialized interventions (e.g., a treatment program for immigrant youth with depression), preventive family support programs (e.g., a program on communication with people from ethnic minorities), psychoeducational programs (e.g., on drug abuse in Turkish youth), programs on participation (e.g., involving immigrant parents in education), and programs on sports (e.g., informing Chinese parents on kids' sport clubs in their neighborhood). Practice shows that these initiatives and projects are "working," but for most of them controlled empirical data on outcomes is lacking, and therefore we do not know what makes them work.

The database of the Dutch Youth Institute does not include specific interventions that are targeted for refugee families or unaccompanied young minors. In mental health care, there is extensive expertise with regard to the treatment of trauma in these groups, however. One example is Centrum 45, a countrywide center with expertise in assessing and treating people with complex trauma symptoms following persecution, war, and violence (www.centrum45.nl). It is recognized as a center of excellence in mental health care for traumatized people. The center also organizes training courses for professionals working with victims of war and violence and coordinates research projects on the assessment and treatment of complex trauma. Another example is a recently started expertise center at the University of Groningen on the assessment of the development and the needs of children from asylum-seeking families, who are under threat to be sent back to their home countries. The assessment results are presented in a report that is used in advocacy. The Children's Rights Convention serves as the judicial framework for the assessments. The Groningen researchers have translated the convention's "in the best interests of the child principle" into a questionnaire that assesses the development and needs of asylum-seeking children (Kalverboer, Zijlstra, and Knorth, 2009; Zijlstra, 2012).

Summarizing the review of evidence-based interventions and good practices for immigrant children and families in the Dutch child welfare system, we conclude that (a) the number of interventions targeted specifically for this group is very limited, as is the number of interventions for the general population, including culturally sensitive elements, and (b) there is very little empirical evidence on the efficiency of interventions.

CONCLUDING REMARKS: HOW TO BETTER REACH CHILDREN AND FAMILIES?

Although during the past two decades the Dutch child welfare system has attempted to make professionals more culturally sensitive and practice more tailored to the specific needs of immigrant clients, including refugees, asylum seekers, and unaccompanied young minors, there still is a ways to go (Eldering, 2012; Van den Broek and Kleijnen, 2009). A major question is how immigrant children and families can gain more access to lower end child welfare services.

The preventive services (e.g., the Youth and Family Centres) at the lower end of the care continuum are open services that provide help "on demand." Parents can turn to these services for advice about the upbringing up and development of children and youth. Children and youth themselves can turn to these services for advice about health, school, relational, or psychosocial problems. First-generation immigrants not only are unfamiliar with the child welfare system and the organization of services, but the "on demand" way of working of services and the face-to-face contact required with Dutch professionals to talk about sensitive issues (relationships, upbringing of children) may put them off. They are not used to this direct way of working in their culture (Kalthoff, 2009; van den Broek and Kleijnen, 2011). Many initiatives to bring services (e.g., family support initiatives) closer to immigrant families and children try to break down barriers by using a group-oriented instead of an individual approach. First, clients chat with each other about more "neutral" issues (e.g., a group of young mothers about the care of their newborn baby), then they are invited to turn to paraprofessionals from their own culture to talk about specific issues related to their questions. Language may be another barrier to be overcome by immigrant clients. A language delay increases the imbalance of power. Again, a group approach and the involvement of interpreters or paraprofessionals from the own culture may help to solve this problem (Eldering, 2012; van den Broek and Kleijnen, 2011).

Ince and van den Berg (2009) reported that professionals focus too much on the externalizing problems of immigrant children and youth. According to these authors, this may be one of the reasons that they are overrepresented in specialized higher end services for children and youth with severe behavioral disorders (e.g., juvenile justice services). At the same time, too little attention is paid to other problems in immigrant children and youth, for instance internalizing problems or trauma symptoms (following child maltreatment or domestic violence). It is important to screen for these problems at an early age and to address them in an early stage. Similarly, more attention is needed for the prevention and the early detection of child maltreatment in immigrant families. Researchers and professionals (MOVisie, 2009a; Zandijk-van Harten and Haarsma, 1996) agree that intrafamilial abuse in immigrant families is still underreported in the statistics of police and Advice and Report Points Child Maltreatment.[6] This is the case for all types of child maltreatment, in particular for sexual abuse, which still is strictly taboo among some immigrant groups (Deug, 1990; www.nji.nl).

In general, services in the child welfare system have been evolving from monocultural (Western focused) to intercultural. Hoogsteder (1996) developed a linear seven-stage model to classify the level of interculturalization of services. The lowest level is that of the monocultural organization, serving only nonimmigrant clients. Reaching immigrant and nonimmigrant clients, employing immigrant professionals, pursuing an intercultural policy, and improving on personnel management adds to the interculturalization of services. Nowadays, only a few services in the Netherlands are totally monocultural and not accessible to immigrant children and families, but only a few reach the highest levels of the ladder. Pursuing a truly integrative intercultural policy and personnel management remains a major challenge to preventive and mental health and child welfare services (Logghe, 1998). One of the problems is a lack of professionals (at the master's level) in social and health sciences from immigrant origin. Non-Western immigrant students are still underrepresented in the Dutch universities. Countrywide, 8.8% of the students registered in Dutch universities in 2011 were non-Western immigrants (behavioral and social sciences: 7.2%; medical sciences: 10.2%; www.trendsinbeeld.minocw.nl/grafieken/3_1_1_23. php). Another problem is the still dominant role in the teaching curricula for students and the training of professionals of Western theories, both on the causal mechanisms underlying problematic parenting and problem behavior in children, and on how to intervene. These theories are based on (implicit) Western norms and values. Social work, social pedagogy, and psychology curricula include courses on intercultural communication, cultural diversity, and culturally sensitive assessment and intervention, but too often they are part of loose and temporary projects and very basic. This has been going on for years, which made some academics conclude that the ambitious project started in the early 1990s to make the Dutch child welfare system a culturally sensitive system has failed (Vollebergh, 2002). Finally, there is a need for more and participatory academic research on intercultural issues regarding child welfare, with professionals, clients, and stakeholders being partners, as well as a need to "translate" knowledge from research to professionals in the field (Eldering, 2012).

NOTES

1 statline.cbs.nl/StatWeb/publication (accessed November 24, 2013).
2 In 2010, 11,392 children in crisis situations received services in the child welfare system; this is 3.4 per 1,000 children.
3 In 2010, 3,819 children received help in *Jeugdzorg Plus* services; this is 1.1 per 1,000 children.
4 This was the number of interventions in the database, June 2013.
5 Several interventions are currently under evaluation, and it can be expected that some of them will reach higher levels of efficiency within the near future.
6 The Advice and Report Points Child Maltreatment are part of the Youth Care Agencies (*Bureaus Jeugdzorg*).

REFERENCES

Baartman, H. (2005). Over de hoeksteen en kindermishandeling als toetssteen. In H. Baartman & R. Bullens (Eds.), *Kindermishandeling: De politiek een zorg* (Child Abuse: A Concern to Policy), 255–279. Amsterdam: SWP.

Bellaart, H., & Azrar, F. (2002). *Inventarisatierapport jeugdzorg zonder drempels: Een inventariserend onderzoek naar de toegankelijkheid en de kwaliteit van Bureaus Jeugdzorg met betrekking tot allochtone cliënten* (Summary Report Youth Care Without Thresholds: A Review Study on the Accessibility and the Quality of Youth Care Agencies). Utrecht: Forum.

Beunderman, R., Savenije, A., Mattheijer, M., & Willems, P. (2004). *Meer kleur in de Jeugd-GGZ* (More Color in Youth Mental Health Care). Assen: van Gorcum.

Broeze, L. (2011). *Ethnische verschillen in zorggebruik (Ethnic differences in the use of care)*. Master's thesis, University of Utrecht.

De Haene, L., Grietens, H., & Verschueren, K. (2007). From symptom to context: A review of the literature on refugee children's mental health. *Hellenic Journal of Psychology*, 4, 233–256.

Deug, F. (1990). *En dan ben je pas echt ver van huis: Turkse en Marokkaanse vrouwen en meisjes over seksueel geweld en de hulpverlening* (And Then You Are Really Far Away From Home: Turkish and Moroccan Women and Girls about Sexual Violence and Care). Utrecht: Uitgeverij Medusa.

Eldering, L. (2012). *Cultuur en opvoeding* (Culture and Upbringing). Rotterdam: Lemniscaat.

Esping-Andersen, G. (1990). *The Three Worlds of Welfare Capitalism*. Cambridge: Policy Press.

Fazel, M., & Stein, A. (2003). Mental health of refugee children: Comparative study. *British Medical Journal*, 327, 134–135.

Grietens, H. (2013). Is there a pan-European perspective on evidence-based practice in child welfare? A critical reflection. *Journal of Children's Services*, 8(3), 1–8.

———. (2014). A European perspective on the context and content for social pedagogy in therapeutic residential care. In J.K. Whittaker, J.F. Del Valle, & L. Holmes (Eds.), *Therapeutic Residential Care with Children and Youth: Developing Evidence-Based International Practice*. London: Jessica Kingsley.

Groark, C., Sclare, I., & Raval, H. (2011). Understanding the experiences and emotional needs of unaccompanied asylum-seeking adolescents in the UK. *Clinical Child Psychology and Psychiatry*, 16, 421–442.

Hodes, M. (2010). The mental health of detained asylum seeking children. *European Child & Adolescent Psychiatry*, 19, 621–623.

Hoogsteder, J. (1996). *Hoe kleurrijk is het welzijnswerk? Een landelijk onderzoek naar de stand van zaken op het gebied van intercultureel beleid* (How Colourful Is Welfare Work? A Survey on the State of the Art Regarding Intercultural Policy). Rijswijk: VOG.

Ince, D., & van den Berg, G. (2009). *Overzichtsstudie interventies voor migrantenjeugd: Ontwikkelingsstimulering, preventie en vroeghulp* (Review Study on Interventions for Immigrant Youth: Promoting Development, Prevention and Early Intervention). Utrecht: Nederlands Jeugdinstituut.

Jap-A-Joe, M., & Jap-A-Joe, M. (2012). *Surinaamse cliënten en hun kinderen in de jeugdbescherming (Surinam clients and their children in the child protection system).* Bachelor's thesis, Fontys Hogeschool Pedagogiek, Den Haag.

Jeugdzorg Nederland. (2010). *Brancherapport Jeugdzorg* (Report on Youth Care). Utrecht: Jeugdzorg Nederland.

———. (2011). *Brancherapport Jeugdzorg* (Report on Youth Care). Utrecht: Jeugdzorg Nederland.

Jurrius, K., Bauer, J., Rutjes, L., & Stams, G.J. (2011). Databank biedt overzicht van cliëntentevredenheidsonderzoek (Database provides overview of client satisfaction surveys). *Jeugd en Co Kennis*, 4, 30–39.

Kalthoff, H. (2009). Opvoedingsondersteuning aan migranten schiet tekort (Parenting support to immigrant families fails). *Jeugd en Co Kennis*, 5, 8–18.

Kalverboer, M., Zijlstra, E., & Knorth, E. (2009). The developmental consequences for asylum-seeking children living with the prospect for five years or more of enforced return to their home country. *European Journal of Migration and Law*, 11, 41–67.

Knijn, T., & van Nijnatten, C. (2011). Child welfare in the Netherlands: Between privacy and protection. In N. Gilbert, N. Parton, & M. Skivenes (Eds.), *Child Protection Systems: International Trends and Orientations*, 223–240. Oxford: Oxford University Press.

Kromhout, M. (2002). *Marokkaanse jongeren in de residentiële hulpverlening: Een exploratief onderzoek naar probleemvisies, interculturalisatie en hulpverleningsverloop* (Moroccan Youth: An Exploratory Study on Perceptions of Problems, Interculturalization and Care Trajectories). Amsterdam: SWP.

Logghe, K. (1998). *De verschillen kun je niet wegpoetsen. . .* (You Cannot Rub Off the Differences. . .). Tilburg: Stichting Zorg & Palet.

McCarthy, C., & Marks, D. (2010). Exploring the health and well-being of refugee and asylum seeking children. *Journal of Health Psychology*, 15, 586–595.

Meijs, L., Roza, L., Baren van, E., & Hoogervorst, N. (2012). De rol van de civil society in de transitie van de jeugdzorg (The role of the civil society in the transition of youth care. *Jeugdbeleid*, 6, 71–79.

MOVisie. (2009a). *Factsheet huiselijk geweld: Feiten en cijfers* (Factsheet Domestic Violence: Facts and Figures). Utrecht: MOVisie.

———. (2009b). *Factsheet jeugdprostitutie: Feiten en cijfers* (Factsheet Girls' Prostitution: Facts and Figures). Utrecht: MOVisie.

Oude Breuil, B.C. (2005). *De Raad voor de Kinderbescherming in een multiculturele samenleving* (The Council of Child Protection in a Multicultural Society). Den Haag: Boom Juridische Uitgevers.

Pels, T., Distelbrink, M., & Postma, L. (2009). *Opvoeding in de migrantencontext: Review van onderzoek naar de opvoeding in gezinnen van nieuwe Nederlanders* (Parenting in the Context of Migration: A Review of Research on Parenting in Families of New Dutch Citizens). Utrecht: Verwey-Jonker Instituut.

Stevens, G., Pels, T., Bengi-Arslan, L., Verhulst, F., Vollebergh, W., & Crijnen, A. (2003). Parent, teacher and self-reported problem behavior in the Netherlands: Comparing Moroccan immigrant with Dutch and with Turkish immigrant children and adolescents. *Social Psychiatry and Psychiatric Epidemiology*, 38, 576–585.

Stevens, G., Pels, T., Vollebergh, W., & Crijnen, A. (2004). Patterns of psychological acculturation in adult and adolescent Moroccan immigrants living in the Netherlands. *Journal of Cross-Cultural Psychology*, 35, 689–704.

Trienekens, S. (2008). *Interculturalisation in mental health care: A qualitative study on the perceptions of and experiences with interculturalisation of professionals in mental health care*. Master's thesis, University of Utrecht.

van de Haterd, J., Poll, A., Felten, H., Vos, R., & Bellaart, H. (2010). *Naar interculturele competentieprofielen in het preventieve en ontwikkelingsgericht jeugdbeleid—Definitief concept* (Towards Intercultural Competence Profiles in Preventive and Development-Focused Youth Policy—Final Concept). Utrecht: Nederlands Jeugdinstituut.

Van den Broek, A., & Kleijnen, E. (2009). Voorzieningen bereiken migranten niet altijd (Services do not always reach immigrant clients). *Jeugd en Co Kennis*, 5, 37–48.

Van der Gaag, R., & Speet, B. (2010). Verschillen tussen allochtone en autochtone cliënten. *Jeugd en Co Kennis*, 4, 34–43.

van der Linden, A., ten Siethoff, F., & Zeijlstra-Rijpstra, A. (2005). *Jeugd en recht* (Youth and Law). Houten: Bohn Stafleu Van Loghum.

Van Yperen, T., & Stam, P. (2010). *Opvoeden versterken* (Strengthening Upbringing). Onafhankelijk advies in opdracht van de Nederlandse Vereniging van Gemeenten. Den Haag: Nederlandse Vereniging van Gemeenten.

Vollebergh, W. (2002). *Gemiste kansen: Culturele diversiteit en jeugdzorg* (Missed Chances: Cultural Diversity and Child Welfare). Nijmegen: Katholieke Universiteit Nijmegen.

Wiegersma, A., Stellinga-Boelen, A., & Reijneveld, S. (2011). Psychosocial problems in asylum seekers' children: The parent, child, and teacher perspective using the Strengths and Difficulties Questionnaire. *Journal of Nervous and Mental Disease*, 199, 85–90.

Zandijk-van Harten, T., & Haarsma, L. (1996). *Grenzen voorbij: Kindermishandeling in allochtone gezinnen*. (Beyond Borders: Child Maltreatment in Immigrant Families). Amsterdam: VU Uitgeverij.

Zijlstra, E. (2012). *In the Best Interests of the Child? A Study into a Decision-Support Tool Validating Asylum-Seeking Children's Rights from a Behavioural Scientific Perspective*. Groningen: Wöhrmann Print Service.

Websites

Centrum 45: www.centrum45.nl

Children's Rights: www.kinderrechten.nl

Dutch Council for Refugees: www.vluchtelingenwerknederland.nl

Dutch Statistics: www.cbs.nl

Dutch Youth Institute: www.nji.nl

Jeugdzorg Nederland: http://prestatieindicatoren.jeugdzorgnederland.nl

Pharos National Knowledge and Advisory Centre on Migrants, Refugees and Health Care Issues: www.pharos.nl

Verwey-Jonker Institute: http://www.nji.nl/eCache/DEF/1/32/051.html)

5

IMMIGRANT CHILDREN AND FAMILIES
IN THE CHILD WELFARE SYSTEM IN AUSTRIA

Christoph Reinprecht

INTRODUCTION

This chapter discusses the significance of child protection services for immigrant children and families in Austria. The country represents a particular case: in recent years, Austria has become one of most important immigration countries in the European Union, and it has also played a key role in the international migration system. Since the 1990s the number of immigrants has risen remarkably; today, around 18% of the population is foreign born. In Vienna and other cities, around one-third of the population is foreign born. However, public opinion and institutional realities lag behind these developments, and the country continues to struggle with the idea of being an immigrant country. At the institutional level, changes are occurring only slowly. In recent years, these changes have become apparent, for instance in the establishment of an Undersecretary of State for "Integration Affairs," in a shift toward a "selected immigration policy" targeting highly qualified immigrants (through the so-called "Red-White-Red-Card"—the colors of the Austrian national flag), or in the establishment of a system that monitors integration in municipalities and public services. This chapter casts light on the fact that the cultural and ethnic diversification of children and families has so far not lead to a substantial adjustment of the family and child protection services in Austria. This is also related to the conservative character of the Austrian welfare system. At the same time, increasing tensions between child welfare services and migration policy can be observed and may point to upcoming institutional reforms.

The terms "immigrant families" and "immigrant children" refer to the category of "a person of migrant background" as defined by the Austrian administrative statistics.[1] With regard to immigrants, Austrian statistics distinguish between three categories: "foreigners" (individuals who are not Austrian citizens in legal terms), the "foreign born" (foreigners and the foreign born together constitute the category "of foreign origin"), and individuals "of migrant background" (parents born in a foreign country) (Statistik Austria, 2012: 22f).

This chapter is organized in four parts: starting with a brief description of the child protection system in Austria, we continue to summarize the main elements of immigration to Austria and the Austrian immigration regime, with specific attention to the situation of children in immigrant families, and the state of the art in research on immigrant families and children in Austria. We then discuss how law- and policy-related aspects frame and influence the situation of immigrant children and outline the functioning of child protecting services and related experiences. The last part of the chapter presents main insights from the survey carried out in Austria in the summer of 2012.

THE CHILD PROTECTION SYSTEM IN AUSTRIA: BASIC LEGAL FRAMEWORK AND PRINCIPLES

The Austrian child protection system (*Jugendwohlfahrt*) represents a specific field of family welfare policy. Child protection targets children and adolescents up to 18 years and their families and social environment. The system's main juridical reference point is the national youth welfare law of 1989 (recently amended in 2013), which defines, in its first paragraph, as its main objective the protection of the expectant mother and the newborn within his or her family environment on one hand and the rights of minors on the other hand. By following *subsidiary principles*, which delegate social welfare provisions not provided by the state to the family, the law reflects the supportive and advisory function of youth welfare. The primary objective of the law is to assist families in fulfilling their responsibilities in the care and education of minors. The state intervenes only if it is necessary for the benefit of the minor. The law defines the tasks of child and youth protection services and social workers by specifying the general objectives of child welfare with regard to safeguarding the child's welfare and the provision of support and protection in interaction with the concerned families and children, and all relevant actors are involved in the respective case. By law, there is no distinction by migration or ethnic background: the agenda of child protection services includes, in principle, all children living on Austrian territory; the set of services is universal. Due to the Austrian *federalism principles*, regional authorities are responsible for implementing and carrying out the law.

As in other domains of social protection, the main challenge for children and youth protection services and social workers is to find a balance between the supporting and the disciplining function of the law: strengthening the subjective rights of minors versus educational interventions if the family system is disorganized (Scheipl, 2011: 555). With respect to immigrant families and children, this mandate is challenged by several factors: on the one hand by the specific needs of immigrant groups, often unknown or even ignored by institutions and services, and on the other hand by the fact that social work, including child and youth protection services as provided by the youth welfare system, is often not (or not sufficiently) known among the client population with a migration background. Beyond that, Austria's *universalist approach* (all children living on the Austrian territory are targeted; there are no immigration-specific measures or interventions) is constantly in tension with the immigration regime and the predominant *ius sanguinis* principle, which postulates that citizenship is handed down by the parents (see Bauböck, Perchinig, and Sievers, 2009). This affects around one-fifth of immigrant children younger than 19 years, particularly children of immigrants with nonnaturalized status, as well as unaccompanied refugees or undocumented migrants. A foreign citizenship status may lead to extremely problematic situations, not only when adolescents get into conflict with the police and juridical authorities but when they are at risk of being repatriated by force. In Austria, children of families with unclear or nonauthorized residence status (this concerns, for instance, refugee-immigrants from Kosovo) are faced with a high risk of deportation, even if they were born in the country and independently of their social integration or educational performance.[2]

ORGANIZATION

To understand the Austrian system of child protection, it is necessary to consider the particular character of the country's welfare regime. Child protection services are embedded in a complex system of interactions between national, regional, and local authorities, social insurance bodies, and private organizations and are deeply anchored in welfare and family policy traditions. Three main characteristics are important: first, Austria is known for a generous and universalist family benefit system. From an international comparative perspective, the public expenses for families are above average (Thévenon, 2011). In 2011, around 10% of total welfare spending went to family support and child protection. Only a small part of 7% of the benefits is demand driven (i.e., dependent on the level of income); the majority of benefits are universal, and only few benefits are specifically targeted at low-income families and their children, and immigrant children do not represent a specific target group. There are three domains of family-related benefits: insurance benefits (coinsurance of children, maternity allowance, etc.), universal transfer payments (child-care payments, family allowance, tax allowances for children and single earners), and public services (free school enrollment, free transport, free university admission). Contrary to these benefits, which are not dependent on citizenship status, the access to social aid—a publically financed pillar of the welfare system targeting protection against poverty—requires citizenship or a particular legal status involving residence status or length of stay. In the intersection of child protection and antipoverty policy, the predominance of diverse principles may produce critical and insecure situations for immigrant children and families.

Second, and following the typology of Esping-Anderson (1990), Austria can be classified as a conservative-corporatist (or Christian-democratic) welfare state with a moderate level of decommodification, an employment-based social insurance system, and strong subsidiarity principles according to which families are given a key solidarity function, whereas the state interferes only when the family's capacity of caring for its members has been exhausted. This long-standing and culturally profoundly embedded system has contributed to upholding traditional family structures and gender roles, for instance by discouraging women from entering the labor market. The increasing employment rate of women, particularly since the 1970s, was constantly contradicted by limited opportunities for full jobs and professional advancement—women are overrepresented in half-time and atypical jobs (see Stier, Lewin-Epstein, and Braun, 2001). The conservative character of the Austrian welfare system is mirrored in principles such as coinsurance and pensions for dependent relatives and tax allowances for single earners. These elements are of specific importance in the field of immigration, for example in the context of immigration in the context of family reunification. Here, women are hampered in accessing the labor market (they do not automatically receive a work permit), one important factor explaining the relatively low employment level among immigrant women in Austria.

The third characteristic of the Austrian welfare system is its federalist and decentralized organization. On the basis of national laws that function as a general framework, child welfare and protection are the responsibility of regional authorities, which "implement legislation". The relative autonomy of the nine federal states (Bundesländer) is reflected in diverging interpretations of the national legal framework (for instance in some states the protection of the expectant mother also covers unborn children) but can also be seen in varying practices both in jurisdiction and service allocation. Each of the nine states is provided with an independent children and youth advocacy office, based on the United Nations Convention on the Rights of the Child, with a mandate to observe and defend interests and rights of children. The operational tasks and concrete interventions are decided at the district and city levels—there are altogether 80 district authorities and 15 statutory cities, which are responsible for establishing child protection services.

Due to its decentralized and regionalized character, the Austrian child protection system has been criticized for its highly fragmented landscape with a variation of regulations in the nine states and an even larger variety of local practices. As a consequence, there are no nationwide quality criteria and no standardized and comparable statistics, as categories of intervention are used differently depending on the state. This unsatisfactory situation has recently (2013) led to an agreement between seven of the nine states regarding the standardization of basic child welfare principles. This new law, which passed the national parliament in April 2013, introduced uniform standards for private providers and foster families, a four-eye principle in complex cases, standardized federal statistics, new regulations for information and data transfer, and efforts toward professionalization. However, this new law will not change the general architecture of competences; the implementation of legislation and operational tasks will remain at the regional and local levels.

Main Axes of Intervention

The main tasks of youth welfare are the protection of children against violence, advice and support for parents in educational matters, placement of children with adoptive and foster parents, legal representation in alimony matters, and methods for determination of paternity. As a basic principle, decisions should be taken in connection with all relevant institutions and in particular in cooperation with the involved families and children.

The Austrian child welfare system provides different types of services and interventions (Scheipl, 2011; Till and Till-Tentschert, 2009; Heizmann, 2007). The main measures are the following:

- *Social (preventive) services:* This voluntary type of service is provided for parents who seek advice (so-called parenting classes); it includes also preventive and therapeutic support for minors and their families.
- *Child care interventions*: If a child is in danger of neglect by her or his parents (e.g., if sporadic school attendance is reported by nursery workers or teachers), the child protection service will try to intervene with the objective to ensure the parents' capacity to take care of their child; such agreements are mandatory and include counseling sessions and different forms of educational aid. Noncompliant parents are forced to accept conditions on the basis of court decision;
- *Educational support:* If parents are not capable of meeting the educational interests and needs of their child, child protection services may intervene in favor of the child by providing educational child guidance services or support for minors provided by mobile services (social and pedagogical support at home);
- *Child removal and external accommodation*: If the safety of a child is compromised, child protection services will remove the child from the

parents' home; a removal may be temporary (e.g., at a crisis intervention center) or longer term (e.g., in a foster family or a children's home);
child removal is based on an agreement with the parents; if they are
noncompliant, a court decision is required.
- *Adoption.*

This classification of interventions reflects a continuum of supportive-voluntary
to mandatory-forced practices (adoption represents a field in its own), although,
in practice, it is often difficult to distinguish between the different types of services and interventions. (Certain services may be used for both voluntary and
mandatory interventions; the nine states also proceed differently in this regard.)

In 2011, Austrian youth welfare services reported around 40,000 "forced
interventions", 27,000 cases of mandatory child care/educational support
interventions, and around 12,000 cases of child removal and external accommodation (BMWFJ, 2012). In the long run, data show stable rates of external
accommodation (including foster parents) but increasing child care and educational support. Increasing demand has been reported for "assisted accommodation" (assisted shared flats) and all forms of social and pedagogic support and
care; in particular the demand for educational support is drastically increasing
(Scheipl, 2011; Heimgartner, 2009). Male children are targeted to a higher extent
by social and pedagogical assistance. The extent of measures and interventions
differs between the states, which is also an effect of incomplete and destandard-
ized documentation. There are no data available concerning the proportion of
immigrant children among child welfare cases.

The Increasing Role of the Third Sector and Nongovernmental Organizations

Since the institutional setting is not coherent, child protection services may
operate in quite different ways. From case to case, social workers try to balance between the requirements of support and control. Following the subsidiarity principle, social workers will evaluate the educational resources of the
family, and in case of intervention they have to privilege the least intrusive
means (*gelindeste Mittel*). Corresponding to the general objective to realize and
achieve child rights and welfare, social workers are obliged to listen to the child.
If a child is less than 10 years old, the assessment will also include other persons. Social workers will become active and intervene only if serious problems
(deprivation, school absence, violence, sexual harassment) have been reported.
The law obliges institutions and employees in social and educational sectors to
communicate their observations to child protection services.

The agenda of youth protection has increasingly been assigned to nongovernmental organizations (NGOs; third-sector, private welfare child protection
organizations). While state and regional authorities keep control, private organizations are (increasingly) mandated with operational tasks. In this regard,

realities are also different in the nine federal states: whereas in some regions the provision of services, including the external accommodation of children in homes or foster families, is primarily run by private (nonprofit) organizations, this is less the case in other countries, such as Vienna. Overall, small and medium-sized organizations are predominant.

Due to its fragmented and strongly regionalized architecture, a nationwide assessment of how immigrant children are addressed and treated by child protection institutions, and how children and their families experience the interactions with these institutions, is impossible and not adequate. Basically, it can be noted that immigrant families and children are not specifically targeted by family welfare and children protection authorities; following its universalist mandate, there are basically no services responding to immigrant-specific needs.[3] In Austria, immigrant-specific measures and interventions have traditionally been designed in the areas of labor market integration and health and social services. Only the educational sector provides specific offers and services for immigrant children, such as language training, target group–oriented information, and support for participation in preschool education and school enrollment.

At the same time, children protection services that do not explicitly target immigrants provide (primarily financial) support to private organizations and NGOs engaged in migration and integration policy implementation, or in the field of child and youth protection. There is a broad range of civil society organizations, including an increasing number of ethnic minority associations that are important engines in advocating, supporting, and defending the interests of migrant families and children. Many of these initiatives are not specifically targeted and respond to a wider audience, for instance in delivering services for parents in general, or in offering multilingual support. Other groups are embedded in the community and deliver services for a group of clients in specific neighborhoods and within certain ethnic boundaries. The obviously precarious situation of minor refugees and undocumented migrants has led to a growing network of initiatives and associations working with children belonging to these groups.

AUSTRIA: A "DE FACTO IMMIGRATION COUNTRY"

In the past decades, Austria was confronted with important international immigration processes such as the immigration of a foreign labor force mainly recruited in former Yugoslavia and Turkey, with a peak at the beginning of the 1970s or, more recently, after the fall of the iron curtain and the war in Yugoslavia. Compared to the 1960s, when foreign citizens represented 1% of the total population in Austria, the number increased to 4% in the 1970s and to 12% in 2011 in absolute terms (the following data are provided by Statistics Austria;

see also Figure 5.1): today, 971,000 foreign nationals live in Austria. The country has a total population of 8,315,000 inhabitants. The population of foreign origin (foreign-born individuals, including naturalized individuals) accounts for 1,493,000 or 18% of the total population; those with migration background (foreign origin and both parents foreign born) account for 1,568,000 or 19%. The population with a migration background is unequally distributed among the nine regions: the highest percentage is reported for Vienna (39%), the lowest for the less industrialized southern and eastern regions—Carinthia and Burgenland (10%).

The fact that in the decades after World War II, Austria has become a "de facto immigration country" has been critically perceived in public discourse and provokes withdrawal reflexes in public debate and politics. In the scholarly literature, Austria has therefore been classified as an "immigration country against will" (Fassmann and Münz, 1995). However, the country's immigration history does not reflect a continuous and regular process, because periods of strong immigration were followed by years of stagnation. In recent decades, migration forms and migration policies have changed, and an increasing diversification of migration patterns has occurred. This has led to growing sociostructural and sociocultural heterogeneity. Basically, postwar immigration passed through three main phases: first, from the active recruitment of a labor force of migrant background in the 1960s and 1970s to family reunification; second, immigration caused by the crisis in (Central) Eastern Europe and the war in former Yugoslavia; third, immigration movements in response both to interregional economic disparities in Europe and to globalization processes, including growing numbers of non-European immigrants, and asylum migration.

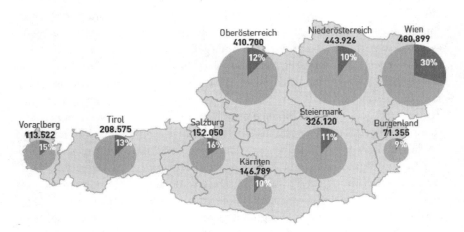

Figure 5.1. Proportion of young people (zero to 25) of foreign origin in the nine Austrian regions. Average value: 16%; definition of foreign origin = foreign born and Austrian born with non-Austrian citizenship. Source: Register of residents, 1.1.2012. Statistics Austria, 2012.

Today, 42% of the population with foreign origin comes from Yugoslavian succession states (without Slovenia) and from Turkey—that is, from the former labor force recruitment countries. The situation of these populations is characterized by economic poverty to a high degree: 45% of the population originating in Turkey is at risk of poverty, compared to an overall risk level of 12%. This population is also characterized by higher unemployment rates, bad housing standards, a lower social and education status, social segregation, and low social mobility rates over generations. Another 20% of immigrants originate in Central Eastern European countries. These immigrants represent a more heterogeneous population, partly with higher social and educational status and often successful in the labor market. Another 21% of immigrants come from (old) European Union countries.

The largest groups of origin are from Germany, Serbia (including Montenegro and Kosovo), Turkey, Bosnia and Herzegovina, Romania, Croatia and Poland, Hungary, and the Czech Republic. Among groups with a longer migration history, around one-third of immigrants have become naturalized. In recent years, immigration from Turkey and former Yugoslavia has slowed down, whereas intra-European mobility (in particular from Germany but also from new accession countries, mostly qualified immigrants) and migration from extra-European regions have become more significant, including an increasing number of refugees and asylum seekers from sub-Saharan Africa and Central Asia. There is also growing relevance of invisible groups such as undocumented seasonal workers and different kinds of informal labor market migration, in particular in the segment of personal and home services.

In the past two decades, migration and integration policies have also profoundly changed. For a long time, Austria's migration policy was influenced by the guest worker ideology—recruitment, no permanent residency, low status, and no societal integration. The country held on to this policy until the 1990s, when new patterns of immigration emerged in the shadow of political and military events in Central Eastern and South-Eastern Europe. This "structural conservatism" of immigration policy in Austria results from the deeply rooted corporatism in Austrian policy (including welfare), where political decisions require a negotiation and balance of organized interests between capital and labor (Kraler, 2011). Since the mid-1990s, immigration and asylum laws, and so-called "laws for foreigners", have been redefined multiple times, by shifting the immigration agenda from labor market services to security authorities. Austria is known for a restrictive immigration and integration regime, and the country pursues this restrictive policy also at the European policy level. Immigration and integration regulations are quite complex today, based on a quota regulation for newcomers, specific regulations for highly qualified professionals and a seasonal workforce (both of increasing relevance), restrictive settlement and naturalization norms, and an integration regime that is based both on a system of administrative and police control and an assimilation paradigm (language assessment, etc.).

The important population shift that has resulted from immigration processes over the past decades has deeply changed Austrian society. On one hand, this can be seen in a changing composition of the social structure. For example, as an effect of immigration, the percentage of the Muslim population has increased from 0.3% in 1971 to 6% in 2011 with an estimated population of 15% in 2050 (Goujon, Skirbekk, Fliegenschnee, and Strzelecki., 2007). Immigration also challenges the functioning of basic welfare institutions and infrastructures in education, health, social security, as well as the everyday life of the people, who are increasingly confronted with immigration issues in their immediate social environment, including their own family; there is a growing number of mixed partnerships and children with one parent who is foreign born. As mentioned previously, the country has troubles in dealing with this changing reality and in translating immigration into a vital element of social change. In recent years, media and public discourse have focused more on issues related to Islam, and, at the same time, there has been an ongoing extension and differentiation of juridical norms and regulations, including decreed integration measures such as language and history courses (Bail, 2008; Perchinig, 2010).

CHILDREN OF IMMIGRANTS

Official statistics use three criteria in relation to immigrant children and youth: foreign origin, migration background, and predominant language spoken. *Foreign origin* includes those who are foreign born and born in Austria with non-Austrian citizenship: around 14% of children younger than 19 years can be counted as of foreign origin (see also Figure 5.1, which includes people younger than 25 years). *Migration background* takes into consideration the origin of the parents: 22% of young people up to 19 years have both parents born outside of Austria. Among them, two out of three count as second generation (i.e., they were born in Austria). In the age category 15 to 19 years, half of young people belong to the first generation (i.e., they have migration history). Among the children up to five years, only 1.3% were born outside of Austria; 19.4% of these children have parents born abroad. Regarding *predominant language,* in the educational context, the categories for defining migration background do not refer to national or immigration status but rather to the native language (i.e., the language of parents and the language that is spoken at home). The average rate of children with non-German native language in Austrian schools is about 19%. In elementary schools (first four classes from 6 to 10 years), this applies to 24%, in high schools to 16%, and in schools for children with learning disability to 29% of all children.

The children of immigrants are not equally distributed among the nine regions (Integrationsfonds, 2012). In Vienna, 40% of the population younger than 19 have both parents who are foreign born. If the category of migration background refers to one foreign-born parent, the number climbs up to more than 70% (Stadt Wien, 2012). Regarding the country of origin, children with former Turkish, Serbian, and German origins are most numerous, followed by young people with Bosnian, Romanian, Croatian, and Polish origins. Two-thirds of children with a migrant background have parents who have immigrated from Turkey and former Yugoslavia. In recent years, immigration from Germany and Central Eastern Europe (in particular from Romania) has significantly increased. At the same time, a relevant numbers of young immigrants from the Russian Federation and Afghanistan, mostly refugees, have been recorded.

More significant than general data regarding the different categories of immigrant children is having knowledge about immigrants' living conditions and family situations. Children in families with Turkish and also ex-Yugoslavian origins live more often in larger households (Turkey: 3.79 persons; former Yugoslavia [without Slovenia]: 2.95 persons; autochthonous Austrians: 2.27 persons), also because immigrant households include more often nonnuclear family members as well. An analysis of EU-SILC data showed that 60% of children in families with Turkish origin live in households with five or more individuals. Among children from families who immigrated from former Yugoslavia, this percentage is 45%. Children in autochthonous families live in households composed by three to four members (Steinwender and Lindinger, 2009). Since the average number of children in immigrant families is higher than in Austrian families, immigrant children more often grow up with siblings, especially in families of guest worker migration background. The average number of children in families originating in Turkey is 2.19, from former Yugoslavia (without Slovenia), 1.91, and in autochthonous Austrian families, 1.63. Statistics also indicate that children from immigrant families move out earlier from their parents' home due to earlier marriage or parenthood (Statistics Austria, 2012).

Risks Related to Growing Up in Immigrant Families

Growing up in Austria as a child in an immigrant family may imply certain risks, in particular for descendants of former guest worker migrants. The most significant risk consists of poverty and social exclusion. In Austria, the risk of poverty is particularly high for immigrants from Turkey. Around 25% of the population with a migration background is confronted with a risk of poverty compared to 12% among the autochthonous population; among immigrants originating in Turkey, this number climbs to 45%. Whereas 16% of immigrants live in poverty (autochthonous population 6%), 20% of Turkish immigrants do. Organisation for Economic Co-operation and Development data indicate that, in Austria, 14% of children (under 18) are at risk of poverty.

One-third of these children have a migration background. Particular problems of poverty-determined life-worlds of immigrant children concern low-quality and overcrowded homes, low social status, insufficient income, debt, and unemployment of parents (Wiesböck, 2011).

As a consequence of poverty, in particular in combination with a marginal and fragile position in society, as is the case for former guest worker immigrants, the likelihood is high that the underprivileged social status of children with a migration background will be passed on to subsequent generations, and social upward mobility is thus impeded across generations (Jenkins and Sieder, 2007). Empirical studies emphasize this risk particularly for the descendants of former labor force migrants (Crul, Schneider, and Heering, 2012; Specht, 2009; Weiss, 2007) and underline the stabilizing role of the educational system in preserving existing inequalities. The risk of a perpetuation of poverty is reinforced by the legal framework and its underlying *ius sanguinis* principle, which defines children of immigrants as foreign nationals.

To summarize main research results (Bacher, 2010; Crul et al., 2012; Unterwurzacher, 2012), immigrant children in the Austrian school system are more likely to achieve poorer results and to attend a lower level secondary school (*Hauptschule*), a polytechnic school or one of the new midlevel schools of general education (*Mittelschulen*), and much less frequently a grammar or high school, that is a school with university entrance qualification (*Matura*). The likelihood of reading university entrance level is around 2% for ex-Yugoslavian children and 1% for children from Turkish families. These percentages reflect not only children's disadvantaged starting position (the low educational level of parents) but also the very selective character of the Austrian school system, which determines a student's educational trajectory at the early stage of transition between primary and secondary schools. Research shows that teachers are more likely to assign immigrant children to lower level secondary schools or even to special-needs schools (*Sonderschulen*), where immigrant children with deficient language skills are particularly likely to be placed. Research also emphasizes an overproportional drop-out risk among immigrant children: after eight years of school attendance, 13% of non-German native speakers have left the school system compared to 4% of German native speakers (i.e., these children failed to obtain a school leaving certificate).

PISA and PIRLS test programs constantly show a lower degree of school achievement among children with non-German first-language background. Research identified a strong influence of socioeconomic factors, deficient German language skills, and the architecture of the school system as the main factors behind these results (Bacher, 2010). Research also demonstrated that parents, in particular those originating in Turkey, share high motivational norms; that is, their expectations regarding the educational performance of their children are high, but at the same time their means for providing their children with educational help (such as tutoring, etc.) are weak. Traditional cultural norms and values, by contrast, play only a minor role. In short, multi-variate analyses emphasize the explanatory power of predictors related to social class, whereas the influence of ethnic orientations remains weak.

Educational disadvantages have long-lasting effects for status achievement, professional careers, life chances, and social mobility. The Austrian case confirms the key role that school systems play in the reproduction of social inequalities. The high level of selectivity in the early stage of education reinforces the specific contribution of the educational system to social reproduction. The educational system has been criticized for doing little to promote social mobility but rather stabilizing the existing social stratification in which labor force migrants occupy the lowest position (Gächter, 2009; Reinprecht, 2006). Under these conditions, the family gains centrality: overburdened and overextended, and consequently weakened in its function as a compensatory resource in migration processes (Reinprecht, 2009; Claus and Nauck, 2010).

The Representation of Migrant Children

Contrary to other European countries, the situation of immigrant families and immigrant children has not yet been the focus of public, political, or scientific attention in Austria (Kraler, Kofman, Kohli, and Schmoll, 2011). There is no official reporting system on immigrant families, and migration remains only a side issue in official reports on families; this is also the case for immigrant children and youth, insofar as it concerns their general living situation. So far, the public (and scientific) debate has followed the dominant integration paradigm and has thus focused on educational problems and issues related to schools, as well as on the problem of poverty. At the same time, there are also no statistics available concerning the situation of immigrant children in child protection services. Some local services provide internal data materials; however, the respective data are not documented or openly reported. At the same time, there are no official strategies specifically oriented toward families with migration backgrounds, which is consistent with the general principles of child protection in Austria.

As already mentioned, the subsidiary character of the Austrian child and youth welfare system implies that the public institution intervenes only if the family does not provide for the child's welfare, regardless of the child's nationality, ethnic origin, or migration status. An exceptional case is that of unaccompanied refugee minors. If an unaccompanied refugee minor is identified and detained, the relevant district authority has to be informed and will take over the legal representation of the minor.[4] This also applies to all other decisions that affect the safety and welfare of unaccompanied refugee minors, including asylum applications. Once an asylum procedure has been started, the minor will be provided with basic supplies (health care system, accommodation, and pocket money). Depending on the individual case, unaccompanied minors are sheltered mostly by private organizations, such as charitable welfare organizations

Table 5.1. Unaccompanied refugee minors (Vienna)

Year	Legal representations	Closed procedures	Positive asylum decisions
2008	194	79	14 (7%)
2009	196	75	26 (13%)
2010	191	85	35 (18%)
2011	196	78	42 (21%)

Source: MA 11 (City of Vienna).

(for instance Caritas) but also by private individuals. Public authorities and child protection institutions provide psychological support, language training, and education.

Between 2002 and 2012, about 7% of all asylum applications accounted for unaccompanied minor refugees, with fluctuating numbers year on year. In total, this represents 14,491 unaccompanied minor refugees. There are no official data on positive decisions throughout Austria, and no data on how many unaccompanied refugee minors are represented by child welfare authorities in asylum proceedings. Table 5.1, with data provided by the municipal department in Vienna responsible for unaccompanied minors (MA 11), includes numbers for legal representations for unaccompanied refugee minors, for closed procedures, and for positive asylum decisions. According to these data, the rate of positive asylum decisions among unaccompanied refugee minors lies only slightly above the average level of 19% in Austria in 2011.

The majority of unaccompanied minor asylum seekers are between 15 and 18 years old (approximately 80%), about 5% are younger; about 15% are assessed as being of legal age (18 years).[5] The statistics count more than 50 countries of origin. In recent years, the percentage of minors coming from Afghanistan increased significantly (from 13% in 2006 to 75% in 2012); other important countries are Pakistan, Russian Federation, Somalia, and, more recently, Syria and Algeria.

Social Work with Children of Immigrants

As in other domains of social intervention, social work in the field of child welfare must fulfill a double mandate: a control function in accomplishing the legally defined objectives of child protection and safety and an empowering function in enhancing the capacity of the target groups. Due to the general principles underlying the system of child rights and child welfare (priority of best interests of the child, participation, antidiscriminatory practice, and securing a child's welfare), child protection services and social workers will implement the previously defined forms of interventions in the same way working with immigrant children and families and nonimmigrant children and families.

In practice, social workers are confronted with a series of specific tasks and problems that are most obvious with regard to language and communication problems and hamper the active involvement of parents and children and the development of co-operative solutions. In one of the rare studies carried out in the field of social work with immigrant children in child protection services (Ranftler, 2012), the author illustrates, on the basis of qualitative interviews with social workers, that major communication and language problems strengthen existing prejudices and mistrust both among social workers and service users. Whereas social workers tend to draw on stereotypic images—the respondents focused on Muslims and attributed problems to cultural differences, represented in images of "traditional" family and gender roles and so on—immigrant families have a tendency to create an enemy stereotype of child protection as a form of institutional violence, often nourished by experiences of discrimination and perceived institutional racism. Social workers mentioned they needed language skills and intercultural competencies; moreover, they are in need of more precise information about the migration and integration regulations and about the diversity of immigrants, including information about migrants' living situation, life course, and the challenges of integration. The existing training offers of educational and professional training institutions do not meet these needs and interests. On the other hand, immigrant families are in need of information about their rights and the functioning of the child protection system. This reciprocal ignorance and unawareness produce particular obstacles and tensions in cases where the institution intervenes with force, for instance if it has been decided to remove a child from the family. Among immigrant families, removals are experienced both as violent and discriminatory acts. Unclear communication on behalf of the institution and a lack of information on the part of the families make the situation worse. There are no other valid data regarding this phenomenon in Austria.

Another particular context is the protection of children in cases where the family is repatriated by force. In recent years this has happened repeatedly to Kosovo or Chechen families who lost their temporary residence status after a negative decision of their asylum application, or sometimes after many years of residence and despite their stable integration in the labor market and educational system. In these cases, child protection services often clashes with the legal norms of migration and asylum policies, especially if the families are put in custody pending deportation. The law does allow putting a child under 14 years in custody under certain circumstances, unless a "soft arrest" is foreseen (e.g., the child is put in the custody of child protection services and accommodated in private households and foster families, often together with the mother). The dual role of child protection services is evident in these cases (Fekete, 2007).

There have nevertheless been cases where children stayed in prison with their parents, and many cases in which one part of the family was deported. Following the Convention of the Rights of the Child, child protection services would normally assess an imprisonment, as well as the separation from parents as a profound threat to child welfare. This assessment would normally also be upheld in cases where families are detained together in an open retention center where children are not provided with school and other services. In these cases, child protection services normally do not define their role in assisting the police (normally they would ask the assistance of the police to protect the safety of a child). However, the practice of child protection services varies between regions and districts and also between social workers.

The independent children and youth advocacy offices place the situation of minor members of refugee families regularly in the midst of public debate. As discussed in the following section, child protection services have been assigned to play a key role in defending the interests and welfare of children in refugee families, including unaccompanied minor refugees. With regard to the latter, child protection services gains custody of the child and then must provide the minor with all the necessary support, including access to education and health services. Asylum-related NGOs criticize the fact that in contrast to the demands of the law and the prohibition of discrimination, child protection services are seldom fully utilized for unaccompanied minor asylum seekers. In reality, a majority of cases of unaccompanied minor refugees remains unresolved since the relevant institutions refuse to undertake the necessary steps to initiate a custody procedure, although child protective services are obliged by law to intervene. Often, financial constraints are cited as a reason. However, there are different practices and local cultures, varying between the nine states but also at the municipal level. A recent court of justice decision that has reconfirmed the responsibility of child protection services gives some hope to believe in future changes in this area.

There are some other situations where the existing child protection system is not sufficiently equipped with legal regulations. This concerns the whole and complex domain of child trafficking (evidenced by the absence of a nationwide system of victim protection and support), and the increasing number of children on the move (e.g., independently migrating individuals younger than 19 years old). There are no specific strategies or contact points for these children. The new federal youth protection law also does not take into consideration migration-related issues.

TRAINING OF THE CHILD PROTECTION WORKFORCE

There is no information about training programs that refer specifically to the situation of immigrant children in Austria. Quality assurance measures, as they are stressed by the intended amendment of youth protection law, do not explicitly concern immigration or migrant family related matters. The curricula of the relevant educational institutions for the qualification of social workers mostly regard migration and integration related issues as a cross-sectional sub-ject, sometimes complemented by practice-oriented instructions in the field of intercultural communication or culturally sensitive social work. Bigger cities and child protection services offer internal trainings, often provided by staff members with a migration background. In recent years, the postgraduate edu-cational market has grown, also in regard to training in migration and integra-tion work, sometimes with a specific focus on family issues.

INSIGHTS FROM THE SURVEY: COMPLEX PRACTICE REALITIES AND LACK OF RESOURCES

In view of the lack of information concerning the situation of immigrant children in the Austrian child and youth protection services, the results of the Austrian survey conducted for this book are of particular significance. In Austria, the survey was answered by 199 social workers from eight of the nine regions, involving 30 of the 80 political-administrative districts, including the main cities and different levels of administration.

A first important insight is the observation that almost one in two respon-dents has worked with families with a migration background (44%). With regard to the origins of the migrant families with whom the social workers had been in contact, 89% of respondents mentioned Eastern Europe, 62% Africa, 43% Middle East, 27% Asia, 16% Western Europe, and 15% other regions. Behind these clusters, the answers indicate that in the everyday practice of child protection services, families and children from former Yugoslavian states (in particular from Serbia and Bosnia) and from Turkey are particularly involved (68% of the respondents mentioned these origins), whereas service users from other countries and regions are less often mentioned: 25% refer to families and/or children from Africa and Chechnya, 12% from Romania, 10% from Eastern Europe, 8% from Afghanistan, 8% from Asia, and 3% from Caribbean countries.

In contrast to the relevance of immigrants in the professional everyday life of social workers, nearly 15% of the respondents said that they speak the language of one of the client groups; a similar percentage indicated to have an immi-gration background (i.e., foreign-born parents); 7% has a history of migration themselves. Language and communication problems were mentioned as one of the main problems in the daily work with immigrant families and their chil-dren. The need for language skills and training was noted particularly often in the context of the two case studies. Altogether, 55% of the surveyed social workers underlined being particularly challenged by working with immigrant families. Eighty-one percent noted that these challenges also concern systemic barriers and that these barriers emerge significantly more often in working with immigrant families. Only one-third of the social workers (35%) received special training for working with immigrant children and families. Thirty-two per-cent reported feeling less competent in working with immigrants. One interest-ing result relates to migration background as a facilitator in social work with immigrant service users. According to this survey, respondents who have an immigration background do not evaluate their work with immigrants as less difficult.

The first case, concerning a couple with a newborn child, was assessed by every second respondent as risky (51%) and by 41% as moderately risky. Poverty and deprivation, bad housing conditions, in particular in relation with insuf-ficient water facilities and resulting hygiene deficiencies, and also aspects con-cerning the conduct of life such as malnutrition and lacking language skills, which hamper access to public and private support infrastructures, were most frequently mentioned. About 85% of the social workers would prefer to leave the child with the parents and provide services; only 3% would remove the child from the parents; and 8% stated that they are not able to decide between the alternatives provided because they would need more detailed information. In this regard, it is interesting to observe that the majority of the social workers suggest looking for social services providing supplementary financial support (79%) and welfare benefits (76%). This result mirrors the structure of the wel-fare system, in particular with regard to social aid, where institutional barriers hamper the access to institutions, in particular for immigrants who are often not in the legal position or find themselves without the necessary skills regard-ing language or information. The other options were mentioned considerably less frequently. The low frequencies for job seeking (16%) and better housing conditions (27%) may be interpreted as a reflection of existing difficulties in the Austrian labor and housing markets; at the same time, the results reflect the limited scope of action of social workers (as mentioned by some). Ninety-three percent of the respondents defined the child protection services as responsible for resolving this case, while 87% said that the interest of the newborn is more important than migration-related aspects; 13% believed that it would be neces-sary to regulate migration-specific issues before an intervention can take place.

The second case, concerning the undocumented child not attending school, was nearly unanimously evaluated as a (very high, high, or moderate) risk case (87%). No single respondent said that the case is a low risk or no risk case. The social workers clearly identified violence and abuse as major problems; the parental situation was evaluated as problematic and as a source of risk, as well as the fact that the child was overburdened with tasks and functions that were attributed to the family system. In spite of this critical evaluation of the family situation, 36% of the respondents would leave the child with the parents and provide services, 38% would immediately remove the child from the parents, and 14% could not decide on the basis of the alternatives provided. In the indi-vidual commentaries, some of the respondents supported a temporary removal from the family. The vast majority of the respondents (83%) definitely viewed the child welfare system as responsible for an undocumented child who is not attending school; only 8% said that this is not the case.

The more ambivalent and less decisive answers regarding the second case may also reflect the constraints respondents felt by filling out the questionnaire. In additional and open statements, the social workers stated that they would need additional and more detailed information about the case and described how they would proceed in the particular case. The first step would be a general assessment aiming to evaluate the family's capacity to change the situation and their will to cooperate with youth services. Language problems and the lack of translation services were defined as main problems at this stage. In an emergency situation, the child would be removed from her or his family for a maximum period of eight weeks. During this period the child would be accommodated in an intervention center (residential housing). This would give the social worker some time to assess the situation and its context and to look for alternative strategies by actively involving the parents and other relevant persons. Besides language problems, mistrust, closeness of the family system, and institutional barriers in particular with regard to the family's residence status were perceived as key obstacles in finding long-term solutions. There is a consensus among respondents that the wide range of factors that may finally lead to a concrete strategy for a solution cannot be anticipated.

An interesting aspect in the survey refers to the imagined migration background of the immigrant client, with different outcomes for the two cases. This is also noteworthy with regard to the findings of previous research, which emphasizes the everyday practices of cultural stereotyping in child protection services (Ranftler, 2012). In both cases, almost half of the social workers reported that they conceived an ethnic or cultural background (40% and 45%). However, a significant difference appears between the first and the second case: whereas in the context of the first case the most frequent representations concern people from former Yugoslavia and the Balkan (37%; other mentioned categories are immigrants from Africa, Chechna, and Roma), in the second case the references veer in a different direction, by focusing primarily on individuals from Turkey and of Muslim religious affiliation (together 38%). According to these results, social representations of poverty and deprivation on the one hand and family-system based violence on the other are attributed to different immigrant groups. Is this an indication of social workers ethnicizing of social problems?

One important set of comments by survey respondents concerns the critique of the existing system of organized social work, which does not give sufficient attention and response to the living situation and needs of immigrant families. Concrete issues that were noted were the lack of provision of adequate child care and education help, the lack of language skills and resulting communication problems, the absence of interpreters, and the lack of specific qualifications and training in intercultural social work and concerning migration and integration-related issues. Some respondents observed a lack of financial and human resources and indicated the necessity of additional resources and appropriate structural changes, citing the complexity of immigrant cases and an overworked social work workforce. But there was also a general critique of the way in which welfare institutions—and the Austrian society in general—deal with immigration and related issues. Respondents also pointed to the dominating problem and deficit orientation in public debate, social policy, and social research.

CONCLUSION

The scholarly literature, empirical research, and survey results highlight the fundamental contradiction that still defines Austria as a "country of immigration against will": the sociodemographic and sociostructural changes, which have been contributing to the transformation and diversification of family patterns, children's life worlds, and their trajectories to adulthood for three decades, challenge the traditional system of child and youth protection, which is far from being adequately equipped to respond to the emerging needs and demands of children in immigrant families in particular. Similar to other domains of Austrian society, the institutional realities of child protection need to overcome their blindness to migration and diversity. This statement goes far beyond the necessity to deliver translation facilities, more differentiated statistics and data documentation, and more scientific research. Rather, innovative forms of organization are needed, as well as a radical questioning of routinized institutional practices, including a reorientation of professional qualifications and training. Finally, one of the most interesting findings is the gap between the vast experience and knowledge gained by social workers in their daily work with immigrant families and the continuous denial of institutions that their own structures and practices have to be changed.

NOTES

1 In Austria, immigration statistics are based on a register of residents and micro-census data; arrivals are counted as immigrants after a period of three months. This includes also particular groups such as unaccompanied minors as long they are registered. In the scholarly literature, the categorization of young migrants and migrant descendants (second and third generation) is a matter of debate (Herzog-Punzenberger, 2003). Second-generation immigrants comprise both young people who were born in Austria as descendants of immigrants and young people who immigrated themselves, mostly at a very young age (i.e., before school enrollment). If they immigrated after the beginning of compulsory school education, children are defined as first

generation; if they have attended only a part of their school career in the country of origin, they are defined as "one and a half generation". In some publications the term "second generation" also includes individuals with only one parent of foreign origin (Stadt Wien, 2012). Another important aspect concerns citizenship: in Austria, descendants of immigrants do not automatically receive Austrian citizenship, even if they were born in Austria. The term "of migrant background" therefore includes both Austrian and foreign citizens.

2 In Austria, around 65% of forced repatriations concern families. In 2010, around 240 children were taken outside the country in this way, mostly families and children whose asylum application had been rejected, from the Russian Federation (Chechnya), Kosovo, Georgia, Serbia, and Turkey (Kurds) (see www.asylkoordination.com).

3 The few services targeting immigrant families concern mainly the field of educational support.

4 This principle had applied since 2005. In the years before, child and youth protection services did not feel responsible. The situation remains nevertheless unsatisfactory. Big differences on regional levels indicate a significance of personal engagement of individual civil servants and social workers.

5 Age assessment will be undertaken by the asylum authorities if the age statement of the refugee is assumed as being incorrect (see Lukits, 2012).

REFERENCES

Bacher, J. (2010). Bildungschancen von Kindern mit Migrationshintergrund: Ist-Situation, Ursachen und Maßnahmen (Educational chances of children with migration background: Status quo, background and measures). *WISO*, 33, 29–48.

Bail, C. (2008). The configuration of symbolic boundaries against immigrants in Europe. *American Journal of Sociology*, 73, 37–59.

Bauböck, R., Perchinig, B., & Sievers, W. (2009). *Citizenship Policies in the New Europe*. Amsterdam: Amsterdam University Press.

Bundesministerium für Wissenschaft, Forschung und Wirtschaft (BMWFJ). (2012). *Jugendwohlfahrtsbericht 2011* (Report on Child Protection). Wien: Federal Ministry of Economy, Family and Youth.

Claus, S., & Nauck, B. (2010). Immigrant and native children in Germany. *Child Indicators Research*, 3, 477–501.

Crul, M., Schneider, J., & Heering, L., eds. (2012). *Second Generation Immigrants in European Cities*. Amsterdam: Amsterdam University Press.

Crul, M., Schnell, P., Herzog-Punzenberger, B., Wilmes, M., Slotman, M., & Aparicio Gómez, R. (2012). Educational achievements of the second generation in Europe. In M. Crul, J. Schneider, & L. Heering (Eds.), *Second

Generation Immigrants in European Cities, 101–164. Amsterdam: Amsterdam University Press.

Esping-Andersen, G. (1990). *The Three Worlds of Welfare Capitalism*. Cambridge: Polity Press.

Fassmann, H., & Münz, R. (1995). *Einwanderungsland Österreich? Historische Migrationsmuster, aktuelle Trends und politische Maßnahmen* (Immigration Country Austria? Historical Patterns, Recent Trends, and Political Measures). Wien: Jugend und Volk.

Fekete, L. (2007). Detained: Foreign children in Europe. *Race Class*, 49(1), 93–104.

Gächter, A. (2009). *Der Integrationserfolg des Arbeitsmarktes* (Succesful Labour Market Integration). Wien: Zentrum für soziale Innovation.

Goujon, A., Skirbekk, V., Fliegenschnee, J., & Strzelecki, P. (2007). New times, old beliefs: Projecting the future size of religions in Austria. *Vienna Yearbook of Population Research*, 237–270.

Heimgartner, A. (2009). *Kompontenten einer prospektiven Entwicklung der sozialen Arbeit* (Components of a Prospective Development in Social Work). Wien: LIT.

Heizmann, K. (2007). *Austria: Tackling Child Poverty and Promoting the Social Inclusion of Children: A Study of National Policies*. Peer Review and Assessment in Social Inclusion. Brussels: European Commission.

Herzog-Punzenberger, B., ed. (2006). *Bildungs/be/nachteiligung und Migration in Österreich und im internationalen Vergleich* (Educational Discrimination in Austria and in International Comparison). Wien: Kommission für Migrations- und Integrationsforschung.

Herzog-Punzenberger, B. (2003). *Die "2. Generation" an zweiter Stelle? Soziale Mobilität und ethnische Segmentation in Österreich—eine Bestandsaufnahme* (Second Place for the Second Generation? Social Mobility and Ethnic Segmentation in Austria). Wien: ZSI.

Integrationsfonds. (2012). *Migration & Integration: Schwerpunkt Jugend. Zahlen. Daten. Indikatoren 2012.* (Migration & Integration: Focus on Youth. Figures, Dates and Indicators). Wien: ÖIF.

Jenkins S.P., & Siedler, T. (2007). The Intergenerational Transmission of Poverty in Industrialized Countries. CPRC Working Paper 75. Essex: Institute for Social and Economic Research.

Kraler, A. (2010). The case of Austria. In G. Zincone, R. Penninx, & M. Borkert (Eds.), *Migration Policy Making in Europe: The Dynamics of Actors and Contexts in Past and Present*, 21–60. Amsterdam: Amsterdam University Press.

Kraler, A., Kofman, E., Kohli, M., & Schmoll, C., eds. (2011). *Gender, Generations, and the Family in International Migration*. Amsterdam: Amsterdam University Press.

Lukits, D. (2012). *Unbegleitete Minderjährige Flüchtlinge im Asylverfahren. Unveröffentlichte Masterarbeit* (Unaccompanied Minor Refugees in Asylum Procedure). Salzburg: Universität Salzburg.

Perchinig, B. (2010). All you need to know to become an Austrian: Naturalisation policy and citizenship testing in Austria. In R. van Oers, E. Ersboll, & D. Kostakopoulou (Eds.), *A Re-Definition of Belonging? Language and Integration Tests in Europe*, 25–50. Leiden: Martinus Nijhoff.

Ranftler, J. (2012). *Kulturspezifische Fragestellungen für Sozialarbeiterinnen in der Jugendwohlfahrt. Unveröffentlichte Diplomarbeit* (Culturally Specific Tasks of Social Workers in the Child Protection System) Berlin: Alice Salomon Hochschule.

Reinprecht, C. (2006). *Nach der Gastarbeit: Prekäres Altern in der Einwanderungsgesellschaft* (After Guestwork: Precarious Aging in a Country of Immigration). Wien: Braumüller.

——. (2009). Migrationsforschung—Familienstrukturen (Migration research—Family structures). In Bundesministerium für Justiz (Ed.), *Lebensform Familie: Realität & Rechtsordnung*, 33–42. Wien: Neuer Wissenschaftlicher Verlag.

Specht, W., ed. (2009). *Nationaler Bildungsbericht. Österreich 2009* (National Education Report Austria 2009). Graz: Leykam Verlag.

Scheipl, J. (2011). Jugendwohlfahrt in Österreich (Youth protection in Austria). In Bundesministerium für Wirtschaft, Familie und Jugend (Ed.), *6. Bericht zur Lage der Jugend in Österreich*, 555–576. Wien: Bundesministerium für Wirtschaft, Familie und Jugend.

Stadt Wien. (2012). *Integrations- und Diversitätsmonitor der Stadt Wien 2009–2011* (Integration and Diversity Monitoring of the City of Vienna). Wien: Magistratsabteilung 17.

Statistik Austria, & Kommission für Migrations- und Integrationsforschung. (2012). *Migration und Integration: Zahlen, Daten, Indikatoren 2012* (Migration and Integration: Figures, Facts and Indicators). Wien: Statistik Austria.

Steinwender, G., & Lindinger, K. (2009). Lebenslagen von Kindern mit Migrationshintergrund (Living conditions of children with migration background). In M. Till & U. Till-Tentschert (Eds.), *In Armut aufwachsen. Empirische Befunde zu Armutslagen von Kindern und Jugendlichen in Österreich*, 39–52. Wien: Institut für Soziologie.

Stier, H., Lewin-Epstein, N., & Braun, M. (2001). Welfare regimes, family: Supportive policies, and women's employment along the life-course. *American Journal of Sociology*, 106, 1731–1760.

Thévenon, O. (2011). Family policies in OECD countries: A comparative analysis. *Population and Development Review*, 37, 57–87.

Till, M., & Till-Tentschert U., ed. (2009). *In Armut aufwachsen: Empirische Befunde zu Armutslagen von Kindern und Jugendlichen in Österreich* (Growing Up in Poverty: Empirical Insights into the Poverty of Children and Youth in Austria). Wien: Institut für Soziologie.

Unterwurzacher, A. (2012). *Vom Kindergarten bis zur Matura: Bildungsstationen von Kindern und Jugendlichen mit Migrationshintergrund. Unveröffentlichte*

Dissertationsschrift (From "Kindergarten" to High School: Educational Careers of Children and Youth with Migration Background). Wien: Universität Wien.

Weiss, H., ed. (2007). *Leben in zwei Welten. Zur sozialen Integration ausländischer Jugendlicher der zweiten Generation* (Living in Two Worlds: Social Integration of Foreign Youth of the Second Generation). Wiesbaden: VS Verlag für Sozialwissenschaften.

Wiesböck, L. (2011). Migration—Exklusion—Armut. Trend- und Strukturanalysen zur Ausgrenzung von MigrantInnen in Österreich. In R. Verwiebe (Ed.), *Armut in Österreich: Bestandsaufnahme, Trends, Risikogruppen* (Poverty in Austria: State of Research, Trends and Risk Groups), 209–231. Wien: Braumüller Verlag.

PART II

FAMILY SERVICE–ORIENTED CHILD WELFARE SYSTEMS WITHIN CONSERVATIVE (AND LATIN) WELFARE STATES

6

CHILD WELFARE SYSTEMS AND IMMIGRANT FAMILIES

THE CASE OF SPAIN

Antonio López Peláez and Sagrario Segado Sánchez-Cabezudo

INTRODUCTION

Over the past 15 years, Spain has become a gateway for immigration to such an extent that it is now regarded as a host country, in contrast to its traditional role as a country of emigrants since the late nineteenth century. This phenomenon has given rise to a wide range of studies on immigration flows in Spain. In this chapter, we analyze some of the key characteristics of immigrant families in Spain, focusing on the specific problems of minors and the institutional support they receive via the social services system. First, we analyze the characteristics of immigration flows in Spain. Second, we discuss the latest data on the immigrant population using as reference data on immigrants with a valid registration certificate or residence permit (Spanish Immigration Observatory, 2012). Third, we present the challenges facing the social services system due to the massive influx of immigrants in recent years. Fourth, we examine the current model for the protection of minors. Fifth, we explore child protection from the perspective of social work, focusing specifically on the main programs offered at Spanish universities and the discourse of professionals working in the field. We believe it is important to consider both the experience and the demands of social work practitioners in this area, since the protection of minors and the design of social services programs that ensure their development have always been a priority of social workers, who play a crucial role in child protection systems (Gilbert, Parton, and Skivenes, 2011). Finally, we analyze the available data on interventions by the social services system with regard to minors and the immigrant population. It should be noted that minors are heavily protected by law and that under the current integration model set out in the Spanish Constitution, social services do not distinguish between immigrant and non-immigrant minors.

IMMIGRATION FLOWS AND CHARACTERISTICS IN SPAIN

The Spanish model for the integration of immigrants[1] is based on the massive influx of unskilled labor, which began in the last decade of the twentieth century. The Spanish model is similar to that of other Mediterranean European Union (EU) countries (Lopez and Krux, 2003) that have a continuous influx of immigrants from other EU countries, as well as immigrants from a third country. It is important to note that, under EU legislation, a third-country national is any person who is not a citizen of a member state of the European Union. In Spain, the term "third-country national" refers to foreign workers who wish to work legally in Spain who are age 16 and over and who are authorized to remain in Spain for a period greater than 90 days but less than five years to engage in gainful employment, either in an employed or a self-employed capacity.

We find two types of immigration flows in Spain. The first comprises a very heterogeneous group of immigrants. These immigrants enjoy high purchasing power and may or may not be retired. They choose to settle in Spain for its excellent climate and generous welfare benefits. The second type comprises mainly first-generation immigrants between the ages of 18 and 50 whose main objective is to seek employment and family reunification. Due to their diverse origins, the main challenges facing these immigrants for over a decade have primarily been related to language skills, gender relations, or family relationship models (Alted, 2006), situations that are further compounded by the heterogeneity of Spain's own territorial model.

Immigration flows in Spain can be analyzed by addressing the following four issues:

- Diverse origins. Romanians are the largest immigrant group in Spain, followed by Moroccans (both groups account for 33.10% of total foreign residents, as of March 31, 2012). Of the 15 most numerous nationalities (Romania, 903,964; the United Kingdom, 238,402; Italy, 183,190; Bulgaria, 172,565; Portugal, 127,852; Germany, 126,095; and France, 101,133), seven are from parts of the EU. Evidently, the challenges faced by the social services system vary widely according to nationality, which, in turn, also gives rise to additional issues relating to the management of such diversity (e.g., language problems, either Spanish or the official language pertaining to an autonomous region, as well as diverse models of behavior toward minors, etc.).

- Geographic concentration. The immigrant population in Spain is concentrated in Madrid and on the Mediterranean coast, primarily in four autonomous regions: Catalonia, Valencia, Andalusia, and Murcia. The fact that the immigrant population is concentrated in specific areas of the country has saturated the social services system (and other welfare state institutions) while simultaneously giving rise to specific situations of vulnerability in areas with dispersed populations (i.e., rural areas in central Spain).

- Minors. The age structure of the EU immigrant population differs from that of the third-country immigrant population. Third-country immigrants are younger than community immigrants, a phenomenon that is particularly marked in the case of minors. There are 191,320 minors age zero to four years from third countries compared to 53,292 from EU countries (as of March 31, 2012). A total of 731,222 immigrants under the age of 16 currently reside in Spain, 68.4% of whom are third-country nationals.

- The legal status of immigrant families. The legal status of immigrant heads of family, whether irregular or otherwise, can also affect other family members, giving rise to a variety of situations. For example, some siblings are legal immigrants, while others are undocumented, or the legal status of one parent could be contrary to that of the other. The risk of social exclusion increases in proportion to the extent of the irregularity, and often an important role of social workers is to establish an appropriate strategy in order to legalize all family members together. Some of the risk factors affecting immigrant families include the impossibility of arranging support for families and minors in an irregular situation; the difficulties involved in enrolling children in school; school dropout (although schooling is mandatory in Spain, irregular families encounter greater difficulties in registering and fulfilling the established requisites); the vulnerability of minors in immigrant families that are in an irregular situation and travel the country seeking resources in order to survive; and the wide diversity of local programs and resources, which, in turn, also favor their displacement in an effort to find the best available resources (Quiroga Raimúndez and Alonso Segura, 2011: 47–49).

Relating to the characteristics of the immigrant population and owing to the implementation of successive immigration amnesties, the undocumented immigrant population is on the decline. In 2010, 810,000 people acquired citizenship in a EU member state; Spain contributed the most to this increase. Indeed, while 80,000 people acquired Spanish citizenship in 2008, that figure rose by 55% in 2010, thus surpassing, for the first time, the total number of people who acquired German citizenship. In the EU as a whole, 9 out of 10 people who acquired citizenship were third-country nationals. "At [the] EU level, about 90% of all those who acquired citizenship were previously third country nationals, that is, citizens of non-EU countries. With the exceptions of Luxembourg and Hungary, in all Member States acquisitions by third country nationals outnumbered those by EU citizens" (Sartori, 2012: 3).

Hence an analysis of the available data on legal immigrants provides a fairly accurate picture of the current situation in Table 6.1.

- The number of foreign residents in Spain (5,294,710 as of March 31, 2012, according to the Spanish Immigration Observatory, 2012) now exceeds 11% of the total population (without taking into account the illegal immigrant population). Spain currently boasts an immigrant population that has established itself primarily over the past 15 years with the intention of staying in the country permanently. Despite the severe economic crisis affecting the Spanish economy, in the first quarter of 2012 the immigrant population rose by 0.83% over the previous

Table 6.1. Data on immigrant and nonimmigrant population

Population of Spain (Nov. 2011)	46,815,916[a]
Child population (Nov. 2011)	8,804,490[a]
Immigrant population (%) (Nov. 2011)	11.22%[a]
Immigrant child population (% of child population) (Nov. 2011)	10.74%[a]
Immigrant children in child welfare system, per 1,000 children[a] per country	NA
Immigrant children, in-home services per 1,000 children[b]	NA
Immigrant children in out-of-home placements (care orders), per 1,000 children[b]	NA
Nonimmigrant children in child welfare system, per 1,000 children[b]	NA
Nonimmigrant children, in-home services per 1,000 children[b]	NA
Nonimmigrant children in out of home placements (care orders), per 1,000 children[b]	NA
Children in child welfare system, per 1,000 children[b] (2010)	14.79[b]
Children in child welfare system receiving in-home services, per 1,000 children	NA
Children in child welfare system receiving out-of-home services, per 1,000 children	NA

NA = Data not available.

[a] *Source*: National Statistics Institute, Government of Spain. Survey: Population and Housing Census 2011. (www.ine.es).

[b] *Source*: Information System of Social Services Users, Ministry of Health, Social Services and Equality, Government of Spain. The SIUSS is the source for Spanish data on general social services activity.

quarter. One of the key issues is to analyze how social services have been redesigned to deal with the increasing immigrant population (both legal and illegal) and child welfare in particular.

- In Spain, immigrants holding a valid registration certificate or residence permit fall into two categories: community residents (those belonging to other EU member states and European Free Trade Association countries) and third-country residents. The immigrant population is distributed between the two categories in a similar manner: the number of third-country immigrants as of March 31, 2012, stood at 2,730,970, accounting for 51.58% of the total number of foreign residents in Spain. The number of community immigrants as of the same date stood at 2,563,803, accounting for 48% of all foreign residents in Spain. Since late 2011, both groups have increased. Specifically, the number of third-country immigrants has increased by 1.28%, while the number of community immigrants has risen by 0.36%.

- For more than a decade, Spanish families have been characterized by a low birth rate (Del Fresno, 2011). In this context, minors with foreign citizenship (born outside Spain or born in Spain to foreign parents) represent a growing percentage of the total number of minors in Spain. In 1998, third-country nationals ages zero to 17 accounted for 2% of all third-country nationals, while in 2009 the figure was 17%. In other words, the percentage of minors within the immigrant population is gradually increasing, thus highlighting their desire to remain in the country, reunify their families, and build a long-term project in Spain (Quiroga Raimúndez and Alonso Segura, 2011).

SPANISH CHILD WELFARE LAW AND POLICY[2]

The fundamental principles underlying the protection of minors are set out under the Spanish Constitution of 1978. These principles have not been grouped under the same heading but have been established throughout the constitution. However, chapter III of Title I refers to the obligation of parents to attend to their children's needs and the obligation of public authorities to ensure the social, economic, and legal protection of children within the family.

The legislation set out in international treaties such as the United Nations Child Rights Convention of November 1989, which was ratified by Spain on November of the following year, marked a major change in terms of child protection. The most important national laws are Act 1/1996 of January 15 on the Legal Protection of Children,[3] which partially amended the Civil Code and the Civil Procedure Act, as well as Act 5/2000 of January 12 regulating the criminal responsibility of minors. These national laws are supplemented by other regional and local laws.

These laws refer to three guiding principles for the provision of social services in relation to children: (a) ensure that the child remains within the family of origin unless it is not in his or her interest to do so, (b) promote family and social integration, and (c) prevent situations that might jeopardize children's personal and social development.

To conclude this section, it is important to clarify two legal concepts that are key to determining what intervention measures should be taken by social services with regard to minors. Specifically, we are referring to the distinction between "risk" and "neglect." "Situations of risk for minors" refers to any situation that could potentially cause personal and/or social harm to the minor yet does not require the assumption of guardianship by operation of law. In such situations, the services provided by public authorities should guarantee the minor's right to assistance and lower the risks faced by the minor while promoting protective measures targeted at the minor and his or her family and monitoring such procedures.

"Neglect" is defined as "what happens due to failure to, impossibility of or inappropriate execution of the duties of protection established by the law for the custody of minors when they are deprived of adequate moral or material assistance" (Article 172, Civil Code). In such cases, the regional governments have jurisdiction to assume guardianship or temporary care of minors by operation of law.

This legal distinction between the two terms gives rise to three types of situations that are addressed by the System for the Social Protection of Minors, which is targeted at minors under the age of 18 who are permanent or temporary residents (whether or not they are registered or have legal residency):

(1) Social difficulty (low risk). This refers to minors who live in family or social environments that could cause significant harm to the minors' welfare and development in the short, medium, or long term (i.e., they run the risk of neglect and suffer from inadequate parental care).

(2) Vulnerability (moderate to high risk and neglect). This refers to children whose basic needs are not fulfilled due to (a) problems or external circumstances beyond the control of their parents or guardians or (b) family circumstances, such as the conduct of the parents or legal guardians or adults living with the family. In the latter case, vulnerability may be moderate to high. When there is a situation of high risk, separation may be imminent or actions can be taken to separate the minor from the family and assign a legal guardian due to neglect.

(3) Social conflict. This situation refers to minors ages 12 to 18 with behavioral problems that have seriously altered the accepted norms of coexistence and social behavior and have caused or are likely to cause harm to others. These situations are assessed as social conflict with

and without criminal legal action and may or may not be associated with vulnerability.

In the event of social difficulties, intervention is preventive in nature, while in the event of vulnerability and social conflict, intervention is orientated toward rehabilitation.

THE WELFARE STATE, ORGANIZATION OF THE SOCIAL SERVICES SYSTEM, AND CHILD PROTECTION

The Spanish welfare state has consolidated its role over the past 35 years of democracy and for the past 10 years has faced a new challenge: the integration of a growing influx of immigrants as Spanish citizens. In what follows, we analyze the main characteristics of the Spanish welfare state from the perspective of social services.

The Spanish welfare state is structured into a highly decentralized model in which various institutional bodies are involved (García-Cuevas, 2012). Social services are regulated at the national level through framework laws, at the regional level through what are known as the "social services laws," and at the local level through local entities. Health and education have also undergone an important decentralization process. While decentralization has some advantages, it has also given rise to issues of coordination, especially in relation to immigrant families who move from one place to another. In doing so, these families become dependent on a variety of institutions, and in many cases minors suffer from a lack of coordination between regional governments. For example, if a family moves from one autonomous region or town to another, children have to be reassigned to a new school, and the family has to reapply for social benefits. On occasion, immigrant families will also change location in an effort to avoid sanctions imposed by a region due to the unacceptable treatment of minors. However, the application of law and the penal institutions have not been decentralized.

In response to this decentralized structure, the government created the Childhood Observatory: "The Childhood Observatory of Spain is a professional advisory body created on 12 March 1999 by the Spanish Council of Ministers as a working group whose aim is to build a centralised and shared data system capable of providing information about the welfare and quality of life of children, as well as the development, implementation and effects of public policies on their wellbeing" (Puyó, 2009: 273). The working groups are organized into the following principal lines of research on the situation of minors in Spain:

- Services targeted at immigrant minors in Spain and their social integration

- Child abuse
- Foster care and adoption
- Childhood, adolescence, and the media
- National Strategic Plan for Children and Adolescents
- Coexistence and social inclusion

As regards immigrant minors, the specific objectives are to

- Obtain ongoing knowledge of the situation of immigrant minors in Spain and encourage communication between public and private institutions for better enforcement of the law and attention to their needs.
- Monitor the implementation of services targeted at unaccompanied minors.
- Promote the social and labor integration of minors in Spanish centers, as well as the development of programs and best practices regarding integration.
- Become acquainted and cooperate with international programs in this area that have been developed in the countries of origin of the minors.

Among its priorities, the National Strategic Plan for Children and Adolescents in Spain 2006–2009 (www.observatoriodelainfancia.msps.es) highlights the need to pay special attention to the children of migrant workers and unaccompanied migrant minors, as well as to fostering coordination between autonomous regions. However, problems of coordination continue to persist as evidenced by the observations and recommendations the United Nations made to Spain in 2010 (Convention on the Rights of the Child, November 3, 2010; www.observatoriodelainfancia.msps.es).

SPANISH SOCIAL SERVICES, CHILD WELFARE MEASURES, AND TRAINING OF CHILD WELFARE WORKERS

The social services system in Spain provides services related to prevention, rehabilitation, and assistance in order to ensure that individuals and families have access to the social services system in response to their need for information, guidance, coexistence, participation, and social integration on a case-by-case basis, as well as through community development. Such actions first require the assessment of a professional who performs the following functions: (a) detect situations of personal, family, and community needs; (b) provide information, assessment, orientation, evaluation, and counseling; (c) perform preventive actions; (d) attend to individuals in situations of dependency; (e) intervene in nuclear families or other family units in situations of social risk, especially when minors are involved; (f) provide home care, tele-home care, temporary accommodation, and support to the family unit or other types of family arrangements; (g) promote social inclusion measures; (h) provide nonresidential social and educational services for children and adolescents; (i) deal with urgent social services needs; (j) promote active participation in the community via the appropriate mechanisms in the search for solutions to situations of social need and improve quality of life and foster coexistence; (k) coordinate specialized social services; (l) collaborate with autonomous regions in exercising their role in authorizing and inspecting social services, (m) provide support, information, and advice to female victims of violence about available resources; (n) collect information about social services users, as well as manage programs and services.

According to the Information System of Social Services Users (SIUSS) the services are provided to different sectors of the population: immigrants, emigrants, individuals who abuse substances, the homeless, ethnic minorities, the disabled, the elderly, women, youth, and children and families. In 2010, the highest number of services (35%) was provided to the elderly, followed by families (25%).

Among the actions targeted at families, two measures are specifically aimed at children: protection and prevention, and behavioral intervention, both of which strive to ensure compliance with the measures imposed by juvenile courts and child protection services.

Protective measures are taken at three levels: first by promoting the rights of children, which involves dissemination and awareness campaigns; second, through prevention at varying levels of the community; and third, through decision making in situations of risk and vulnerability. The latter could include preservation of the family unit with the corresponding provision of support through day care centers, basic benefits, and so on; temporary separation in foster care or residential care; and permanent separation and integration in another family arrangement such as permanent foster care, adoption, or guardianship.

Behavioral intervention falls under the control of the basic social services system, which is responsible for child welfare. This measure includes specialized foster care, educational intervention, psychiatric care, and substance abuse treatment. In adherence to a Spanish court ruling, each autonomous region has a youth reformatory system that operates with open and closed conditions of internment.

Training

As far as the provision of specific training on children (designed to enhance the skills of social workers in Spain) is concerned, we can distinguish three main areas: universities, professional schools, and institutions where social workers carry out their professional activity (whether public institutions, where the vast majority of social workers develop their professional activities or other private companies).

The formal education offered in universities is offered in specialized master's and doctoral programs. In this regard, there are specific master's degrees that address the protection of children from a perspective related to the professional activity of social workers and also taking into account the conditions of the immigrant population (e.g., the Master's in Mediation and Intervention with Children in Situation of Vulnerability and/or Social Conflict, offered by Deusto University; the Master's in Contemporary International Migration, from Comillas Pontifical University; the Master's in Social Work, Welfare State and Social Intervention Methodologies, from National University of Education Distance; the Master's in Methods and Techniques in Applied Social Research, from the Complutense University of Madrid; or the Master's in Immigration Management, Universitat Pompeu I Fabra).

In relation to the specific training programs that the public schools of social work offer in Spain, social workers can enter into *Colegios,* which are professional associations that develop a key role in coordinating their professional and training demands. Many professional associations publish their own journals and organize both training courses and lectures and symposia, giving special attention to the training needs requested by social services professionals. In the field of child protection, they design specific courses geared to professional intervention. For example, the Colegio Oficial de Diplomados en Trabajo Social y Asistentes Sociales in Sevilla organizes a series of annual training courses, among which the course "Systems of Child Protection" stands out (November 2013). The Colegio Oficial de Trabajo Social en Málaga offers an online training course on "Gender Violence and Child Abuse" (See http://www.trabajosocialmalaga.org/html/FORMACION_detalles_cursos_formacion.php?c=69).

Finally, in the professional environment, social workers develop their knowledge and skills to a very high degree in public institutions. In the field of local government, city and county councils, which are the primary institutions responsible for social services, social workers design specific training programs on the aforementioned topics.

We can also highlight the annual meetings of the teams of family and childhood workers in the municipalities of fewer than 20,000 inhabitants organized by many councils. An example is that being organized by the Council of Cadiz, with the aim of developing a *Handbook of Family and Childhood Teams Intervention* to deal with the new social challenges of the twenty-first century in an environment marked by high levels of immigration (see http://www.dipucadiz.es/servicios_sociales/REUNION-DE-EQUIPOS-DE-FAMILIA-E-INFANCIA/).

Some other institutions, including foundations and private companies that specialize in the field of social work and social intervention, such as the Red

Cross or Group 5, also offer training courses. For example, various training programs such as the conference "Good Practices with Children, Parenthood, and Community Resources" (November 29–30, 2013, Grupo 5, Madrid) have been developed.

REPRESENTATION OF IMMIGRANT FAMILIES AND CHILDREN: CHALLENGES FOR THE SOCIAL SERVICES SYSTEM

Migration dynamics can also be regarded as family dynamics in the broadest sense of the extended family. Immigrants migrate in what might be termed "migration networks", in which kinship ties and geographical origin play a fundamental role. In a context in which highly diverse migration networks, geographical origins, family strategies, and relational models with minors coincide in time and space, social services have to deal with a more complex assessment of the needs and risks faced by immigrant families in relation to their origin and cultural norms (Segado Sánchez-Cabezudo, 2011). To study this phenomenon in greater depth, the first National Immigrant Survey was conducted between November 2006 and February 2007. From the perspective of our research, the survey highlights an important fact about the family structure of immigrant families: immigrant families are larger than Spanish families and evidence a more complex internal structure (i.e., denser domestic relationships between family and nonfamily members; Requena and Sánchez Domínguez, 2011: 84).

From the perspective of social work, research on immigration flows must take into account issues concerning the protection of the rights of minors (Villagrasa and Ravetllat, 2009). In this regard, we must examine the principal problems detected by the social services system on the one hand and how those issues are dealt with on the other, taking into account the characteristics of the decentralized Spanish welfare system. To achieve this goal, we begin by exploring the most relevant issues and then analyze the characteristics of the Spanish welfare state, focusing on the most important actions undertaken by the social services system regarding minors.

The welfare of immigrant families in developed countries, and specifically in Spain, faces a number of challenges (Arango, 2004; Alted, 2006; Villagrasa and Ravetllat, 2009), which are common and urgent:

- Poverty. This is the foremost challenge, especially in the context of the current economic crisis. The economic downturn, the reduction in the available income of immigrants (evidenced by the drop in remittances sent to their countries of origin [www.remesas.org]), long-term unemployment, and the loss of family structure have meant that a large number of immigrants find themselves in a particularly precarious situation. As we will see later, this precariousness is reflected in the social services targeted at resolving situations of extreme hardship.

- Education and school dropout. Providing minors with education is crucial to achieving social integration. The concentration of immigrants in certain areas of the country, problems of truancy, lack of parental support in school activities, and the underground economy in which minors work on a par with adults demand more and better state support.
- Minors with disabilities. Disability is an acute problem among immigrant families due to their general lack of awareness regarding state support and also due to the specific problems in relation to the children with the disabilities themselves.
- Unaccompanied minors. This is a group of children that suffers a high risk of social exclusion. According to the report *Neither Illegal nor Invisible: The Legal and Social Reality of Foreign Minors in Spain* (UNICEF, 2007), the number of unaccompanied minors in Spain is estimated to be 6,475, although statistics are not available nationwide and mobility is high between regions. The number of invisible minors (i.e., those who live in the streets, domestic workers, or those exploited by their compatriots) must also be added to the total.

All these serious problems faced by immigrant families in Spain are addressed by the social services system. Some of the main services provided to overcome these difficulties are shown in Figure 6.1. As can be observed, the greatest share

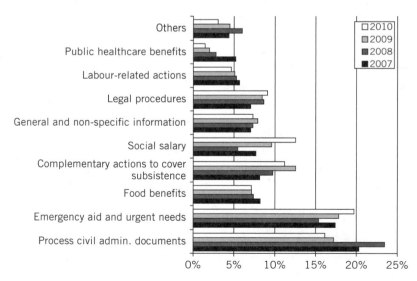

Figure 6.1. Social services provided to the immigrant population. Source: Information System of Social Services Users, Ministry of Health, Social Services and Equality (2007–2010).

of services provided by the social services system consists of "processing civil administrative documents" and "emergency aid or urgent needs."

When social workers initiate contact with minors and their families, they first perform an assessment of the service user's demands and needs. One of the current and major problems when registering child welfare services in the SIUSS is that the system does not distinguish between minors belonging to immigrant and nonimmigrant families. The reason for this is that the system is designed to promote integration and treat and protect all citizens as equals.

Thus if a social worker assigns a service user to the "nationality" category in the SIUSS register, it is not possible to also mark the subcategory of "minor." However, if a social worker first selects the category "family" (instead of "nationality"), they can then select the following subcategory of "minor." In short, the specific details relating to "minors of immigrant families" are virtually nonexistent in the official database handled by the social services system with regard to the services and interventions on a national scale. As a consequence, resources targeted specifically at the "immigrant population" are very rare, following the logic that the population of immigrant minors can potentially benefit from any of the services provided by social services.

However, it can provide data about the services provided to minors. As can be seen in Figure 6.2, most services delivered are related to food benefits and education.

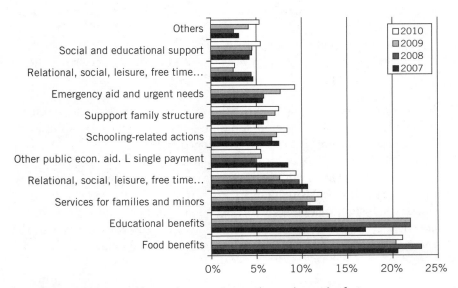

Figure 6.2. Resources used by social services in attending to the needs of minors.
Source: Information System of Social Services Users, Ministry of Health, Social Services and Equality (2007–2010).

AN OVERVIEW OF SOCIAL SERVICE PRACTICE

The current social services system is organized into two main coordinating structures aimed at the protection of minors in Spain. Their names vary from one region to another, but to explain this common structure, we focus on the case of the Autonomous Region of Madrid (Figure 6.3).

    (1) Social Services Centers (*Centros de Servicios Sociales* [CSS]). The CSSs are public, multipurpose centers. There is at least one center per district, and they are usually the first port of call for all types of service demands, including those of immigrant families. The centers are staffed by a team of multidisciplinary professionals.

    (2) Child Care Centers (CAIs). The CAIs comprise another more specific structure. These centers are designed to meet needs and deal with situations requiring technical expertise or specific types of resources. These centers are used as a first port of call only in exceptional circumstances (i.e., for particularly urgent cases).

Often there are also other bodies or agencies that perform a coordinating role between these two institutions, although this varies by region. For example, in Madrid, there are two bodies that engage in coordination tasks:

    (A) Working Groups assigned to Minors and Families (ETMFs). These groups intervene when the CSSs are uncertain about the need for intervention. The CSSs send cases to the ETMFs, where a decision is made.

    (B) Family Support Commissions (CAFs). The CAF is the other coordinating support structure. The CAFs deal with cases deemed moderate to high risk by the CSSs.

In order to provide a general picture of how these structures operate, we offer a brief and very general overview of the main steps involved in processing a case from intake to closure via the above-mentioned bodies.

The first stage in service assessment is always case intake. In general, the CSSs are responsible for this step of the process. In exceptional circumstances, the CAIs may also deal with high-risk cases. If a case is deemed to be urgent, it can be dealt with by either body. The main issues that arise during case intake are whether the social services are the competent body for dealing with the case, which services ought to be provided, and whether the case is urgent.

- When a case is screened in, a global assessment is performed. At this stage in the process, it is usually the ETMFs that decide if the case pertains to a CSS or a CAI. The questions that arise during the assessment

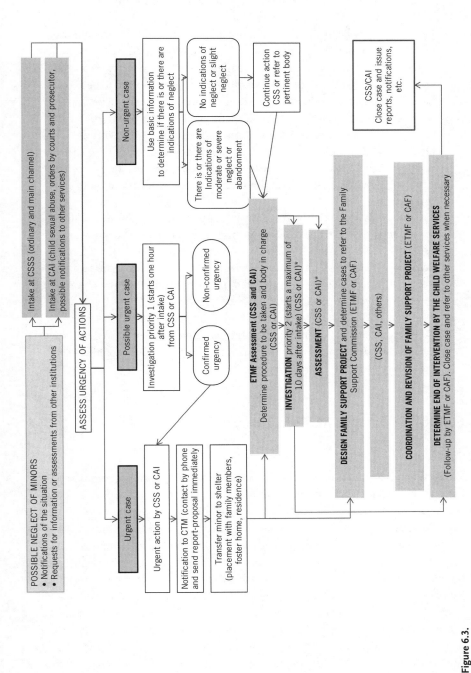

Figure 6.3.

Source: Madrid Town Hall, Family and Social Services Division, *Intervention Manual of Social Services Protection of Minors* (2008), p. 19.

are: What factors have led to the situation of vulnerability? What are the family's strong points? What are the consequences of the minor's state of vulnerability? Which types of support and services do the minor and his or her family need? What is the prognosis regarding parental capacity?

- Once the assessment is complete, a proposal is made and a support project is designed for the family. Proposals are prepared by the center dealing with the case. Proposals usually respond to such issues as the purpose and objective of the intervention; which actions need to be taken (i.e., what protection measures, services, and resources need to be implemented); how long the services will be needed; which body will be in charge of coordinating the intervention; and periodicity of revisions.
- Once again, during the implementation and coordination of the Family Support Project, the ETMF and CAF coordinating structures decide whether the CSSs or the CAIs should be in charge of carrying out the intervention.
- The successive reviews of the Family Support Project are again submitted to the ETMF and CAF coordinating structures. The issues that arise in this stage of the process are whether the initial objectives are being reached, the current situation of the minor, whether the Family Support Project needs to be modified, the date of the next review, and whether or not the service should be discontinued.
- The final stage of the intervention is resolution and closure. In order to close a case, all the technical and administrative actions, as well as any notifications and reports must be registered, along with the resolution that led to the closure.

SURVEY OF FRONTLINE PRACTICE

Sample

We conducted a survey of frontline workers. The survey sample comprised 98 child welfare social workers. Two different surveys were prepared (Survey 1 and Survey 2). In order to compare the results of the surveys, each social worker was administered only one of the two surveys. The surveys asked respondents questions of a general nature and presented two child welfare cases involving immigrant families. The surveys were identical in all aspects, with the exception of the employment status of the parents (this difference is explained later). The survey was sent to several universities throughout Spain and to regional-level government institutions responsible for the protection of minors. Hence the survey respondents were from the north (Vigo and Pontevedra), south (Jaen and Huelva), east (Alicante, Valencia, and Murcia), and central (Madrid and Guadalajara) regions of Spain. All the workers surveyed had experience working with immigrants and their families. In 37% of the cases, the respondents were working with immigrants and their families at the time the survey was administered. Of the total sample, 33% of the workers spoke the language of the immigrant family with whom they worked. Moreover, 72% held either a bachelor's degree, a master's degree, or a PhD in social work, while 64% had undergone specific training to work with immigrants. The respondents had worked with minors in the public social services system for an average of 10 years. All of the respondents (100%) were born in Spain, and 99% had Spanish parents (only one respondent had immigrant parents).

The main tasks and duties that the social workers perform in the organizations in which they work are shown in Table 6.2.

The origin of the immigrants with whom the social workers practiced most often was South America (86%), Africa (82%), and Eastern Europe (67%). In descending order, the immigrants' countries of origin were Morocco (64%), Ecuador (47%), Romania (45%), and Colombia (26%).

Survey Analysis

When the respondents were asked whether the social services system in Spain would take charge of an undocumented minor who was not enrolled in school, 87.1% of the workers answered "yes," compared to 3.5% who responded "no" and 9.4% who stated "I don't know."

In a first step, all of the respondents were shown a vignette of a marginalized migrant family with a newborn baby (see methodological appendix for a full description of the vignette). They were then asked to assess the risk level of the baby appearing in the vignette. Twenty-eight percent of the respondents stated that the baby was at "very high" risk, 38% said that the baby was at "high" risk, and 28% said the baby was at "moderate" risk, while only 6% responded that the baby was at "low risk." The respondents were also asked what actions they would take regarding the baby's future.

The results are shown in Table 6.2 and discussed in further detail in the following.

Table 6.2. Tasks and duties of social workers

Emergency response	5.9%
Investigations and/or risk assessment	18.8%
In-home services	1.2%
Out-of-home services	2.4%
All or most of the above tasks and duties	52.9%
Other tasks and duties for the child welfare services	11.8%
Management tasks	7.1%

- 28% of the workers stated that the baby was at "very high" risk. Of these, 93% answered that they would leave the baby with his or her parents, while 2% said that they would not leave the baby with his or her parents or remove the baby from them.
- Of the 38% of workers who stated that the baby was at "high" risk, 74% responded that they would leave her or him with its parents, 10% said that they would begin procedures to remove the baby from his or her parents, and the remaining 6% stated that they would take neither of the two options presented to them in the survey.
- Of the 28% of workers who assessed that the baby was at "moderate" risk, the majority (96.5%) stated that they would leave him or her with the parents, while 3.5% said they would not take either of the actions.
- Finally, the 6% who responded that the baby was at "low" risk stated that they would leave him or her with the parents.

The workers who said they would leave the baby with the parents were shown a list of possible actions they could take. Most of the respondents (97.3%) said they would refer the family to other community services, and 91.9% stated they would refer the parents to the general welfare service system. Moreover, 81.1% said they would help the parents find a job, while 75% stated that they would provide them with other services available in Spain. When the workers were asked if they would find the family a place to live with amenities and running water, 58.1% said they would.

The questionnaire also included an item that asked the social workers if they would encourage the parents to return to their home country. Twenty-three percent of the respondents said "yes," compared to 40.5% who said "no" and 8.1% who said that this was not an option for the Spanish welfare services.

Finally, following the words of our Norwegian colleague, "to explore how the borders between immigration and child welfare are drawn," we asked the social workers to respond to three statements regarding this case, specifically, the authority of the welfare services to act, the child's welfare versus immigration issues, and immigrant status. Seventy-seven percent of the workers said that this was a case in which the welfare services had authority to act, 87% said that the interest of the newborn prevailed over immigration issues, and only 10% said that aspects related to the family's "immigrant" status must be addressed first.

In a second step, we showed the workers another vignette about a marginalized migrant family with a daughter who suffered abuse. Again, the social workers were asked to assess the daughter's risk level and state the actions they would undertake. In this second phase, however, the two surveys were different. In Survey 1, both parents were employed, while in Survey 2 both parents were unemployed. Approximately half of all the respondents were shown Survey 1, while the other half were shown Survey 2 (see the methodological appendix for a full description of the vignette). It is interesting to note that more workers (44%) stated that they would remove the child from her parents in the first case (if the parents were employed) than those who would remove the child from her parents in the event that they were unemployed (32%). The results are shown in Figure 6.4, Figure 6.5, and Figure 6.6 and discussed in further detail in the following.

Survey 1 (employed parents):

- Of the 35% of social workers who assessed the case as "very high" risk, 11% stated that they would leave the child with her parents, while 49% said they would begin procedures to remove the child from her parents. Moreover, 29% stated that they would remove the child from her parents without prior preparation, and the remaining 11% of the workers said that they would not undertake any of the above actions.

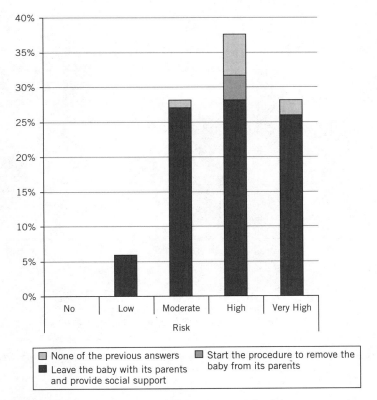

Figure 6.4. Actions of social workers involving an immigrant family living in precarious conditions with a baby.

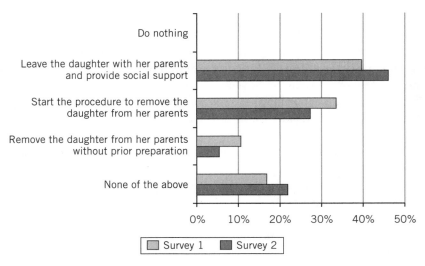

Figure 6.5. Actions of social workers involving a family with a daughter who suffers abuse: Survey 1 (employed parents) and Survey 2 (unemployed parents).

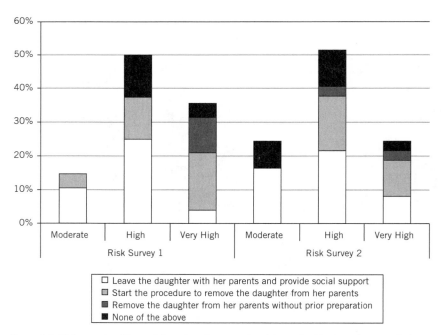

Figure 6.6. Risk perceived by social workers in a case involving a family who mistreats their daughter: Survey 1 (employed parents) and Survey 2 (unemployed parents).

- Of the 50% of social workers who assessed the case as "high" risk, half (50%) stated they would leave the child with her parents, while 25% would begin the procedure to remove the child from her parents, and the remaining 25% said they would not undertake any of the actions proposed in the survey.
- The remaining 14% of the respondents assessed the case as being of "moderate" risk. Of these, 71% said they would leave the child with her parents, while 29% stated they would begin the procedure to remove the child from the family.

Survey 2 (unemployed parents):

- 25% of respondents assessed the case as "very high" risk. Of these respondents, 32% said they would leave the child with her parents, 44% would begin procedures to remove the child from her parents, and 12% would remove the child from the parents without prior preparation. The remaining 12% said they would not undertake any of the above actions.
- Of the 51% of social workers who assessed the case as "high" risk, 42% stated they would leave the child with her parents, 31% would begin procedures to remove the child from her parents, and 6% would remove the child from her parents without prior preparation. The remaining 21% of respondents stated that they would not take any of the above actions.
- Twenty-four percent of the social workers assessed the case as "moderate" risk. Of these, 67% stated they would leave the child with her parents, while the remaining 33% would begin procedures to remove the child from her parents.

These results and percentages reveal an underlying notion that goes beyond and takes precedence over any ideals or even benefits: the utmost, first priority of the welfare services of Spain is to protect minors. However, this does not occur solely in Spain; there is an evidence basis for a governmental imperative to protect minors in every county (Lee and Svevo-Cianci, Hart, and Rubinson, 2011; Werkeley, 2013).

The literature on child abuse has long emphasized the importance of the cultural context in which abuse takes place, especially attitudes to parental abuse. Some authors, such as Corby (2006) and O'Hagan (2006), point out that what may be considered abuse in one culture may be simply unpleasant behavior in another. However, the fact that certain abusive practices are not subject to penalty in certain cultures does not mean we have to remain impassive to abuse (Idil, Gul, Yildirim, and Oney, 2010).

In Spain, research has been conducted within the social services field on how to change the perceptions and practices of parents who mistreat their children (Byrne, Rodrigo, and Martin, 2012). They conclude that both formal and informal social support (the last of which is more powerful) can be a very effective means of preventing child abuse by promoting changes in parental beliefs and practices related to "at-risk" parenting. As we have mentioned, this is a pressing issue in which research can play a role by improving the tools used by the social services system to assess situations of maltreatment (Arrubarrena and De Paúl, 2012) and highlighting the importance of social services as facilitators of positive adaptation when children are the subject of abuse (Ungar, 2013).

CONCLUSIONS

The number of third-country minors in Spain is forecast to increase in the near future, and the integration of immigrant families and minors is now a key challenge that needs to be addressed in order to ensure the long-term sustainability of the Spanish population. As highlighted in this chapter, the challenges faced by the social services system are threefold:

First, the increasing number of minors, as well as their diverse living conditions and origins, require ever-increasing resources in a context of economic downturn. In this respect, the increasingly larger number and more specific demands made by this particular population group stand in stark contrast to the current saturation of the social services; a situation that has arisen as a direct result of budget cuts and lack of adequate specialized programs targeted at the new challenge of integrating immigrant minors and their families. Specialization must go hand in hand with the constant retraining of social services professionals.

Second, decentralization and the variety of programs and resources available per municipality, province, and autonomous region have given rise to new processes of social exclusion and can only be addressed through greater coordination to ensure the adequate and homogeneous implementation of rights anywhere in Spain. In turn, the lack of coordination or the lack of effective collaboration, and the varying protocols carried out by different professionals and institutions involved in the protection of minors, also demand greater coordination. Better coordination is needed not only in a legal sense or with regard to the available services but also, and more important, among the professionals involved: social workers, legal services, psychologists, and so on.

Third, more and better preventive strategies and programs must be developed based on a thorough analysis of the living conditions of the immigrant population. These programs and strategies must take into account the key factors that lead to the exclusion and vulnerability of immigrant minors and their families, as well as risk situations suffered by minors within the family. For social workers, the foremost barrier against social exclusion is the family, but we also know from experience that many situations of vulnerability and abuse arise or are created within the family.

ACKNOWLEDGMENTS

This chapter has been possible thanks to the support of several institutions. We especially thank María del Rosario Sanz Cuesta, head of the Department of Families of the Family and Social Services of the City Hall of Madrid, for her help and the access she gave us to various printed materials related to this study. We are also grateful to the social workers of the Family Support Services (CAI) of the City Hall of Madrid, as well as all the other social workers in Spain who have participated in the survey. Special thanks go to Marcos Urabayen, the social worker and PhD student who provided us with access to both the data and social workers from Castilla-La Mancha.

NOTES

1   People who move across national boundaries for any reason (out of free will or as refugees, displaced persons, etc.).
2   Based on Madrid Town Hall, Family and Social Services Division, *Intervention Manual of Social Services Protection of Minors* (2008).
3   The general principles of action set out in this law has led to the following categorization (Madrid Municipal Council, 2008): (1) the supremacy of the child's interest over any other legitimate interest that could coincide; (2) the educational character of all measures taken under the law; (3) the restrictive interpretation of the limitations on the legal capacity of minors; (4) the maintenance of the child in the family of origin unless it is not in the interest of the minor; (5) the family and social integration of the minor; (6) the prevention of all situations that may impair the minor's personal development; (7) public awareness of situations relating to vulnerable minors; (8) the promotion of social participation and solidarity; (9) the objectivity, impartiality, and legal security of protective actions to ensure the shared responsibility and interdisciplinary character of any measures undertaken; and (10) the endeavor, in any intervention, to obtain the cooperation of the minor and his or her family, with minimal interference in his or her school life.

REFERENCES

Alted, A., ed. (2006). *De la España que emigra a la España que* acoge (From the Emigrant Spain to the Host Spain). Madrid: Fundación Largo Caballero.

Arango, J. (2004). La inmigración en España a comienzos del siglo XXI (Immigration in Spain at the beginning of the 21st century). In J. Leal (Ed.), *Informe sobre la situación demográfica en España*, 161–186. Madrid: Fundación Fernando Abril Martorell.

Arrubarrena, I., & De Paúl, J. (2012). Improving accuracy and consistency in child maltreatment severity assessment in child protection services in Spain: New set of criteria to help caseworkers in substantiation decisions. *Children and Youth Services Review*, 34(4), 666–674.

Byrne, S., Rodrigo, M.J., & Martín, J. C. (2012). Influence of form and timing of social support on parental outcomes of a child-maltreatment prevention program. *Children and Youth Services Review*, 34, 2495–2503.

Corby, B. (2006). *Child abuse: Towards a knowledge base* (3rd ed.). New York: Open University Press.

Del Fresno García, M. (2011). *Retos para la intervención social con familias en el siglo XXI: Consumo, ocio, cultura, tecnologías e hijos* (Challenges for Social Work with Families in the 21st Century: Consumption, Leisure, Culture, Technology, and Children). Madrid: Trotta.

García-Cuevas Roque, E. (2012). Decentralisation and social welfare policy in Spain's autonomic state. *Comunitania: Revista Internacional de Trabajo Social y Ciencias Sociales* (Comunitania: International Journal of Social Work and Social Sciences), 4, 63–84.

Gilbert, N., Parton, N., & Skivenes, M. eds. (2011). *Child Protection Systems: International Trends and Orientations*. Oxford: Oxford University Press.

Idil Uslu, R., Gul Kapci, E., Yildirim, R., & Oney, E. (2010). Sociodemographic characteristics of Turkish parents in relation to their recognition of emotional maltreatment. *Child Abuse & Neglect*, 34(5), 345–353.

Lee, Y., & Svevo-Cianci, K. (2011). General comment no. 13 to the convention on the rights of the child: The right of the child to freedom from all forms of violence. *Child Abuse & Neglect*, 35, 967–969.

López Peláez, A. (2006). Inmigración, educación y cohesión social (Immigration, education, and social cohesion). *Sistema. Revista de Ciencias Sociales*, 190–191, 291–308.

———. (2012). Profesión, ciencia y ciudadanía: retos para el Trabajo Social y los Servicios Sociales en el siglo XXI (Profession, science and citizenship: Challenges for social work and social services in the 21st century). *Portularia. Revista Internacional de Trabajo Social y Bienestar*, 1, 61–72.

———, ed. (2010). *Técnicas de diagnóstico, intervención y evaluación social* (Diagnostic Techniques, Intervention and Social Assessment). Madrid: Universitas.

López Peláez, A., & Krux, M. (2003). New technologies and new migrations: Strategies enhance social cohesion in tomorrow's Europe. *The IPTS Report*, 80, 11–17.

Moreno Márquez, G., & Aierdi Urraza, X. (2008). Inmigración y servicios sociales. ¿Última red o primer trampolín? (Immigration and social services: A last network or first trampoline?) *Zerbitzuan*, 44, 7–18.

Observatorio de la Inmigración. (2012). *Extranjeros residentes en España* (Foreign Residents in Spain). Madrid: Ministerio de Empleo y Seguridad Social.

O'Hagan, K. (2006). *Identifying emotional and psychological abuse.* Berkshire, UK: Open University Press.

Puyó Marín, M.C. (2009). El Observatorio de la infancia (The Childhood Observatory). In C. Villagrasa Alcaide and I. Ravetllat Ballesté (Eds.), *Por los derechos de la infancia y la adolescencia* (For the Rights of Children and Adolescents), 269–276. Barcelona: Bosch.

Quiroga Raimúndez, V., & Alonso Segura, A. (2011). *Abriendo ventanas: Infancia, adolescencia y familias inmigradas en situaciones de riesgo social* (Opening Windows: Infancy, Adolescence and Immigrant Families in Situations of Social Risk). Barcelona: Fundación Pere Tarrés—Universidad Ramon Llull.

Reher, D.-S., ed. (2008). *Informe Encuesta Nacional de Inmigrantes* (National Immigrant Survey Report) (ENI 2007). Madrid: Instituto Nacional de Estadística (Ministerio de Trabajo e Inmigración).

Requena, M., & Sánchez-Domíguez, M. (2011). Las familias inmigrantes en España (Immigrant families in Spain). *Revista Internacional de Sociología (RIS),* 1, 79–104.

Sartori, S. (2012). Population and Social Conditions. Eurostat: Statistics in Focus 45/2012. Luxembourg: Eurostat. http://epp.eurostat.ec.europa.eu/cache/ITY_OFFPUB/KS-SF-12-045/EN/KS-SF-12-045-EN.PDF

Segado Sánchez-Cabezudo, S. (2011). *Nuevas tendencias en trabajo social con familias: una propuesta para la práctica desde el empowerment* (New Trends in Social Work with Families: A Proposal from the Empowerment Practice). Madrid: Trotta.

Ungar, M. (2013). Resilience after maltreatment: The importance of social services as facilitators of positive adaptation. *Child Abuse & Neglect,* 37(2–3), 110–115.

UNICEF. (2007). *Ni ilegales ni invisibles. Realidad jurídica y social de los menores extranjeros en España* (Neither Illegal nor Invisible. Legal and Social Reality of Foreign Minors in Spain). Madrid: UNICEF.

Villagrasa Alcaide, C., & Ravetllat Ballesté, I., eds. 2009. *Por los derechos de la infancia y la adolescencia.* Barcelona: Bosch.

Werkeley, C. (2013). Resilience in the context of child maltreatment: Connections to the practice of mandatory reporting. *Child Abuse & Neglect,* 37, 93–101.

7

PUBLIC SERVICES AND MIGRANT MINORS IN ITALY

REDEFINING SKILLS FOR SOCIAL WORK

Roberta Teresa Di Rosa

INTRODUCTION

The presence of minors of foreign origin in Italy began to stand out in the 1990s and has become an increasingly significant phenomenon in recent years. The number of underage children (aged zero to 17 years) of noncitizen parents was numbered at only 20,000 in the 1990s; currently, there are approximately 1 million. Before describing the laws and services dedicated to these children, it is necessary to provide some clarification about the terminology used here. In this chapter, the term "foreigner" is used alternately with the term "migrant." Migrant people in Italy are defined as foreigners according to Italian law (first in the Constitution of the Italian Republic, Article 10), in everyday language, in statistical data, and in the welfare system, which evidences the difficulties of dealing with migrants in Italian society. Consequently, we also use the phrase "foreign minors," as it occurs in Italian law and services, to define "minors with non-Italian nationality" or those children and teenagers who are "non-Italian citizens involved in migration processes, personally or through family relations" (Save the Children Italy, 2011: 17). The category "foreign minors" constitutes a large and varied category that comprises both children from European Union (EU) countries and those who are citizens of non-EU states. This group of children includes minors accompanied by a parent (or by an adult with primary responsibility for their care) and unaccompanied minors (children who voluntarily emigrate and children who are victims of forced migration), as well as children in other kinds of situations. Also included are children born in Italy by migrant parents who continue to be "foreigners" to the Italian state due to citizenship rules, although these children represent 13% (one out of eight) of all the children born in Italy (Idos/Caritas, 2011). Another necessary clarification relates to social services. In Italy, social services are characterized by variations between regions and municipalities, due to political and administrative decentralization. There is profound fragmentation on the legislative and welfare fronts and in the planning and implementation of interventions. This is essential to keep in mind when examining the organization of social services and interventions for migrants, especially for minors.

The first issue we address is the magnitude of the migration phenomenon and the various characteristics of foreign minors in Italy today. Before discussing the legislation and social policies pertaining to foreign minors, we summarize the legislative dimensions of the migration sector that have characterized Italy in the past 30 years. During this period, Italy has made a transition from a country of emigration to a country of immigration, alternating between periods of political openness to integration and other periods that were centered on issues of immigration control. These periods emerge from legislative provisions. After examining the laws and social policies on immigration, we reflect on public social services and the impact that immigration control has had on their organization, as well as on the protection of, and service offered to, foreign minors and families. Then we discuss issues related to the quality of services and the professional competence of social workers, namely, their education and training. Subsequently, we examine the challenges presented to the entire social system by the still new multicultural experience in Italy (Spinelli, 2005). Finally, we present the results of a survey that examines the wider context of the provision of law, migration policies and social services for migrants in Italy.

THE PRESENCE OF MIGRANTS IN ITALY

The increasing presence of foreigners (the population without Italian citizenship present for various reasons in the state territory) is a highly noticeable trend in Italian society as the overview in Table 7.1. In the past decade, the foreign population has increased by 294%: the number of foreigners living in Italy increased from 1,270,533 in 2002 to about 5,011,000 at the beginning of 2012 (Idos/Caritas, 2012).

The migrant population is increasingly characterized by stabilization processes: more than half of all migrants have lived in Italy for more than five years and 20% own the homes they live in. Fifteen percent of resident immigrants were born in Italy. The number of families with at least one foreign member is 2,074,000 (over 8% of the total number). The number of foreign minors has

Table 7.1. Summary table of immigration in Italy, 2011

		Source
Total population of Italy	60,820,764	2011 census provisional data
Non-EU foreigners legally present in Italy	3,865,385	Ministry of the Interior—Istat 2011
EU residents in Italy	1,334,820	Ministry of the Interior—Istat 2011
Estimated number of legally present foreigners	5,011,000	Caritas Migrantes 2011 Estimate
Percentage of the total foreign population	8.2	Caritas Migrantes 2011 Estimate
Percentage of women out of total foreign residents	49.5	Caritas Migrantes 2011 Estimate
Foreigners born in 2011	79,587	Caritas Migrantes 2011 Estimate
Foreign minors from non-EU countries	867,890	Caritas Migrantes 2011 Estimate
Percentage of minors in population of non-EU foreigners	23.9	Ministry of the Interior 2011
Minors enrolled at school	755,939	Ministry of Education 2011
Acquisitions of citizenship	56,001	Istat 2011 Estimate
Marriages with a foreign spouse	21,357	Caritas Istat data 2009
Territorial distribution of foreign residents (%)		**2011 Census provisional data**
Northwest	35.8	
Northeast	27.6	
Centre	23.8	
South	9.0	
Islands	3.8	
Total	100.0	
Continent of origin (%)		**Idos/Caritas migrantes 2011 (estimate)**
Europe	50.8	
Africa	22.1	
Asia	18.8	
America	8.3	
Oceania	0.0	
Total	100.0	
Top five countries of origin		**Idos/Caritas migrantes 2012 (estimate)**
Romania	997,000	
Morocco	506,369	
Albania	491,495	
China	277,570	
Ukraine	223,782	
Total five countries	2,496,216	(50.6% of the total foreigners)

increased at a fast pace (this is proof of the growth of the phenomenon of immigration in general and of the stabilization of family groups) increasing from 277,976 in 2002 to 993,238 in 2012 (Idos/Caritas, 2012).

There is a clear distinction between the places where migrants arrive and the places where they settle, as is revealed by an analysis of their regional distribution. 70.8% of minors (aged 0–14) live in the north west. The situation is the opposite in the south of Italy. This information reflects the socioeconomic imbalance between the north and the south of Italy; even the nonforeign Italian population is involved in migratory processes from the South and the Islands—characterized by high unemployment and a fragile economy—to the industrialized and economically leading North. For migrants, the South is a territory of first reception and transit, from which they move to the North in search of work, as shown by their concentration in the areas of greater economic and productive development of the country.

With regard to their origins, minors under 14 years old are primarily Moroccans (19.2%), Albanians (16.1%), and Chinese (8.3%). These figures are tied to the longstanding presence of these groups in Italy, as well as to the presence of families that are part of these communities. Just as important but less represented are Filipinos, Peruvians, Ecuadorians, and Moldavians. Within these established migrant communities, minors are more numerous in the age bracket of 15 to 17 years. This is due to the fact that we do not always see entire families arrive from these countries; in some cases women leave their younger children in the country of origin.

As for children born in Italy, approximately one-fifth have a foreign mother: out of 561,544 recorded births in 2010, newborn children with two foreign parents numbered 78,000, and those with just a foreign mother numbered 24,000, together representing 18.8% of all new births. In 1993, there were 7,000 newborn children with two foreign parents. That figure doubled in 1998, tripled in 1999, was seven times as great in 2004, and was more than 10 times as great in 2010. In turn, minors who have reunited with their families—with one or both parents already residing in Italy—are estimated to constitute 40,000 social service cases per year (Istat, 2011). With respect to enrollments in schools, in recent years the largest increases in student population have been in nursery school, following new births, and in upper secondary school because of families reuniting, as well as the growing age of immigrant children (Table 7.2). There are 188 nationalities represented in the Italian school system, with some nationalities represented in higher concentrations. There are 126,441 Rumanians, 99,421 Albanians, and 92,620 Moroccans—groups of students who represent, respectively, 17.8%, 14%, and 13% of the total of non-Italian students (Ministry of Education, 2012).

Among adolescents, a specific subgroup consists of unaccompanied foreign minors, defined as such for their characteristics and their legal status. Unaccompanied foreign minors are those for whom reception, assistance, and

Table 7.2. Students with non-Italian citizenship by school level, school year 2011/2012

	Total enrolled	Percentage of total enrolled
Nursery school (3–6 yrs.)	156,701	9.2
Primary school (6–11 yrs.)	268,671	9.5
Secondary I grade school (11–14 yrs.)	166,043	9.3
Secondary II grade school (14–18 yrs.)	164,524	6.2
Total enrolled	755,939	8.4

Source: Ministry of Education, 2012: 8.

Table 7.3. Main statistical sources on the presence of foreign children in Italy

Statistical source	Group of children on whom information has been recorded
Municipal population registers	Resident minors, information developed and published by Istat (Demoistat)
Ministry of Education	Enrolled in schools
Ministry of the Interior Ministry of Labour and Social Affairs	Children with a residence permit; information developed and published by Istat (Demoistat) Reports of unaccompanied foreign minors—Committee for Foreign Minors
Ministry of the Interior Department of Equal Opportunities	Unaccompanied minors seeking international protection minors victims of trafficking included in the paths of assistance (pursuant to ex art. 18 of Legislative Decree 286/1998)

Source: Save the Children Italy, 2011: 14.

support for integration are performed by municipalities. In 2012, 7,370 minors were recorded as unaccompanied and were assisted by social services. Between 2009 and 2010, 845 municipalities (14.2%) took responsibility for unaccompanied foreign minors, serving a total population of 10,467: 5,879 in 2009 and 4,588 in 2010 (ANCI-Cittaitalia, 2012). The unaccompanied foreign minors fostered by social services are mainly males (91.7% compared to 89.7% in 2008), slightly under adult age (55% are 17 years old), coming primarily from Afghanistan (16.8%), Bangladesh (11%), Albania (10%), Egypt (8.7%), Morocco (8.7%), and Kosovo (5.9%) (ANCI-Cittaitalia, 2012).

With regard to their distribution in Italy, more than half of the unaccompanied foreign minors who arrived in the country in 2010 are concentrated in the municipalities of Lazio, Emilia Romagna, Lombardy, and Puglia. In fact, these are the local entities that have invested the most in the reception of unaccompanied minors. The autonomy that is granted to municipalities in Italy allows for discretion in the type and extent of social services offered. Therefore to better understand the role of foreign minors in Italy it is important to analyze various sources and to crosscheck the data of the different systems that record foreign minors' presence (Save the Children Italia, 2009).

Foreign minors—accompanied and unaccompanied, from the EU or not— are affected by each region's social service systems. The region's administrative position influences the kind of paths that are available to foreign minors, as we shall see in the section dedicated to the organization of services.

LAWS AND SOCIAL POLICIES

Until the mid-1990s, national laws regarding immigration focused on emergency measures. The main aim of such measures was to legalize the presence of foreign immigrants, but this process left their rights undefined. At that time, immigration was perceived as a social problem, and the immigrant population was considered solely a source of labor. Among the laws passed in Italy, some have offered a glimmer of hope for integration: for example, Law 40/1998 of the Unified Code on Immigration (Legislative Decree 286/1998), passed by center-left governments, introduces the right to health care for all immigrants regardless of their legal status. It also establishes the right of immigrants to be integrated into Italian society without forsaking their original cultural heritage. Now migrants are no longer considered simple economic entities but social subjects.

In regard to social policy that addresses families, of notable interest is Title V of the Legislative Decree 286/1998 called "Right to Family Unity and the Protection of Minors." Before 1998, a "right to family unity" did not exist. In 1998, family unity became a right, and the conditions in which it could be applied were broadened. This law also addressed health and social assistance, education, and primary and secondary assistance. In these laws, particular protection is given to minors (Article 29), who are guaranteed the right to education and to health services, even if they are in the country as undocumented migrants.

Over the years, however, this "opening" has been reduced (until being practically *de facto* closed) by subsequent laws, especially Law 189/2002 and Law 94/2009, passed by a center-right government. With these laws, immigration has become a matter of public order. The entry of immigrants to Italy is strongly hindered in regard to access to social and public services, as well as procedures for reuniting families and for requesting political asylum. Here it is possible to see a utilitarian line of reasoning: the more advantageous migrant for the receiving society is the one who is healthy and active in the labor market, not the one who requires expenditures for education, health and accommodation for relatives (Ambrosini, 2009). The prevailing (and rather short-sighted) opinion is that the advantage to the Italian economy derived from foreign workers (in terms of cheaper labor and contributions paid to the welfare system) is offset by the presence of nonproductive family members who, once legally present, have the right to access public services, thus increasing the cost of public spending.

Recently, the provisions and conditions necessary for obtaining residency and work permits have been tightened. The "crime of clandestity" has been introduced: any non-EU citizen who enters Italy without a residency permit, or who remains in Italy after losing a permit, commits a criminal offense. These recent changes demonstrate that the political will of some governments makes it difficult for immigrants to become a permanent feature of the Italian social landscape. The previously mentioned practices constitute "a plan that proposes exclusion instead of inclusion, inequality instead of equality, hospitality instead of citizenship" (Spinelli, 2002: 2). In 2012, an important cultural step in the opposite direction was taken with the National Plan for the Family, approved by the Council of Ministers in June of 2012. The plan specifically addresses the protection of immigrant families and their integration into society: immigrant families with a residency permit are able to access all the same public social services available to Italian citizens. For migrants, the plan offers inclusion, inspired by social pluralism and respect for different cultures within the limits of constitutional principles and the Italian legal system. The approval of the plan marks the first time that a provision was adopted in Italy that contains consistent guidelines with regard to family policy, guaranteeing centrality and social citizenship to the family. It must be noted, however, that previous laws, and all their limitations, also remain in force. Those who encounter difficulties in legalizing their position will remain without any protection for their family rights.

A brief period of opening and political commitment to the integration of foreign migrants led to the establishment of many services designed to make integration possible. However, since the new millennium, Italy has followed a migratory policy aimed more at stopping migration flows than absorbing and integrating them. This policy has been influenced by the European context and the need to uphold policies of immigration control (Sciortino, 2000). It leaves the implementation of actions and initiatives to manage immigrants to various agents at the local level (Tognetti Bordogna, 2004).

With regard to protection from discrimination and racism, in Italy today, however, foreigners—limited not only to migrants but also to asylum seekers and the Roma and Sinti populations, along with other minorities with a long historical tradition in Italy, such as the Jewish population in Italy—are often victims of acts of racism and discrimination. For these individuals, protection through the penal code is often difficult to access and is typically ineffective against racist acts (Vassallo Paleologo, 2002). Laws prohibiting acts of discrimination on the basis of one's ethnic or racial origin, religion, language, or nationality were introduced in 1998. Successive laws (Decree 215/2003, Decree 216/2003, Legislative Decree 150/2011) provide victims with an opportunity for recourse in courts of law, although socially disadvantaged victims cannot easily access this kind of protection.

Consequences for the Protection of the Rights of Foreign Minors

Italy recognizes the status of the child as "a holder of rights as an individual and inside the family and the social community in which he lives, grows and matures" (Istituto degli Innocenti, 2009: IX) and guarantees with its laws (Law 285/1997; Law 451/1997) an important protection of childhood. The country also guarantees to foreign minors all the rights enacted by the 1989 Convention on the Rights of the Child. These include the right to education, to medical assistance, and to placement in a safe environment. Placement in a safe environment may entail protection when their parents are not in a condition to exercise their parental authority or to fostering if children are considered deprived of a fit family environment. Additionally, children have the right to the unity of the family (even if, as we have seen, over the years there have been restrictions placed on the right to family unity).

Unfortunately, lack of access to health care—despite legal provisions—remains a critical problem. At the local level, due to the decentralization of the administration, the application of national norms regarding access to health services by foreign minors and their families has not been homogeneous, and this has had negative repercussions on foreign minors' health conditions (Geraci e Bonciani, 2011). Further, the issue of health care for immigrants was ignored in the last national health-care plan (Lai-momo/Idos, 2012). Politically, there is resistance to approve a change in citizenship laws that would safeguard the rights of children born in Italy. The present Law 91/1992, which follows the principle of *ius sanguinis* and not that of *ius soli*, makes it extremely difficult for migrants to acquire Italian citizenship. The present law does not recognize the social and cultural bonds that minors born in Italy have with the country. Rather, it forces them to live officially as foreigners until they become adults, which risks jeopardizing their future processes of integration and social inclusion.

At the end of the 1990s, the government established a permanent Commission for Foreign Minors. Its aims were to protect the rights of foreign minors (over the age of six) who were temporarily admitted into Italy, to monitor their conditions, and to coordinate the activities of the various administrations involved in these processes. This Commission was dissolved in 2012 by the Decree on Spending Review, and the Commission's functions were transferred to the Directorate-General of Immigration and Integration Policy at the Ministry of Labour and Social Policy. With regard to prevention and protection from abuse, violence, and exploitation, current laws (Law 66/1996, Law 269/1998, Law 38/2006) are applied both to Italian and foreign minors. Particular attention is given to foreign minors in cases when they are in Italy without their families.

The Italian legislature, in keeping with international and European practices, has issued numerous laws that protect minors from violence and abuse (Decree of the President of the Republic of May 13th 2005, Law 7/2006 and Ministerial Decree of December 17th 2007). These laws are designed to prevent, oppose, and repress practices of abuse—including female genital mutilation—and also to provide guidelines for professionals working with foreign families.

In summary, there are contradictory elements between the policies that protect children and adolescents and those designed to control immigration. This contradiction hinders the recognition of some fundamental rights, which have become more difficult to define due to the modification of both the eligibility requirements for receiving social benefits and the mechanisms for their allotment.

ORGANIZATION OF CHILD WELFARE SERVICES

The organization of public social services working with migrants must be examined in light of the previously-mentioned evolution of laws and social policies over the past thirty years (Gui, 2009). Until the mid-1990s, national laws were focused on emergency measures that aimed to legalize the presence of foreign migrants but that left their rights undefined. In those years, religious and secular organizations took on an active role in providing assistance. Social interventions were concentrated on providing temporary shelter, education, and employment. Public social services have also diversified over the years because of the various reforms introduced at the end of the 1990s. Social services provided by municipalities have been integrated with health services offered by public health authorities (Law 328/2000). Local social, health, and juvenile justice services take on cases of both Italian and migrant minors. Cases involving minors are handled by child welfare services (which have different names and organization, depending on the regional or local system).

Territorial social services (those services guaranteed by the social workers of the local authorities—the municipalities and the regions) range from actions that have a supportive and preventive nature to those that safeguard minors, including removing them from their families when necessary. The supportive and preventive measures (which have developed since the issuing of Law 285/1997) have taken on various forms in different territorial contexts. Two such forms involve the creation of socioeducational centers, where teenagers can spend leisure time together, and initiatives that develop parenting skills. Various services exist to support minors within their families, including economic assistance, home-schooling services, and family centers. Territorial social services collaborate with the judicial authority (Juvenile Court) in cases where there is a risk of danger to a minor's safety or psychophysical development, including the most serious situations of mistreatment and abuse (Tilli, 2013). There is also an Office of Social Service for Minors that reports to the Ministry of Justice. This office assists minors between the ages of 14 and 17, who encounter judicial problems (in Italy minors under 14 years of age cannot be charged), with the aim of preventing them from heading down criminal paths and instead promoting processes of growth (Mastropasqua, 2013).

REPRESENTATION OF MINORS IN THE CHILD WELFARE SYSTEM

Migrant minors can interact with Italian institutions in different ways based on the paths of action open to them. These paths are determined most significantly by the reasons for the minors' presence in Italy and their legal status. If minors are legally present with their parents or relatives who act as their guardians, they are offered the same services as Italian minors and their families. These services include home help, economic assistance, fostering, and community care. Because these minors are registered on their parents' residency permit, they have access to national health services and to local social and educational services. There are some limitations to these assistance services, in particular with regard to economic assistance (ex art. 41 T.Us. 286/98). Minors whose parents are undocumented migrants are only able to access health-care and educational services.

Unaccompanied foreign minors—those who are refugees or are applying for international protection and minors who are victims of slavery—are assigned a tutor, hosted in a community center, and given support for their social and educational integration (Save the Children Italia, 2011). Minors belonging to the Roma and Sinti minorities (even if they are Italian citizens) have access to special integration services and projects, both at educational and social levels.

It is difficult to find specific data regarding the services provided to migrant children within their families, but table 7.4 shows the complete list of services and interventions for families with minors, alongside a list of the services dedicated to immigrants and "nomads" (as the Roma and Sinti are called in service-sector language).

At the local level, the kinds of social services available depend on the political and social will of public administrators. Research shows that over the years municipalities have intervened in different ways toward the migrant population depending on the current culture of that municipality, which determines how social services are planned and managed (Spinelli, 2005). Even with regard to the protection of minors (both Italian and migrant), we see great heterogeneity in the organizational systems adopted in the various regions of Italy (CISMAI, 2009).

Table 7.4. Services provided by municipalities by area of intervention

All families and minors in Italy	Immigrants and nomads (all non-Italian individuals residing in Italy)
INTERVENTIONS AND SERVICES	

Professional social service activities:
Professional social service
Housing intermediation and/or allocation of accommodation
Service for the custody of minors
Service for the adoption of minors
Service for mediation in families
Activity of parent support

Social integration:
Interventions for the social integration of subjects who are weak or at risk
Recreational, social, and cultural activities

Interventions and educational-welfare services and work placement:
Socioeducational schooling support
Territorial and/or domiciliary socioeducational support
Support for work placement

In-home assistance for families with minors:
In-home social welfare assistance
Vouchers, therapy benefit, continuing care benefit
Distribution of meals and/or home laundry service

MONEY TRANSFERS

Money transfers for the payment of interventions and services:
Financial contributions for health services and treatment
Costs for nursery schools
Costs for integrative or innovative services for the early childhood
Costs for residential services
Financial contributions for the education services
Financial contributions given as loans
Financial contributions for accommodation
Financial contributions for work placement
Financial contributions to supplement family income
Financial contributions for foster care
General contributions for social associations

Activity of professional social service:
Professional social service
Housing intermediation and/or allocation of accommodation

Social integration:
Interventions for the social integration of subjects who are in social fragility condition or at risk
Recreational, social, and cultural activities
Services of cultural mediation

Interventions and educational-welfare services and for work placement:
In-home assistance
In-home social welfare assistance
Vouchers, therapy benefit, continuing care benefit
Distribution of meals and/or home laundry service

Emergency social intervention (mobile units, etc.)

Money transfers for the payment of interventions and services:
Expense vouchers and meal vouchers
Financial contributions for health services and treatment
Cost for semiresidential services
Cost for residential services
Financial contributions given as loans
Financial contributions for accommodation
Financial contributions to supplement family income
General contributions to social associations

All families and minors in Italy	Immigrants and nomads (all non-Italian individuals residing in Italy)
STRUCTURES	
Daytime or semiresidential structures: Nursery schools Integrative or innovative services for early childhood Day care centers (permanent or temporary, i.e., during summertime) Playrooms/laboratories Youth centers or social centers Family centers	*Community and residential structures:* Residential structures "Equipped areas for nomads" (areas designed for the settlement of Roma and Sinti provided with some basic services such as energy and water)
Community and residential structures: Residential structures Summer or winter centers	

Source: Istat, 2009.

Table 7.5. Data on minors under the responsibility of the child welfare system in Italy (away from family)

	Number	%
Total number of minors out of family	29,309	100
In foster families	14,528	49.57
In residential care	14,781	50.43
Foreign minors away from home	6,448	22.0
Unaccompanied minors	1,290	4.4

Source: Istituto degli Innocenti, 2012.

Alongside the emergency services that offer immediate assistance to migrants, there are an increasing number of other structures. Some are organized like territorial ones but are open only to migrants; others are open to the entire population. At the institutional level, there is a tendency to follow a model of "subordinate integration": a type of integration characterized by the recognition of certain rights but also by enduring discrimination, social inferiority, and racism (Jabbar, 2003).

As for residential services, we can draw some interesting conclusions based on the latest published data on the subject (Table 7.5). On December 31, 2010, there were 29,309 minors placed in residential care or temporarily hosted in families; this amounted to a little more than three infants and children between zero and 17 years of age per 1,000 children (Istituto degli Innocenti, 2012).

Among those taken into care, the number of unaccompanied foreign minors represents 22% of the total amount of migrants, or around 4% of all those who do not live with their family of origin. This particular group of migrants, almost all of whom are adolescents, is placed mainly in residential centres (88%). The most recent orientation of services for families and minors consists of working with the services to which the migrants and the local population already have access (Tognetti Bordogna, 2004). It seems more useful to give adequate resources to communal services for infants and toward schools, health centers, and hospitals that offer flexible and diversified solutions and projects, rather than creating ghetto services for migrants (Liaci and Luison, 2000). The most effective services have proven to be those that do not address migrants as a generic category but that serve individuals, families, and groups in their complexity and unique context (Bramanti, 2010).

TRAINING OF SOCIAL WORKERS

The nascent needs of the migrant population are decidedly challenging to social services. It is evident that traditional solutions—as has been proven quantitatively and from the point of view of the typology and the method of intervention—are not adequate (Tognetti Bordogna, 2004). The needs of migrant individuals and families, belonging to cultures that are not only different from the native ones but also very different from each other, require the redefinition of methodologies used and the necessary competencies required for the analyses of needs and the planning of interventions (Campanini, 2002). Given that this competency is not always provided in university courses for social workers, at least not specifically or in a uniform way throughout the country, social workers must acquire competency in the field in other ways. Apart from direct experience, many professionals have personally invested in professional training and refresher courses, which are necessary for orienting services toward an intercultural point of view.

Training for social workers in Italy includes a three-year degree course followed by an exam to acquire a professional qualification, after which graduates may be employed professionally in the social services sector. However, it is increasingly becoming the norm to integrate these three years of coursework with other courses, both at university and outside university. Today, there are master's courses (theoretical/practical training courses that take one or two years to complete) and master's degree courses (which take two years in addition to the bachelor's degree courses), which deal specifically with interculturality and the integration of migrants. These courses are offered by both public and private universities and other training centers. However, they are taught differently throughout the country, depending on the budgetary and training priorities of the universities.

Recognizing the importance of training is an essential next step in the evolutionary process of responding to migrants' various social needs. However, it is difficult to implement this step because of the economic difficulties of social service agencies and due to the lack of training provided by employers for social work professionals. Most times, in fact, social service agencies do not (for budgetary reasons) offer training and refresher courses for professionals. For the same reason, they do not even grant their employees the opportunity to have time off work to attend these courses, even if they decide to attend them at their own expense. It often happens that professionals have to use their holiday time to attend courses, seminars, and conferences. Within the field of social services, the difficulty of offering adequate services to foreign children and families is at best dealt with by using intercultural mediators (translators with social competencies) alongside professional social workers. However, this creates an unclear role for both parties, as there is no precise definition of what each role entails, both with regard to norms and duties and functions of the position (Di Rosa, 2005).

These deficiencies are only partially compensated for by the existence of international organizations and research and training institutions, both public and private, that regularly publish research reports. These reports serve as essential points of reference for social workers to deepen their knowledge of the migratory dynamics affecting minors. Fortunately, the need for specific training is becoming increasingly clear, as can be seen from the National Plan for the Family, approved in 2012. The plan calls for "the institution of a specialized local service for dealing with the problems of migrant families (. . .) These important functions will have to be provided through the presence of adequately trained [social workers] in order to facilitate the relationship that foreign citizens have with organisations and institutions, facilitate access to public services and the processes within them, and manage the allocation of responsibility for foreigners" (National Plan for Family, 2012: 36).

The increased presence of foreign minors in Italy has forced the country to rethink and undertake a general reorganization of public social services. Migrants can access public services only with difficulty. For many reasons social services are still responding more often to emergency situations rather than promoting preventive interventions. The methods of action are often based on extremist presuppositions that are not focused on the general reality of migrants' situations (Spinelli, 2005).

WORKING WITH MIGRANTS: A VIEW FROM CHILD WELFARE PRACTICE

In our sample of 98 Italian social workers,[1] 90% of them had some experience working with immigrant families. The number of years of experience in working with minors ranged from a minimum of a few months to a maximum of 35 years, with the greatest concentration of experience being between three and six years. The age of social workers who responded to the survey indicates a significant presence of young professionals in the sector. However, we must also bear in mind the greater propensity of younger colleagues to participate in this study and their greater professional motivation to report on this subject. With regard to the linguistic abilities of our sample, more than half of the respondents did not know a language spoken by the ethnic groups with whom they worked (namely English, French, and Arabic). The study of foreign languages is not part of the university curriculum for degree courses in social services. In Italy, even in schooling prior to university, not much consideration is given to the acquisition of foreign languages. This fact heavily affects social workers' relationship with migrants and results in the risk of aggravating the negative effects of linguistic distance (Mazzetti, 2003). Even when a language can be counted on to transmit basic concepts, this does not mean that social workers are able to pick up on cultural codes, the ways of life, the models of social organization and the cultural worlds of those who utilize the services (Di Rosa, 2010).

With regard to the functions performed by social workers, the most prevalent were those concerning checks and/or risk evaluation (13%), residential services (8%) and addressing emergencies (4.2%). Managerial functions were also undertaken: 7% of respondents who reported that they perform managerial duties did not have an exclusive mandate or clear division of roles with regard to these functions. Rather, all these functions were performed within the same office by the same personnel (57.3%).

With regard to training, all the social workers in the Italian sample held a bachelor's degree, a master's degree, or a PhD degree in social services, and more than 60% stated that they had recently attended specific professional refresher courses for working with immigrants. Regarding the nationalities and origins of the social workers in the sample, it is noteworthy that they were all almost exclusively Italian nationals or children of Italians. Only a very small percentage (2%) claimed to have immigrated or to be the child of immigrant parents, but it cannot automatically be inferred from this that they are of foreign origin. It seems more plausible that they are children of Italians who migrated abroad and then returned. In Italy today, professional social work is almost exclusively undertaken by people of Italian nationality. This derives above all from regulatory factors, given that Italian citizenship is a prerequisite for access to public competitive exams. This considerably penalizes second-generation migrants, even if they were born in Italy, and prevents them from accessing jobs in the public sector and in professions that are subject to these statutes.

Characteristics of Service Users and Proposals for Change

The immigrants that access the services provided by the social workers in our sample mostly come from Africa, Eastern Europe, Asia, and Latin America. This is in keeping with the aforementioned statistics on the presence of foreigners in

Italy per size of national groups. Only 16.7% of respondents had worked for services dedicated exclusively to migrants. The other respondents indicated that migrants represented between 20% and 30% of their workload. The type of interventions used in the cases ranged from the so-called "canonical interventions," such as economic help (95%) and housing policy (85%), to more preventive interventions that could be considered a means to further integration, such as helping parents to find a job (89.7%) and putting people in contact with community services (89.3%). Only 27% considered it important to encourage the family to return to their country of origin. This percentage undoubtedly denotes a certain evolution of national social models.

With regard to the perception of risk faced by minors, it is important to distinguish between two types of cases contained in the survey, referred to as Cases 1 and 2. In Case 1, the level of perceived risk goes from moderate to high, but given that the difficulties are considered to be purely economic in nature, social workers support measures that sustain the whole nuclear family. Respondents were almost all in favor of preserving the family unit, which is seen both as a resource that cannot be renounced and as a right of the minor. This ideology fits within a system of welfare in which the family has a central role and is considered a fundamental resource that must be used to overcome the state of need. In Case 2, the level of perceived risk goes from high to very high because the minor has been physically abused. In this case, the percentage of workers who were in favor of separating the minor from the family was greater. The separation is deemed preferable regardless of the parents' work situation (employed or unemployed). A comparison between the results obtained in the two versions of the questionnaire shows that, regardless of the work situation of the parents, the fact that the minor is subjected to abuse is reason enough to initiate processes that protect the child, even at the expense of family ties. This evaluation of risk seems to be influenced by elements that are markedly linked to cultural characteristics, since the notion of abandonment and the interests of the minor are far from being objectively defined. The evaluation of the interest of the minor becomes a critical consideration in situations of serious economic distress, which can lead to the separation of the minor from his or her family, in accordance with provisions established by the authorities.

The data reveals that no matter how much importance is given to the family unit, this comes in second when the fundamental rights of the minor are threatened, as seen in the responses to Cases 1 and 2. In order to protect the rights of minors, responsibility should lie with the services that deal specifically with minors rather than those that deal with families or with migrants in general. This is confirmed by the fact that a high percentage (78.6%) of the surveyed sample stated that in cases where migrant minors (belonging to families illegally present in Italy) do not meet the requirements of compulsory education, the matter should be addressed by national services for minors and not by services for migrants.

In cases when social workers would specifically direct their services to minors, the survey respondents reported that they would still consider the cultural dimensions of the cases in question. The professionals believe that it is necessary to address the interests of the minors by considering the family dynamics that derive from their social groups and backgrounds. Despite the evident efforts of social work professionals to adopt egalitarian policies of intervention toward the non-immigrant population and the immigrant population, the presence of foreign families was considered to be more problematic by about 60% of respondents.

With regard to the perception of risk, there seems to be a tendency to consider migrant families to be more at risk and more problematic than nonmigrant families. This assumption manifests in the difficulties that social workers encounter when faced with people who may be more "difficult" to manage and who have unusual parameters of need. However, it cannot be overlooked that there may also be a certain degree of prejudice that tends to remain in the collective consciousness of social workers. Proof of this could be the fact that 61% of the sample declared to have imagined the cultural or ethnic origin of the minors in the cases examined. This piece of data could be linked to the tendency of principal media agencies and national policies to treat immigration as an alarming problem, in particular with regard to minors.

Professional Competencies and Adequacy of Services

Finally, the topic of social workers' self-perception is significant, in particular with regard to their own competency in dealing with immigrant families. 47% of social workers in the sample declared that they felt "less competent," 42% said they felt "equally competent," and only 11% claimed to feel "more competent." These data indicate that the profession has a real need for specific training. It is no longer considered feasible to improve organizations by providing social workers with assistance from cultural mediators. Now, despite attempts to safeguard the right of cultural mediators, more value has been given to social workers, through an upgrading of competencies that allows them to face on their own the most frequent and common problems that characterize social work with foreign people (Cohen, 2011). Setting aside respondents' self-perceived level of professional competency, it should be noted that immigrant families are considered to be more demanding than Italian families (56%), or, at least, equally as demanding (42%). Only a small percentage considered them to be less demanding (2%). The sense of inadequacy does not only regard the individual professional and his or her competencies, however, but is also expressed toward the existing services: 66% of respondents ascertain that it is necessary to create a public service responsible specifically for managing cases involving migrant families and minors.

FINAL CONSIDERATIONS

Observing the system of services that a country creates for interacting with members of other cultures and responding to their needs is in some way analogous to taking a snapshot of that society with regard to its conception of nation, state, citizenship, and who should have the right to be included (Gozzoli and Regalia, 2005). In terms of the future of integration of migrant minors in Italy, much will depend on the development of migration policy. The recognition and protection of the fundamental rights of migrant minors will require a significant investment in the training of social workers (Fumagalli, 2007) and the reorganization of public services (Tarsia, 2010). The significant presence of migrant families with minors forces local welfare services to devise effective integration paths both for adults and minors (Di Rosa, 2010; Tarsia, 2010). The difficulties perceived by social workers can also lie in role conflicts that they may experience. They continuously have to mediate between institutional mandates (which require them to select the service users and reduce the service expenses, in order to maintain the process of standardization) and their professional (ethical) mandate, which calls for respect and responsibility toward the specific characteristics and needs of each client (Spinelli, 2005). There is no doubt that migrants require that social work professionals reorganize their competencies and their procedures; their work models—linked to Western history and tradition—can no longer adequately interpret and respond to all the requests that they face. Rather than seeing this as a problem, it should be viewed as an opportunity to create social services that are more in tune with the contemporary, globalized age.

NOTE

1   All the survey work in Italy was carried out by Dott. Gabriella Argento.

REFERENCES

Ambrosini, M. (2009). Introduzione: Separate e ricongiunte: Le famiglie migranti attraverso i confini (Introduction: Separated and reunited: Migrant families beyond borders). *Mondi Migranti*, 3(1), 37–44.

ANCI-Cittalia (2012). *Quarto Rapporto ANCI sui Minori stranieri non accompagnati* (Fourth ANCI Report on Unaccompanied Foreign Minors). Rome: ANCI.

Bramanti, D. (2010). *Welfare community e servizi di prossimità: analisi di una buona pratica per le famiglie fragili* (Welfare Community and Services of Proximity: Analysis of Good Practices for Fragile Families). National

Conference on the Family, November 8–10:"Family: History and Future for All." Retrieved December 8, 2013, from http://www.conferenzafamiglia.it/media/7174/bramanti%20relatore%209%20gruppo.pdf

Campanini, A. (2002). *Il servizio sociale nella società multietnica* (The Social Service in the Multiethnic Society). Milan: Unicopli.

Cohen Emerique, M. (2011). *Pour une approche interculturelle en travail social. Theories et pratiques* (For an Intercultural Approach to Social Work: Theories and Practices). Rennes: Presses de l'EHESP.

Di Rosa, R.T. (2010). Oltre discriminazione e razzismo: verso una competenza professionale transculturale (Beyond discrimination and racism: Toward a professional transcultural competence). In M. Mannoia and M.A. Pirrone (Eds.), *Il razzismo in Italia: Società, istituzioni e media* (Racism in Italy: Society, Institutions and Media), 291–301. Rome: Aracne.

———. (2005). *Mediazione tra culture. Politiche e percorsi di integrazione* (Mediation Between Cultures: Policies and Integration Paths). Pisa: Ed. Plus.

Fumagalli, M. (2007). Servizi sociali, operatori, cittadini stranieri: cambiamenti ed opportunità (Social services, operators, foreign citizens: changes and opportunities). In M. Tognetti Bordogna, (Ed.), *Arrivare non basta: Complessità e fatica dell'emigrazione* (Arriving Is Not Enough. The Complexity and Effort of Migration), 273–282. Milan: FrancoAngeli.

Geraci, S., & Bonciani, M. (2011). Servizi sociali, operatori, cittadini stranieri: cambiamenti ed opportunità (Laws on assistance in pregnancy and postpartum for foreigners). In L. Lauria and S. Andreozzi (Eds.), *Istisan Reports 2011/12: Birth and Immigration in Italy: The 2009 Investigations*, 48–62. Rome: ISTISAN.

Gozzoli, C., & Regalia, C. (2005). *Migrazioni e famiglie: Percorsi, legami e interventi psicosociali* (Migration and Families. Paths, Ties and Psychosocial Interventions). Milan: FrancoAngeli.

Gui, L. (2009). *Organizzazione e servizio sociale* (Organization and Social Work). Rome: Carocci.

Idos/Caritas Migrantes. (2011). *Statistic Dossier on Immigration 2010*. Rome.

———. (2012). *Statistic Dossier on Immigration 2011*. Rome.

Istat. (2009). *Report on Social Work Interventions and Social Services of Municipalities*. Rome: Istituto nazionale di statistica.

———. (2011). *National Census of the Population*. Rome: Istituto nazionale di statistica.

Istituto degli Innocenti. (2009). *Diritti in crescita: Terzo-quarto rapporto alle Nazioni unite sulla condizione dell'infanzia e dell'adolescenza in Italia* (Rights during Growth: Third-fourth Report of the United Nations on the Conditions regarding Infancy and Adolescence in Italy). Florence: Istituto degli Innocenti.

———. (2011). *Bambini e adolescenti fuori dalla famiglia* (Children and Teenagers Out of Their Family). Presidency of the Council of the Ministers, Ministry of Labour and Social Policy, Centre of Documentation and Analysis for Infancy and Adolescence. Florence: Istituto degli Innocenti.

Jabbar, A. (2003). Immigrati: riconoscimento, partecipazione e percorsi di cittadinanza (Immigrants: Recognition, Participation and Paths to Citizenship). Retrieved December 8, 2013, from http://www.didaweb.net/liste/leggi.php?a=552&lista=040

Lai-momo/Idos. (2012). *Comunicare l'immigrazione: Guida pratica per gli operatori dell'informazione* (Communication and Immigration. Practical Guide for Operators in the Field of Information). Rome: Ministry of Labour and Social Policy and the Interior Ministry.

Liaci, S., & Luison, L., eds. (2000). *Mediazione sociale e sociologia: Riferimenti teorici ed esperienze* (Social Mediation and Sociology. Theoretical References and Experiences). Milan: FrancoAngeli.

Mastropasqua, I. (2013). Servizio sociale e giustizia minorile (Social service and juvenile justice). In A. Campanini (Ed.), *Nuovo dizionario di servizio sociale* (New Dictionary of Social Work), 609–612. Rome: Carocci.

Mazzetti, M. (2003). *Il dialogo transculturale* (Transcultural Dialogue). Rome: Carocci.

Ministry of Education. (2012). *Statistical Report October 2012*. Rome: Ministry of Education.

Ministry of Labour and Social Policy. (2012). *Bambine e bambini temporaneamente fuori dalla famiglia di origine: Affidamenti familiari e collocamenti in comunità al 31 dicembre 2010*. (Children Temporarily out of their Family of Origin: Foster Families and Placements in Residential Care up to December 31st 2010). Rome: Ministry of Labour and Social Policy.

Save the Children Italy. (2009). *I minori stranieri in Italia: Identificazione, accoglienza e prospettive per il futuro* (Foreign Minors in Italy: Identification, Reception and Perspectives for the Future). Rome: Save the Children Italy.

———. (2011). *I minori stranieri in Italia, L'esperienza e le raccomandazioni di Save the Chidren* (Foreign Minors in Italy: The Experience and the Recommendations of Save the Children). Rome: Save the Children Italy.

Sciortino, G. (2000). Towards a political sociology of entry policies: Conceptual problems and theoretical proposals. *Journal of Ethnic and Migration Studies*, 26(2), 213–228.

Spinelli, E. (2002). Immigrazione e razzismo: Ostacoli ad una buona prassi professionale (Immigration and racism: Obstacles to the "good practice" of social work). *Risorse Sociali*, 2, 2–4.

———. (2005). *Immigrazione e Servizio sociale* (Immigration and Social Work). Rome: Carocci.

Tarsia, T. (2010). *Prendersi cura del conflitto: Migrazioni e professionalità sociali oltre i confini del welfare* (Taking Care of Conflict: Migration and Social Professionalism beyond the Confines of Welfare). Milan: FrancoAngeli.

Tilli, C. (2013). Servizio sociale e minori (Social work and minors). In A. Campanini (Ed.), *Nuovo Dizionario di servizio sociale* (New Dictionary of Social Work), 622–626. Rome: Carocci.

Tognetti Bordogna, M. (2004). *I colori del welfare: Servizi alla persona di fronte l'utenza che cambia* (The Colors of Welfare: Services in Light of Changing Service Users). Milan: FrancoAngeli.

Vassallo Paleologo, F. (2002). *Studio analitico sulla legislazione italiana e sulle prassi applicative contro gli atti di discriminazione razziale* (Analytical Study on Italian Law and Practice Application against Acts of Racial Discrimination). Florence: CO.S.P.E.

PART III

CHILD PROTECTION–ORIENTED CHILD WELFARE SYSTEMS WITHIN LIBERAL WELFARE STATES

8

THE UNITED STATES

CHILD PROTECTION IN THE CONTEXT OF COMPETING
POLICY MANDATES

Ilze Earner and Katrin Križ

INTRODUCTION

In common parlance, the United States is often referred to as "an immigrant country." This is an accurate epithet if one considers the country's migration history,[1] increasing levels of immigration in the past decades (Waters et al., 2008), and the number of foreign-born individuals in the United States, which is the highest of any country in the world (Pison, 2010): in 2010, 40 million people, out of a total population of 309,350,000, were foreign born. However, can the United States also be called "a country *for* immigrants"—especially a country supportive of the well-being of immigrant children, youth, and families? In this context, the evidence is ambivalent and contradictory when it comes to the country's public policy environment. For instance, deportations of undocumented immigrants have risen to record levels under the Obama administration (Lopez & Gonzalez-Barrera, 2013), while more people are immigrating using the so-called "E-B5 immigrant investor visa" program—a program that awards special visas to people who invest a minimum of $1 million in the US economy (National Public Radio, 2013; USCIS, 2013). On the other hand, in 2012 President Obama issued an executive order that protected those young people from deportation who migrated to the United States before they were 16 years old through "deferred action for childhood arrivals" (Majorkas, 2012). This chapter highlights the challenges that the US child welfare system faces as it seeks to protect immigrant children, youth, and families in a public policy environment that spans contradictory policies often not in children's best interest.

In this chapter, we use the term "immigrants" to refer to foreign-born individuals. In US scholarship on migration and child welfare services, in which the term "immigrants" is widely used, and in national statistics such as the US Census, "immigrants" are considered "foreign-born" individuals, defined as individuals who were not US citizens when they were born. The "foreign born" include a range of migrants, including refugees, permanent residents, undocumented immigrants,[2] international students, and naturalized US citizens. Someone who was born inside the United States or US territories or who was born outside the United States and had at least one parent who was a US citizen is defined as "native born." Seven percent of the foreign-born population are children under 18, compared to about 27% of the native population (Grieco et al., 2012). The children of foreign-born parents are referred to as "children of immigrants"[3] (Fortuny et al., 2009) or "the second generation" in the US literature on this population (Kasinitz et al., 2009). Children of immigrants constitute a growing number of children in the United States overall: more than one in five children (23%), or 16.4 million children, out of a total population of 74 million children under 18 (US Census, 2009) have a foreign-born parent (Fortuny et al., 2009). It is important to note that regardless of their parents' immigration status, children of immigrants who are born in the United States automatically acquire US citizenship. Immigration status is an important consideration in the United States since it directly determines the scope and extent of public services, including child welfare, that are offered to individuals.

CHILD PROTECTIVE SERVICES: LEGAL AND POLICY FRAMEWORKS

We use the plural "child protective services" interchangeably with "child protection system," even though a centralized national child welfare system does not exist in the United States. While there are federally mandated regulations and minimum standards to address child abuse, services, out-of-home placement, and adoption, each state interprets and implements this legislation locally (Berrick, 2011). The largest federally funded programs that support state and tribal child welfare services are authorized under Title IV-B and Title IV-E of the Social Security Act.[4] Policy that determines how children are protected is outlined in the Child Abuse Prevention and Treatment Act of 1974 (PL 93-247), the Adoption Assistance and Child Welfare Act of 1980 (PL-96-272), the Multi-Ethnic Placement Act of 1994 (PL103-382), the Interethnic Adoption Provisions of 1996 (PL104-188), and the Adoptions and Safe Families Act (ASFA) of 1997 (PL-105-89).[5]

Despite numerous efforts at reform beginning in the 1990s, child protective services in the United States still largely embrace a child protection orientation. This approach stands in stark contrast to the family services approach that predominates in the Nordic and continental European countries and that provides universal services designed to prevent family dysfunction and disintegration (Gilbert, 1997). The child protection orientation in the United States is characterized by an investigative and legalistic response in the assessment of abuse that creates an adversarial framework in which caseworkers practice (Gilbert et al., 2011b). While there has been movement over the past decade to incorporate a more family-service and preventive orientation—as evidenced by the implementation of "differential response systems" (American Humane Association, 2005)—there are still over 400,000 children in care of the state throughout the United States, and family reunification (i.e., returning a child once removed due to abuse or neglect) can take, on average, two years (USDHHS, 2012). Equally problematic is the fact that while official efforts focus on keeping families together, the needed long-term support services may not exist or may be subject to time limits, thereby placing children at risk.

The guiding principles of child welfare services as defined by federal law focus on what is termed "children's safety, permanency, and well-being" to ensure that the "best interests of the child" are met. First, "safety" refers to children's protection from abuse and neglect and emphasizes the importance of children being safely cared for in their homes when possible. Second, children should reside in stable living situations where family connections and continuity in relationships with a caregiver is maintained ("permanency"). When a child is not safe and removed from his or her family, then the primary permanency goal according to the law is to reunify the child with his or her birthparent or other extended family caregivers (Berrick, 2011). Third, children should receive appropriate services to meet their educational, physical, and mental health needs, and their families should have access to services to ensure their capacity to take care of them ("child and family well-being") (Reed and Karpilow, 2009; Berrick, 2011).

COMPETING POLICY MANDATES

The child welfare system continues to be an important arena for the interaction of immigrant families and the social services sector. However, when an immigrant family or child enters the child welfare system, a number of policy streams such as immigrant policy (the set of legislative initiatives at both federal and state levels affecting immigrants' access to government services and benefits), child protection policy, immigration policy, and child welfare policy that focuses on ensuring the "best interests of the child" all create a collision course of competing mandates. This problem has only recently been documented and examined in the literature (Dreby, 2012; Lincroft et al., 2006), and while model programs do exist in many parts of the United States, they are the exception, not the rule. In this section, we identify major legislation and competing mandates and discuss how they impact immigrant children, youth, and families.

Access to needed or required social services by immigrant children, youth, and families is a basic problem, but it can have serious ramifications when there is child welfare involvement. In 1996, the US Congress passed landmark legislation known as the Personal Responsibility and Work Opportunity Reconciliation Act (PRWORA) that fundamentally changed how individuals and families could access government-funded social services and benefits. While most Americans understood PRWORA as "welfare reform," few realized that it also created for the first time a nascent "immigrant policy"; that is, in order to be eligible for many government benefits, immigrants now have to prove that they are "qualified" based on their immigration status. Legal permanent residents, foreign-born individuals who have been granted the right to live and work permanently in the United States, are eligible for government-funded social services except that they now have a waiting period of five years in order to qualify for certain benefits; refugees and asylees are automatically qualified, whereas other categories of immigrants, such as the undocumented, are entirely excluded from any benefits except for access to emergency medical care, public education, and prenatal care (Borjas, 2011). PRWORA applies to federal benefits (i.e., those funded by the federal government), which include substance abuse services, disability benefits, Medicaid (the federal government program of health care for the poor), and nutrition support programs (Weaver and Hackman, 2009). In the intervening years since the adoption of PRWORA, many states have implemented legislation that likewise curtails immigrants' access to similar state-funded programs.

Child protection services to resident families are entirely funded by the federal government; however, no child is denied emergency child protective services based on his or her immigration status. It is after a report of child abuse or neglect is filed or children wind up in foster care on account of immigration enforcement when problems arise. We depict three scenarios to demonstrate how competing mandates can affect immigrants. A fourth scenario involves minors who cross the US border on their own without a parent or guardian and are apprehended by immigration officials. This population, referred to as "unaccompanied alien minors," represents a very small portion of the population of immigrant children, and they are not served within the normal child welfare services delivery system. Rather they remain under immigration authority jurisdiction, the US Office of Homeland Security, and are placed in facilities operated by the US Office of Refugee Resettlement pending the outcome of their immigration status hearing. These facilities are sometimes contracted with local child welfare services providers.

Normally, if a child is removed from the home and placed in out-of-home care in the United States, the federal government pays for foster care services under Title IV-E, which reimburses the individual states for these services. If a child is an undocumented immigrant, the state cannot draw down Title IV-E reimbursements for those services. Under most circumstances, the state will pay for foster care services out of state discretionary funds (Vericker and Capps, 2007). If an undocumented immigrant child must remain in foster care and there is no possibility of family reunification, the state may move to apply for immigration relief for that child under the Special Immigrant Juvenile Status process. This allows the child who is undocumented to become a legal permanent resident prior to exiting foster care. The state must absorb the entire cost of this legal immigration process. Some states with large undocumented immigrant populations such as California have model programs to identify undocumented immigrant children who come into the foster care system so that their need for immigration relief can be identified and addressed (Saco, 2008). This is not uniformly true of all states; there are many cases in which an undocumented immigrant child exits foster care only to realize afterward that they have no legal right to live and work in the United States. Many state juvenile or family courts are unaware or confused about this status and therefore fail to identify or encourage young people who would be eligible to apply for Special Immigrant Juvenile Status (Lincroft et al., 2006). There is no immigration relief available for these youth after they leave foster care.

A second scenario that creates problems for immigrants is a situation in which an undocumented family referred to child welfare is then mandated for services that are necessary to address specific problems that place children at risk of harm. For example, if a parent is identified as having a substance abuse or mental health problem, the child welfare service plan for family reunification would include mandatory treatment and counseling for the parent. However, an undocumented immigrant parent would not be eligible for state-funded substance abuse or mental health treatment services. Unless a parent paid for these services out of pocket, which would be prohibitively expensive, child welfare caseworkers might then deem the parent "noncompliant" with the service plan goal of family reunification. Under the ASFA, a parent who fails for 12 out of 18 months to comply with necessary service goals in order for family reunification to take place is automatically subject to termination of parental rights proceedings. This has, in fact, happened to immigrant families; in some instances they have lost children for failure to comply with service plans solely because their immigration status prevented them from accessing required services (Bernstein, 2000).

A third scenario involves immigration enforcement activities and what happens when undocumented immigrant parents are subject to deportation proceedings. In response to political pressure to address the large numbers of undocumented immigrants flooding into the United States, Immigration and Customs Enforcement, an arm of the Department of Homeland Security, began to rapidly step up enforcement activities beginning in 2001 (Dettlaff and Phillips, 2007). Parents swept up in these Immigration and Customs Enforcement raids are often jailed in secure immigration facilities awaiting their deportation proceedings; there is no requirement to notify next of kin or anyone else, for that matter. Child welfare caseworkers often become involved when minor children are left behind when a parent is arrested. Immigration law does not recognize or operate under the "best interests of the child" principle, and there is no provision for allowing detained or deported parents access to their minor children who may be placed in foster care. Again, under the ASFA, lack of contact between a parent and child in care results in the eventual termination of parental rights, in this case for no other reason other than a parent (or parents) being unable to contact their children. These cases, and there have been several, are especially egregious as there is no allegation of neglect or abuse on the part of the parent(s) (Dreby, 2012).

As indicated previously, a fourth scenario involves a minor child who is foreign born, crosses the US border without a parent or guardian, and has no legal right to do so. These children are identified as "unaccompanied alien children" at the discretion of the Border Patrol and may be placed in facilities operated by the Office of Refugee Resettlement Division of Unaccompanied Children Services. Approximately 8,000 children per year are apprehended and served in facilities across the United States. Seventy-five percent of these children are deported to their country of origin; a minority is reunified with existing family members or kin already present in the United States. There is usually no legal way to remedy their undocumented immigrant status once in the United States (Women's Refugee Commission, 2009).

This contradictory and chaotic policy environment also acts in ways to inhibit the initial process of child welfare caseworker–client engagement with less dramatic but nevertheless significant outcomes. Numerous studies have documented immigrant parents' fear of all government authorities, as well as social services providers, who they suspect may turn over information about their immigration status to immigration authorities. This "chilling effect" has resulted in immigrant parents' reluctance to enroll (or not enrolling) their children in early childhood education programs, after-school programs, or nutrition support programs and otherwise not accessing services they or their children are eligible to receive (Lincroft and Resner, 2006; Yoshikawa, 2011). Križ et al.'s (2011) study showed that during the engagement process, child welfare caseworkers experience several engagement barriers, including immigrants' fear of detention and deportation, fear of child removal, and, based on experiences in their country of origin, fear that caseworkers are potentially representatives of repressive government authority. Furthermore, specific legislation such as the Violence Against Women Act and the Trafficking Victims Protection Act (2000, 2013) allows immigrants special legal protections in instances where they are either the victims of crime, trafficking or domestic violence; however, without specialized training, many child welfare caseworkers are unaware of these benefits and fail to refer eligible clients (Workgroup on Safety and Well-Being for Immigrant and Refugee Children and Families, 2010).

IMMIGRANTS IN THE UNITED STATES

Recently most immigrants overall and most recent arrivals have been from Latin America and the Caribbean. Table 8.1 shows the specific regions of birth of the foreign-born population in 2010.

The nine countries of birth of the most recent arrivals between 2008 and 2010 included Mexico (19.3%), China (8.6%), India (7.7%), the Philippines (4.1%), Korea (3.2%), Cuba (2.8%), the Dominican Republic (2.8%), Vietnam (2.4%), and El Salvador (2.0%) (Walters and Trevelyan, 2011). We also know that the fertility rate is higher among immigrant than native-born women and that immigrant households are larger, include more children, and are more likely to contain several generations than nonimmigrant households. The immigrant population is also more likely to participate in the labor force and to live in poverty and less likely to have health insurance compared to the native-born population (Grieco et al., 2012).

In 2010, 29 million of the foreign born were documented immigrants: of these documented immigrants, 14.9 million were naturalized citizens, 12.4 million permanent residents, and 1.7 million legal temporary migrants (Passel and Cohn, 2011). Of the 40 million foreign-born individuals, 11.2 million were

Table 8.1. Regions of birth of foreign-born population, 2010

Region of Birth	%
Africa	4
Asia	28.2
Europe	12.1
Latin America and the Caribbean	53.1
Mexico	29.3
Other Central American countries	7.6
South America	6.8
Caribbean	9.3
Northern America	2
Oceania	0.5
Total	100

Source: Grieco et al., 2012.

"undocumented" or "unauthorized" in 2010—3.7% of the population over-all. Undocumented immigrants are foreign-born noncitizens who may have entered the country using invalid documents, or those who used valid documents and then overstayed visas, crossed the border illegally, or otherwise violated their terms of admittance. In the United States, 58% of all unauthorized immigrants are from Mexico, representing approximately 6.5 million individuals (Passel and Cohn, 2011). California is the state with the highest percentage of undocumented immigrants: 2.45 million in 2004 (Fortuny et al., 2007). As of January 2011, 264,574 individuals were registered as refugees and 6,285 as asylum seekers (UNHCR, 2012). In 2011, the United States admitted 56,384 individuals as refugees and 24,988 as asylees (Martin and Yankay, 2012). Since 1975, the United States has settled over 3 million refugees (Refugee Council USA, 2012).

Among the estimated 5.5 million children born to undocumented immigrants in 2010, 4.5 million were born in the United States (and were thus US citizens); 1 million children were foreign born and, like their parents, also undocumented immigrants. The number of children who were born into households in which there was at least one parent who was an undocumented immigrant amounted to 350,000 by March 2010 (Passel and Cohn, 2011).

CHILDREN OF IMMIGRANTS

Compared to children of native-born parents, children of immigrants face several unique challenges, such as a higher poverty risk, which may adversely affect their well-being. It is well documented that children who are poor and members of a racial minority are overrepresented among children referred for investigation of maltreatment (National Clearinghouse on Child Abuse and Neglect Information, 2005). Fortuny et al. (2009: 1) note that "children of immigrants [. . .] face many universal risk factors to children's well-being, such as lower parental education and family incomes, but they are also affected by factors unique to immigration, such as lack of parental citizenship and English proficiency." Despite the comparatively higher parental work effort by immigrants compared to native-born individuals, children of immigrants are more likely to be poor and have low income: in 2006, 22% of children of immigrants lived in poverty compared to 16% of children of native parents. On the positive side of the ledger, children of immigrants are more likely to live with both parents (Fortuny et al., 2009). Children of Mexican immigrants, who comprise 39% of all children of immigrants, face higher health risks in childhood than most other children as a result of their families' low socioeconomic status, limited English proficiency, high levels of food insecurity, unauthorized legal status, and the climate of reception in the new destination communities where Mexican families have been settling (van Hook et al., 2013).

Table 8.2. Children's poverty level and health insurance coverage, by immigrant and legal status, 2004

Demographic information	Children of undocumented immigrants (%)	Children of documented immigrants (%)	Native children (%)
Children in poverty	37	21	17
Children without health insurance	53	23	10

Source: Fortuny et al., 2007.

Undocumented children and children of undocumented parents face additional challenges because their (or their parents') legal status bars them from access to many public benefits and services and public health insurance (Fortuny et al., 2007; Ku and Jewers, 2013). Table 8.2, which shows that children of undocumented parents are more likely to live in poverty and lack health insurance than children whose parents are documented, illustrates the implications of legal status on a child's well-being.

In addition, children of undocumented immigrants may be adversely affected by the fact that that for undocumented immigrant parents, fear of deportation, avoidance of financial aid programs, isolated social networks, and poor working conditions result in parental stress, economic hardship, and inadequate access to healthcare (Križ and Skivenes, 2012; Yoshikawa, 2011). According to the Patient Protection and Affordable Care Act or ACA, which passed into law in 2010, undocumented immigrants and young people who were granted deferred action on deportation through the Deferred Action for Childhood Arrivals program (DACA) are excluded from the private health insurance and the subsidies the government provides to make this type of insurance more affordable (National Immigration Law Center, 2013). Further, undocumented immigrant women who were abused by their partners may not seek help because they fear deportation or because they fear showing disloyalty to and shaming the family (Martin & Mosher, 1995).

REPRESENTATION OF IMMIGRANT CHILDREN, YOUTH, AND FAMILIES IN CHILD PROTECTIVE SERVICES

There are significant research gaps related to the representation of immigrant children, youth, and families in the child welfare system because it is impossible to identify in state and national-level datasets which children in the child welfare system are immigrant children or children of immigrants because "data on the immigration status or the country of origin of parents is not collected uniformly at a local, state or national level" (Dettlaff, 2012: 5). There are, in fact, good reasons to not collect these data as it protects the confidentiality needs of immigrants who may otherwise face deportation if readily identified (Dettlaff, 2012). We do know that immigrant families face unique challenges when interacting with the child welfare system (Earner, 2007; Velazquez and Dettlaff, 2011). There is evidence of multiple systemic barriers that may adversely affect the outcomes of immigrant children, youth, and families who become involved with child welfare (Ayón, 2009; Velazquez and Dettlaff, 2011). These barriers include language access, immigration status, and cultural competency and skills of agency staff, including knowledge about the unique challenges of immigrant children, youth, and families and of eligibility requirements for public services (Dettlaff and Phillips, 2007; Earner, 2007; Križ et al., 2012; Križ and Skivenes, 2012; Johnson, 2007).

Ayón, Eisenberg and Erera (2010: 612), who studied Mexican parents' interactions with child protective services in Southern California, showed that Mexican immigrant families "experienced different paths to services based on documentation status, their need for Spanish language services, and the family's and worker's knowledge of systems of care and the department's resources." Immigrant parents did not feel well informed about the expectations, goals, and processes of child protective services. Service barriers for both documented and undocumented immigrant families included long waiting lists, services provided by less experienced providers, and location and transportation (Ayón et al., 2010). Child welfare workers may not have training on immigration issues and cultural differences and therefore lack awareness of the unique challenges resulting from immigration and acculturation. There may be a lack of quality bilingual and bicultural services; language barriers may result in miscommunication and service delivery delays, which can prevent children from reunifying with their families. Immigrant children in foster care may not receive the services they need because of a lack of culturally or linguistically appropriate services. Further, as a result of public funding limitations for immigrant children who are undocumented and need substitute care, as discussed in the section on law and policy, states may not be able to provide adequate care for these children. Working effectively with immigrant families may also involve transnational cooperation, which, however, may not exist. When parents are deported, they are unable to complete services; and undocumented status creates barriers to kinship placements (Ayón, 2009; MCWNN, 2009; Ayón et al., 2010; Dettlaff and Cardoso, 2010; Dettlaff and Lincroft, 2010; Velazquez and Dettlaff, 2011).

There are only a handful of studies analyzing the representation of immigrant children and youth in the child welfare system. Based on the National Survey of Child and Adolescent Well-Being (NSCAW; 2005), which gathered data on a nationally representative sample of children who were subject to maltreatment reports with child protective services between 1999 and 2000, we know that less than 3% of all children who come into contact with the child welfare system are foreign-born immigrant children. The NSCAW is a voluntary longitudinal, nationally representative survey of children and families who have been the subjects of child protective investigations that was developed under the auspices of the Children's Bureau. This survey made it possible for the first time to research the immigration status of families, children, and youth involved with the child welfare system. The findings presented were based on a sample of 3,717 children (Dettlaff and Earner, 2012).

The share of children of immigrants who came to the attention of the system was 8.6% (Dettlaff and Earner, 2012; Lincroft and Dettlaff, 2010). Among the second generation in the child welfare population, 82.5% were US-born citizens. There are racial and ethnic disparities in terms of the representation of the second generation: Hispanic and Black children of immigrants are over-represented and non-Hispanic Asian and white children are underrepresented in the child welfare population: for instance, while Hispanic children represent 55% of all children in the general population, they represent 67.2% in the child welfare system (Dettlaff and Earner, 2012).

There was no significant difference between the number of (substantiated and not substantiated) child maltreatment investigations for children of immigrants and children of native parents. However, as Table 8.3 shows, the types of substantiated maltreatment differ significantly: children of immigrants are more likely to experience physical abuse, sexual abuse, and emotional abuse, whereas children of native-born parents are more likely to experience physical neglect and neglectful supervision. The less likelihood of physical neglect among children of immigrants may be explained by the greater likelihood of two-parent families and the lower likelihood of substance abuse and intellectual and cognitive impairments in these families (Dettlaff and Earner, 2012).

A comparison of the characteristics of children in families of native-born parents and immigrant parents who come to the attention of child welfare systems based on NSCAW data shows that there are no significant differences in the child's age, caregivers' marital status, income, and education levels. In

Table 8.3. Types of substantiated maltreatment of children of immigrants and native parents

Type of substantiated maltreatment	Children of immigrants (%)	Children of native parents (%)
Emotional abuse[a]	25.1	11.1
Physical abuse	32.6	25.6
Sexual abuse	15.8	12.1
Physical neglect [a]	2.1	16.4
Neglectful supervision	21.4	27.0

[a] Significant difference at 95% confidence level.
Source: Dettlaff and Earner, 2012.

families with an immigrant parent, biological fathers were more likely to be present than in families with native-born parents (45.9% versus 28.5%); it was also significantly less likely that there would be a grandparent present in the home and significantly more likely the family would use a language other than English at home and would be uncomfortable using English. Children of immigrant families are more likely to live in two-parent families and less likely to experience a change of primary caregiver in the past 12 months—two protective factors (Dettlaff and Earner, 2012).

There are several significant differences between children in families of immigrant and native parents when it comes to risk factors at the individual family and community level. At the family level, active alcohol abuse, active drug use, intellectual or cognitive impairments, physical impairments, and a recent history of arrest were significantly more likely among native parents. In terms of community-level risk factors, immigrant parents were significantly less likely than native parents to report living in a safe neighborhood and report parental involvement in the community (Dettlaff and Earner, 2012).

TRAINING OF THE CHILD WELFARE WORKFORCE

Recruitment, training, and retention of child welfare staff has been of considerable concern since the enactment of the ASFA of 1997. Contained within this act were provisions that held states accountable for ensuring measureable and timely outcomes for children and families; this legislation also expanded training and technical assistance funding to raise the qualifications of the child welfare workforce. Currently, 11 National Resource Centers under the auspices of the Children's Bureau provide specialized training to the states on topics designed to improve practice and program outcomes (Children's Bureau, 2013). While standards with regard to the education, experience, and training requirements of child welfare workers vary across states, national studies suggest that workers typically hold a bachelor's degree in a human service field, receive up to 52 hours of annual training, and have an average 9.5 years of experience (GAO, 2006; NASW, 2004).

It is unknown how much specialized training child welfare workers receive about the unique needs of immigrant children, youth, and families. The ASFA requires that child welfare outcomes demonstrate cultural sensitivity, but this does not typically include specific training or information on, for example, how immigration status may affect access to services. Some states, including California, Georgia, New York and Texas, have formed partnerships with universities and schools of social work to develop specialized training curricula for their child welfare workers on immigrant issues, and the National Resource Center for Family-Centered Practice and Permanency Planning provides a webinar on immigrants and the child welfare system (NRC, 2008).

ORGANIZATION: MODEL PRACTICE APPROACHES

Organizational and evidence-based practice responses to immigrant children, youth, and families in the child welfare system are sporadic and locally based developments across the United States. Beginning in 2000, the growing recognition that immigrant and refugee families, children, and youth who became involved with the child welfare system were poorly or ineffectively served prompted initiatives in several states with large immigrant populations to rectify the situation. Promising practices with immigrant and refugee populations in child welfare over the past decade have included training caseworkers on cultural competency, improving language access, developing handbooks and guidelines on how immigration status affects access to services and benefits, and training caseworkers to refer immigrants for legal services if there is indication that they could benefit through Special Immigrant Juvenile Status, Trafficking Victims Protection Act, and Violence Against Women Act. In model programs that have been developed, the focus has been on integrating immigration services into the overall child welfare service delivery system through collaboration between care providers and the development of specialized units, departments, task forces, and advisory committees or liaisons. Emphasis has also been placed on recruiting targeted foster families with outreach to the community to build partnerships (Earner, 2010).

One example is the New York City public child welfare agency known as the Administration for Children's Services (ACS). In response to vociferous advocacy and newspaper reports of egregious treatment of immigrant families, ACS established an Advisory Task Force on Immigrant Issues comprised of community representatives and child welfare staff in 2001. In 2003, the Annie E. Casey Foundation stepped in and provided substantial private funding to incorporate this task force into a program of systemic change within ACS to address immigrant issues. With this additional funding, ACS was able to hire a full-time Director of Immigrant Services, develop a training curriculum for caseworkers on immigrant issues, and publish a handbook on immigrant access issues. It is now identified as a "model" program (Lincroft and Resner, 2006).

In Santa Clara County, California (also known as Silicon Valley), there is a large and extremely diverse population of immigrant families and children who are drawn to the area for similar reasons of economic opportunity but land on opposite sides of the socioeconomic spectrum, either as professionals in the high-end technology firms or in the low-end service sector industries as domestics, restaurant workers, landscapers, and other support services. In response to the diverse needs presented by immigrants, as well as to recognize immigrants' invaluable contribution to the local economy, Santa Clara County undertook a unique endeavor to develop a comprehensive countywide response that focused on integration as the central focus of all service provision in the county; this included child welfare services. Immigrant Relations and Integration Services strives to improve all human services to immigrants by fostering collaborations between government and community-based service providers to ensure that safety net services remain available to support all families (County of Santa Clara, 2012). It is an unusual, encompassing approach to addressing problems that can affect families.

PRACTICE: SURVEY FINDINGS

What do the responses of 103 child welfare workers, roughly 80% of who practice in the state of California, suggest about child welfare practice with immigrant children, youth, and families in the United States? First, the survey findings show that while the child workers surveyed generally felt well prepared to practice in a culturally competent way with immigrant children, youth, and families, they also reported facing more system barriers working with immigrant than with nonimmigrant families. This, we believe, is a reflection of the challenges that workers face when practicing in a migrant and immigration policy context that contradicts the mandates of the child welfare system and the best interests of the child in ways we have discussed here. While child welfare workers—two-thirds (67%) of whom reported speaking the language of the immigrant children, youth, and families they work with—perceived themselves as competent in and comfortable working with immigrant families, many said they experience working with this population as challenging, and almost all of them reported encountering system barriers: 43% considered it more challenging to work with immigrant families compared to nonimmigrant families, and 91% said they experienced more system barriers when working with immigrant families than nonimmigrant families.

Second, the survey findings also give evidence of the child protection orientation of the US child welfare system, as discussed by Berrick (2011) and Gilbert et al. (2011a). However, we see this child protection focus less so in the responses on risk assessments than we had anticipated, which, especially in Case 2, were clearly tilted toward the high risk end of the risk spectrum. We had anticipated the risk assessment levels to be lower than this, given the high risk thresholds of child protection-orientated systems such as the United States (Križ and Skivenes, 2013). In fact, most respondents assessed Case 1 as a moderate risk case (41%), 22% assessed it as high risk, and 22% as low risk. Over half of the respondents assessed Case 2 as a high risk case (51%); 25% assessed it as moderate, and 20% as very high risk. Over half of the respondents (54%) would let the girl in Case 2 stay in the home with her parents and provide services, and 43% would either start preparations for an out-of-home placement or remove the girl from the home at once. The guiding principles of "permanency" and "child and family well-being" are reflected in the high proportion of survey respondents who would let the baby in Case 1 stay with her parents while providing services, as well as in the high number of workers who suggested in-home services despite high risk assessments in Case 2.

What was interesting about Case 1 was that all of the respondents indicated that they would link the family with community services. This was a larger share than those who said that they would help find the family a place with amenities and running warm water, and those who responded that they would provide other public services. This could suggest that workers seem to rely more so on community services than statutory services. This speaks to the "residual" character of the US welfare state (Esping-Anderson, 1999), where community services play a large role in welfare provision, especially at a time when public child welfare service budgets are being cut. The fact that a large proportion of workers also reported experiencing systemic barriers tells a story of the lack of access to services needed as experienced by immigrant children, youth, and families, as discussed by Earner (2007), Ayón (2009), Ayón et al. (2010), and Križ and Skivenes (2012).

While over half of respondents (55%) thought that an undocumented child who is not attending school is the responsibility of the child welfare system, almost one-third (32%) felt that the child welfare system was *not* responsible. Of the latter group, 73% indicated that there was another state authority that was responsible. This could be interpreted to mean that while most workers see it as the role of the system to protect children regardless of their legal status, they actually do not see it as the role of the child welfare system to enforce school attendance.

The survey responses about the origins of the immigrant groups that respondents work with reflect the prevalence of immigrants from Latin America, primarily Mexico, in California. Most respondents indicated that they worked with immigrant families from South America or the Caribbean (71%) and Asia (40%). Interestingly, many of the respondents indicated that they were either immigrants themselves (34%) or the children of immigrants (63%). Over two-thirds of respondents (68%) reported speaking the language of one of the immigrant groups they work with. These figures evidence a high number of bilingual workers who are assigned to work with immigrant children, youth, and families in the agencies we surveyed in California. This is testimony to the fact that child welfare agencies in California operate within the framework of the 1973 Dymally-Alatorre Bilingual Services Act. The goal of this law is to provide equal access to services to those who do not speak or write English or whose primary language is not English. The law requires state agencies to employ qualified bilingual staff in positions where employees interact with the public (CACSS, 2012).

The fact that a large proportion of respondents (83%) reported having received training relevant to working specifically with immigrants speaks to the system's support of cultural competent service provision (at least in California). In terms of competency, almost one in every five respondents stated that they felt *more* competent working with immigrants; 59% felt equally competent and 19% less competent—the size of this group roughly corresponds to the proportion of those who reported not having received any training.

CONCLUDING REMARKS

To conclude, the survey findings were encouraging with respect to child welfare caseworkers' perceptions of their competency and comfort levels when working with immigrant families—a reflection of the high level of bilingual and bicultural workers in California. On the negative side of the ledger, the findings of the survey corroborate previous research studies that suggest that the child welfare system faces serious challenges when working with immigrant families—challenges that are systemic and institutional and lie in the competing policy mandates of child welfare, migrant, and immigration policies, as we have discussed in this chapter.

NOTES

1   However, the term "immigrant country" obfuscates the eliminationist policies of the colonizers towards the Native American population.
2   Undocumented individuals are, however, undercounted in Census data (Fortuny et al., 2009). The terms "undocumented immigrant," "unauthorized immigrant," or "illegal immigrant" refer to foreign-born individuals who presently do not have the right to reside in the United States. These individuals are difficult to officially track and are the subject of contentious policy debates about US immigration laws.
3   "Children of immigrants" are children who have at least one parent who is foreign born (Fortuny et al., 2009).
4   For a comprehensive timeline of all US child protection legislation, see USDHHS (2013).
5   For an extensive discussion on child protection policies, recent policy debates, and child protection-related statistics, see Berrick (2011).

REFERENCES

American Humane Association. (2005). *Differential Response in Child Welfare, Protecting Children* 20(2–3). Retrieved January 3, 2013, from http://www.americanhumane.org/assets/pdfs/children/differential-response/pc-20-2-3pdf.pdf.

Ayón, C. (2009). Shorter time-lines, yet higher hurdles: Mexican families' access to child welfare mandated services. *Children and Youth Services Review*, 31, 609–616.

Ayón, C., Aisenberg, E., & Erera, P. (2010). Learning how to dance with the public child welfare system: Mexican parents' efforts to exercise their voice. *Journal of Public Child Welfare*, 4, 263–286.

Bernstein, N. (2000). Family law collides with immigration and welfare rules. *The New York Times* (November 20). Retrieved January 3, 2013, from http://www.nytimes.com/2000/11/20/nyregion/family-law-collides-with-immigration-and-welfare-rules.html?pagewanted=all&src=pm

Berrick, J.D. (2011). Trends and issues in the U.S. child welfare system. In N. Gilbert, N. Parton, and M. Skivenes (Eds.), *Child Protection Systems: International Trends and Orientations*, 17–35. Oxford: Oxford University Press.

Borjas, G. (2011). Welfare reform and immigrant participation in welfare programs. *International Migration Review*, 36(4), 1093–1123.

California Department of Child Support Services (CACSS). (2012). Bilingual services. Retrieved March 31, 2013, from http://www.childsup.ca.gov/Home/BilingualServices.aspx.

Children's Bureau. (2013). National Resource Centers. Retrieved March 29, 2013, from http://www.acf.hhs.gov/programs/cb/assistance/national-resource-centers.

County of Santa Clara. (2012). Immigrant Relations and Integration Services (IRIS). Retrieved January 3, 2013, from http://www.sccgov.org/sites/ohr/immigrant%20relations%20and%20integration%20services/Pages/Immigrant-Relations-and-Integration-Services-(IRIS).aspx.

Dettlaff, A.J. (2012). Immigrants and refugees: The Intersection of Migration and Child Welfare. Webcast retrieved January 3, 2013, from http://www.hunter.cuny.edu/socwork/nrcfcpp/webcasts/index.html.

Dettlaff, A.J., & Cardoso, J.B. (2010). Mental health need and service use among Latino children of immigrants in the child welfare system. *Children and Youth Services Review*, 32, 1373–1379.

Dettlaff, A.J., & Earner, I. (2007). The intersection of child welfare and migration: Emerging issues and implications. *Protecting Children*, 22(2), 3–7.

———. (2012). Children of immigrants in the child welfare system: Findings from the National Survey of Child and Adolescent Well-being. *Migration and Child Welfare National Network Research Brief*. Retrieved January 3, 2013, from http://www.americanhumane.org/assets/pdfs/children/pc-childofimmigrantpdf.pdf.

Dettlaff, A.J., & Johnson, M. (2011). Child maltreatment dynamics among immigrant and U.S. born Latino children: Findings from the National Survey of Child and Adolescent Well-being (NSCAW). *Children and Youth Services Review*, 33, 936–944.

Dettlaff, A.J., & Phillips, S. (2007). The ICE-man cometh. Immigration enforcement considerations for child welfare systems. Retrieved January 3, 2013, from http://www.f2f.ca.gov/res/pdf/ImmigrationEnforcement.pdf.

Dreby, J. (2012). How today's immigration enforcement policies impact children, families, and communities. A view from the ground. Center for American Progress. Retrieved January 3, 2013, from http://www.americanprogress.org/wp-content/uploads/2012/08/DrebyImmigrationFamiliesFINAL.pdf

Earner, I. (2007). Immigrant families and public child welfare services: Barriers to services and approaches to change. *Journal of Child Welfare*, 86(4), 63–91.

———. (2010). Immigrant issues and child welfare. Paper presented at the Annual Foster Care Manager's Meeting, US Department of Health and Human Services, Children's Bureau, Washington, DC, October 6.

Esping-Anderson, G. (1999). *The Three Worlds of Welfare Capitalism*. Princeton, NJ: Princeton University Press.

Fortuny, K., Capps, R., & Passel, J. (2007). The characteristics of unauthorized immigrants in California, Los Angeles County, and the United States. Washington, DC: Urban Institute. Retrieved January 3, 2013, from http://www.urban.org/UploadedPDF/411425_Characteristics_Immigrants.pdf.

Fortuny, K., Capps, R., Simms, M., & Chaudry, A. (2009). Children of immigrants: National and state characteristics. Washington, DC: Urban Institute. Retrieved January 3, 2013, from http://www.urban.org/uploadedpdf/411939_childrenofimmigrants.pdf.

Futures Without Violence. (2012). The Facts on Immigrant Women and Domestic Violence. Washington, DC: Futures Without Violence. Retrieved January 3, 2013, from http://www.futureswithoutviolence.org/userfiles/file/Children_and_Families/Immigrant.pdf.

Gilbert, N., ed. (1997). *Combatting Child Abuse: International Perspectives and Trends*. New York: Oxford University Press.

Gilbert, N., Parton, N., & Skivenes, M. (2011a). Changing patterns of response and emerging orientation. In N. Gilbert, N. Parton, and M. Skivenes (Eds.), *Child Protection Systems: International Trends and Orientations*, 243–257. Oxford: Oxford University Press.

Gilbert, N., Parton, N., & Skivenes, M. (2011b). Introduction. In N. Gilbert, N. Parton, and M. Skivenes (Eds.), *Child Protection Systems: International Trends and Orientations*, 3–13. Oxford: Oxford University Press.

Grieco, M., Acosta, Y., De la Cruz, P., Gambino, C., Gryn, T., Larsen, L., Trevelyan, E., & Walters, N. (2012). *The Foreign-Born Population in the United States: 2010*. Washington, DC: US Census Bureau. Retrieved January 3, 2013, from http://www.census.gov/prod/2012pubs/acs-19.pdf.

Johnson, M.A. (2007). The social ecology of acculturation: Implications for child welfare services to children of immigrants. *Children and Youth Services Review*, 29, 1426–1438.

Kasinitz, P., Waters, M., Mollenkopf, J., & Holdaway, J. (2009). *Inheriting the City: The Children of Immigrants Come of Age.* New York: Russell Sage Foundation.

Križ, K., & Skivenes, M. (2012). How child welfare workers view their work with undocumented immigrant families: An explorative study of challenges and coping strategies. *Children and Youth Services Review,* 34(4), 790–797.

———. (2013). Systemic differences in views on risk: A comparative case vignette study of risk assessment in England, Norway and the United States (California). *Children and Youth Services Review,* 35(11), 1862–1870.

Križ, K., Slayter, S., Iannicelli, A., & Lourie, J. (2012). Fear management: How child protection workers engage with non-citizen immigrant families. *Children and Youth Services Review,* 34(1), 316–323.

Ku, L., & Jewers, M. (2013). *Health Care for Immigrant Families: Current Policies and Issues.* Washington, DC: Migration Policy Institute. Retrieved November 30, 2013, from http://www.migrationpolicy.org/pubs/COI-HealthCare.pdf.

Lincroft, Y., & Dettlaff, A.J. (2010). Children of Immigrants in the U.S. Child Welfare System. Washington, DC: First Focus. Retrieved January 3, 2013, from http://www.firstfocus.net/library/fact-sheets/children-of-immigrants-in-the-us-child-welfare-system.

Lincroft, Y., & Resner, J. (2006). Undercounted and Underserved: Immigrant and Refugee Families in the Child Welfare System. Baltimore, MD: Annie E. Casey Foundation. Retrieved January 3, 2013, from http://www.aecf.org/KnowledgeCenter/Publications.aspx?pubguid=%7BA6A32287-6D6B-4580-9365-D7E635E35569%7D.

Lopez, M.H., & Gonzalez-Barrera, A. (2013). High Rate of Deportations Continue under Obama depsite Latino Disapproval. Pew Research Center. Retrieved on August 4, 2014, from http://www.pewresearch.org/fact-tank/2013/09/19/high-rate-of-deportations-continue-under-obama-despite-latino-disapproval/.

Majorkas, A. (2012). Deferred Action for Childhood Arrivals: Who Can Be Considered? Washington, DC: The White House. Retrieved March 31, 2013, from http://www.whitehouse.gov/blog/2012/08/15/deferred-action-childhood-arrivals-who-can-be-considered.

Martin, D.C., & Yankay, J.E. (2012). Refugees and Asylees: 2011. Washington, DC: Department of Homeland Security. Retrieved January 3, 2013, from http://www.dhs.gov/refugees-and-asylees-2011.

Martin, D.L., & Mosher, J. (1995). Unkept promises: Experiences of immigrant women with the neo-criminalization of wife abuse. *Canadian Journal of Women and the Law,* 8, 3–44.

Migration and Child Welfare National Network (MCWNN). 2009. Immigrant Families and Child Welfare: The Texas Learning Laboratory. Paper presented at the Council on Social Work Education Annual Program Meeting,

November. Retrieved January 3, 2012, from http://www.americanhumane.org/assets/pdfs/children/pc-mwcnn-09-learning-lab-abstract.pdf.

National Association of Social Workers (NASW). (2004). Assuring the Sufficiency of a Frontline Workforce. Washington, DC: NASW. Retrieved March 29, 2013, from http://workforce.socialworkers.org/studies/children/children_families.pdf.

National Clearinghouse on Child Abuse and Neglect Information. (2003–2005). Racial Disproportionality in the Child Welfare System: What We Know. Washington, DC: National Information Clearinghouse. Retrieved January 3, 2013, from http://www.hunter.cuny.edu/socwork/nrcfcpp/downloads/bib/Disproportionality_whatweknow.pdf.

National Immigration Law Center. (2013). Frequently Asked Questions: The Affordable Care Act & Mixed-Status Families. Los Angeles: National Immigration Law Center. Retrieved November 30, 2013, from http://www.nilc.org/immigrantshcr.html.

National Public Radio. (2012). Investing in Citizenship: For the Rich, a Road to the U.S. *All Things Considered*, January 26, 2013. Retrieved March 31, 2013, from http://www.npr.org/2013/01/26/170358985/investing-in-citizenship-for-the-rich-a-new-road-to-the-u-s.

National Resource Center for Family-Centered Practice and Permanency Planning (NRC). (2008). Immigrants and Refugees: The Intersection of Migration and Child Welfare. New York: NRC. Retrieved March 29, 2013, from http://www.nrcpfc.org/webcasts/archives/14/WebcastAgenda.pdf.

National Survey of Child and Adolescent Well-Being (NSCAW). (2005). CPS Sample Component Wave 1: Data Analysis Report. Washington, DC: Administration for Children & Families. Retrieved January 3, 2013, from http://www.acf.hhs.gov/programs/opre/abuse_neglect/nscaw/reports/cps_sample/cps_toc.html.

Passel, J., & Cohn, D.V. (2011). Unauthorized Immigrant Population: National and State Trends, 2010. Research Report. Washington DC: Pew Research Center.

Paxson, C., & Waldfogel, J. (2003). Welfare reforms, family resources, and child maltreatment. *Journal of Policy Analysis and Management*, 22(1), 85–113.

Pison, G. (2010). The number and proportion of immigrants in the population: International comparisons. *Population and Societies* 472. Retrieved January 3, 2013, from http://www.ined.fr/en/publications/pop_soc/bdd/publication/1520/.

Reed, D.F., & Karpilow, K. (2009). Understanding the Child Welfare System in California: A Primer for Service Providers and Policymakers. California Center for Research on Women and Families. Berkeley: California Center for Research on Women and Families. Retrieved January 3, 2013, from http://ccrwf.org/wp-content/uploads/2009/03/final_web_pdf.pdf.

Refugee Council USA. (2012). History of the U.S. Refugee Resettlement Program. Washington, DC: Refugee Council USA. Retrieved January 3, 2013, from http://www.rcusa.org/index.php?page=history.

Saco, C. (2008). An Overview of Immigration Issues and Child Welfare from a Social Worker's Perspective. Retrieved January 3, 2013, from http://www.f2f.ca.gov/res/pdf/BeyondTheBench.pdf.

United Nations High Commissioner for Refugees (UNHCR). (2012). 2012 Regional Operations Profile—North America and the Caribbean. Washington, DC: UNHCR. Retrieved January 3, 2013, from http://www.unhcr.org/cgi-bin/texis/vtx/page?page=49e492086&submit=GO.

United States Census Bureau (US Census). (2009). Children. Washington, DC: US Census Bureau. Retrieved March 31, 2013, from http://www.census.gov/hhes/socdemo/children/.

United States Department of Health and Human Services (USDHSS). (2012). The AFCARS Report. Washington, DC: USDHSS. Retrieved March 31, 2013, from http://www.acf.hhs.gov/sites/default/files/cb/afcarsreport19.pdf.

———. (2013). Major Federal Legislation Concerned with Child Protection, Child Welfare and Adoption. Washington, DC: USDHSS. Retrieved March 31, 2013, from https://www.childwelfare.gov/pubs/otherpubs/majorfedlegis.cfm.

United States Citizenship and Immigration Services (USCIS). (2013). E-B5 Immigrant Investor Visa. Washington, DC: USCIS. Retrieved March 31, 2013, from http://www.uscis.gov/eb-5-investor.

United States Government Accountability Office (GAO). (2006). Child Welfare. Washington, DC: GAO. Retrieved March 31, 2013, from http://www.gao.gov/new.items/d0775.pdf.

Van Hook, J., Landale, N.S., & Hillemeier, M.M. (2013). *Is the United States Bad for Children's Health? Risk and Resilience among Young Children of Immigrants.* Washington, DC: Migration Policy Institute. Retrieved November 30, 2013, from http://www.migrationpolicy.org/pubs/COI-ChildHealth.pdf.

Velazquez, S., & Dettlaff, J. (2011). Immigrant children and child welfare in the United States: Demographics, legislation, research, policy, and practice impacting public services. *Child Indicators Research*, 4(4), 679–695. doi: 10.1007/s12187-011-9111-9

Vericker, T., Kuehn, D., & Capps, R. (2007). Title IV-E funding: Funded foster care placements by child generation and ethnicity: Findings from Texas. Urban Institute Child Welfare Research Program, Brief 3. Washington, DC: Urban Institute.

Walters, N., & Trevelyan, E. (2011). *The Newly Arrived Foreign-Born Population of the United States: 2010.* Washington, DC: United States Census Bureau. Retrieved January 3, 2013, from http://www.census.gov/prod/2011pubs/acsbr10-16.pdf.

Waters, M., Ueda, R., & Marrow, H., eds. (2007). *The New Americans: A Guide to Immigration since 1965*. Cambridge: Harvard University Press.

Weaver, R., & Hackman, R. (2009). A new era for legal immigrants? Rethinking Title IV of the Personal Responsibility and Work Opportunity Reconciliation Act. *Journal of Policy Practice*, 8, 540–568.

Workgroup on Safety and Well-Being for Immigrant and Refugee Children and Families. (2010). Serving Immigrant and Refugee Families. Rhinelander: Wisconsin Department of Children and Families. Retrieved January 3, 2012, from http://dcf.wisconsin.gov/children/immigrant_refugee/pdf/child_welfare_report.pdf.

Women's Refugee Commission. (2009). U.S. Faces Challenges in the Protection of Unaccompanied Children. New York: Women's Refugee Commission. Retrieved January 3, 2013, from http://womensrefugeecommission.org/press-room/716-unaccompanied.

Yoshikawa, Hirokazu. (2011). *Immigrants Raising Citizens: Undocumented Parents and their Young Children*. New York: Russell Sage Foundation.

9

CHILD WELFARE SYSTEMS AND IMMIGRANT FAMILIES

CANADA

Sarah Maiter and Bruce Leslie

In this chapter we discuss child welfare service provision to immigrant families and children in Canada. We begin with a brief discussion of historical and current immigration policies and public responses to these policies in order to provide an understanding of the broader political and societal contexts and discourses within which services are provided to immigrant families. These discourses influence law, policy, services, and the overall organization of child protection services to immigrant families. This is followed by a discussion of the general organization of the child protection system in Canada; data from the available research on representation of immigrant families and children in the system; and a discussion of legal, policy, and service provision as it relates to immigrant children. We then provide some relevant statistics to show which countries immigrants come from and under what circumstances/categories they are accepted into Canada, social work practice findings from the survey, and a concluding section.

HISTORICAL AND CURRENT IMMIGRATION POLICIES AND ISSUES

Aside from its Aboriginal people, Canada is a country made up of immigrants. The early settlers in Canada, however, established racist immigration policies with the blatant attempt to keep Canada Anglo-Saxon and French and then later a white country (Matas, 1985: 8). The early Canadian Immigration Act (1910) gave the cabinet the power to exclude immigrants belonging to particular races to enter the country. Over the years the wording of these acts changed, but the essential power to reject settlers on the basis of race remained. These sentiments were captured in various government acts throughout the early twentieth century that attempted to restrict immigration based on race along with angry reactions by locals to the immigration of ethnically diverse people with numerous examples existing of attempts to exclude people from diverse ethnic countries from entering Canada (Canada and the World, 2011). To an extent these discriminatory immigration policies continue in the present (Pratt and Valverde, 2002: 137). Thus any discussion of immigrants in Canada includes the pervasive racist policies that have made up Canadian immigration law.

THE CANADIAN CHILD WELFARE SYSTEMS

Canada is a vast country comprising 10 provinces of varying size and population and three northern territories that are large and sparsely populated. Over three-quarters of its highly diverse population of 33 million reside in urban areas, with Vancouver, Toronto, and Montreal, its three largest cities, attracting immigrants from all over the world. More and more immigrants are now also moving out to other cities in search of employment. Legally, Canada's governing powers have been divided between the federal and provincial/territorial governments with health, education, and welfare, including child welfare, being the responsibility of the provinces and territories. Although at one time national standards for welfare policies were enshrined through the provinces/territories receiving guaranteed matching federal funds spent on social welfare programs based on need, this changed in 1995. The federal government, in a debt reduction strategy, changed its model of funding to the provinces and territories to a block transfer of combined funds for health, education, and social welfare to each province. Provinces are now virtually left on their own to fund social welfare programs as they see fit, resulting in many lowering their spending considerably (Swift, 2011) and essentially eroding the national standards of service provision of previous times.

Each of the 10 provinces and the three territories has different organizations and legislation governing child welfare. Provincial/territorial services for children and youth are provided either by a branch of the provincial government or by a private or nonprofit agency under the auspices of provincial child welfare laws. For example, in the province of British Columbia, child protection services are provided by the Ministry of Children and Families, a branch of the provincial government under the terms of the 1996 Child, Family and Community Service Act. The Ministry states that its role is to ensure a child-centered, integrated approach that promotes and protects the healthy development of children and youth while recognizing their lifelong attachment to family and community (British Columbia Ministry of Children and Family Development, 2012). Amendments to the act were made in 2002 to expand the option of placing children with family members, friends of the family, and other community members when taken into the custody of the government. In the province of Ontario, child welfare services are provided through 51 separate Children's Aid Societies under the terms of the Child and Family Services Act (1990), the Children's Law Reform Act (2002), and the Family Law Act (2002). These agencies investigate allegations of abuse and neglect and provide some direct services but primarily refer families to support services for protecting children. Adoption and foster care services are also provided through Children's Aid Societies. The provincial Ministry of Community and Social Services funds Children's Aid Societies in Ontario. Child welfare services for First Nations/Aboriginal children and families are provided by either the provincial agency on behalf of the federal government or directly by First Nations agencies as negotiated under the federal government's policy on Aboriginal self-government. For more details on the child protection system in Canada see Swift (2011).

A number of critiques have been noted about Canada's child welfare system. Perhaps the central concern is a frustration with a child welfare mandate that is described as "narrow, limited and residual" (Zapf, 2004: 413). Indeed, the state becomes involved only when absolutely necessary, when parents have exhausted their resources and their ability to care for their children. The focus of the work of social workers within the child protection system is on the investigation of complaints, determination of neglect and abuse, and the assessment of the level of risk for these behaviors. This residual approach is highly problematic as it is occurring within an overall residual approach to social welfare where the social safety net is being eroded and the neoliberal agenda of the provincial and federal government is on reducing the cost and scope of the state with an emphasis on individuals taking responsibility for their own fate. With the severe cutbacks to the welfare system and social services, the general approach of government policy is to an even greater residual view of the role of social welfare in the lives of people (Hicks, 2009). Social welfare is thus targeted to only those in extreme need, and benefits are provided at low levels so as to discourage their use and to make social welfare less desirable. This neoliberal agenda to social welfare has considerable impact on the lives of children and families, oftentimes resulting in child welfare concerns and involvement. For example, researchers (Thoburn, 2007) have identified inadequate resources for child health and well-being, especially income support, housing, and child care, as among the reasons why children may be brought into state care. Inadequate housing was identified in one in five cases in a 2000 study of cases in which decisions were made to place or keep children in care (Chau, Fitzpatrick, Hulchanski, Leslie, and Schatia, 2001; Leslie, 2005). A close association between poverty and child welfare intervention, especially neglect, has also been shown (Leschied, Chiodo, Whitehead, and Hurley, 2003; Trocmé, MacLaurin, Fallon, Daciuk, Tourigny, and Billingsley, 2001). Furthermore, higher placement rates are reported when child welfare investigations find "neglect as the primary category of maltreatment, benefits or employment insurance as the primary source of income, or public rental as the type of housing accommodation" (MacLaurin, Trocmé, and Fallon, 2003: 39).

THE CHILD WELFARE SYSTEM AND IMMIGRANT FAMILIES

In Canada, immigration, racial, ethnic, or cultural data are not routinely gathered by social service agencies. In the province of Ontario, the eligibility spectrum used to assess whether the child protection system should intervene or not does not contain any categories relating to immigration, nor does the risk assessment used by the system. These variables show up at some time in the process of the intervention as workers gather more information on families for service provision and could show up as early as the first contact when it is learned that language issues are a struggle and interpreter services are required. Yet adding a category in these two tools relating to immigration can also be problematic as it could result in increased surveillance of immigrant families given current social service emphasis on risk management rather than on examining service needs.

Disproportionality in the Child Welfare System

Within the child welfare context in other countries such as the United States, the overrepresentation of racial minority and immigrant families, based on robust research data, has been well identified (Dettlaff and Rycraft, 2010), and considerable effort has been made to understand these findings in order to develop appropriate intervention and prevention strategies and to work at preventing bias throughout the system. In Canada, despite a discussion of and anecdotal concern of overrepresentation of racial and ethnic minorities and immigrant families in the child protection system, there is still a dearth of research-based data. Three relatively recent studies (Blackstock, Trocmé, and Bennett, 2004; Lavergne, Dufour, Sarmiento, and Descoteaux, 2009; Lavergne, Dufour, Trocmé, and Larrivee, 2008) note that racial minority immigrant children and families are overrepresented in the Canadian child protection system compared to their proportion in the general census. Blackstock et al. conducted an analysis of data from a 1998 Canadian incidence study of child maltreatment (Trocmé et al., 2001), the first national study of investigated child abuse and neglect. They found that maltreatment was more often substantiated for Aboriginal children (50%) and visible minorities[1] (VM; 41%), compared to non-Aboriginal "white" children (38%). When differentiating by type of maltreatment, VM cases (35%) were much more likely to be identified for physical abuse, most notably punishment-related abuse, compared to non-Aboriginal (22%) and Aboriginal groups (8%). Lavergne et al.'s. (2008) report of data from a later maltreatment incidence study (CIS, 2003; Trocmé et al., 2005) noted similar trends. Asian children reported for physical abuse accounted for 14% of the sample, a proportion that is 1.6 times greater than their proportion in census data. Asian children also had the highest substantiation rate for physical abuse. In both reports the authors suggest caution in evaluating these findings, noting that higher rates of substantiation does not necessarily mean higher incidence of maltreatment. They raise possibilities of racial bias in reporting and substantiating abuse and struggles on the part of workers when working with families from diverse ethno-racial backgrounds and who are immigrants. This is of note as in both studies workers did not identify parental concerns, housing issues, or child functioning as contributing to the problems in the families—areas for assessment that may be missed. Further research on the process of assessment, worker understanding of parent and child issues, worker–client relationship, and language challenges is warranted as workers may not be able to clearly understand the problems that these parents may be experiencing and may therefore only be able to assess the incident of abuse but not the context of the parents' situation. For example, the struggles of immigrant parents, such as difficulty finding employment, settlement problems, financial problems, and mental and physical health issues, have been identified elsewhere (Maiter, Stalker, and Alaggia, 2009). Indeed, Lavergne et al. (2008) are cognizant of this, suggesting that there are struggles in assessing culturally diverse parents. They note that child protection workers may lack "cultural competence" that is required to work with family structures and immigrants from "non-Western" countries.

A recent study (Lavergne et al., 2009) analyzed children reported to and assessed by the child protection system in Montreal to examine representation of VM children and compare individual and family characteristics, types of reports, and protection services provided to black, other minorities (South and East Asian, Arabs, and so on), and non-VM children. The authors note disproportionate representation and overrepresentation of black children at the reporting stage and further on in the system; non-VM children often live in higher risk situations; professionals proportionately report more VM (black and other) children; and a larger proportion of reports for VM (black and other) children concern physical harm, with most being related to different disciplinary or childrearing methods from those generally used by the majority culture (Lavergne et al., 2009: 7). Overall, then, these findings echo the findings noted earlier from the CIS studies. Disproportionality appears to be prevalent for ethnoracial/immigrant families in the system at reporting and at different stages of service; these families have higher reports of and substantiation of concern regarding physical harm, mostly as related to discipline and childrearing methods. Researchers (Euser, van IJzendoorn, Prinzie, and Bakermans-Kranenburg, 2011) in the Netherlands note the impact of socioeconomic differences on maltreatment rates. They found that when correcting for education level of the parents of two sets of immigrant families in their study, risk disappeared for the traditional group but remained for the nontraditional group. The authors suggest the refugee families in their study are still exposed to considerable stress after their arrival in the Netherlands, and for most of them this is subsequent to a history of severe traumatization. They conclude that "In sum, elevated rates of child maltreatment in immigrant families should not be automatically ascribed to race or ethnicity before lack of educational and material resources implied in low SES has been taken into account as a major risk factor for child maltreatment" (Euser et al., 2011: 70–71). Such insights are also needed for the Canadian situation. Indeed in Canada, researchers (Maiter, Alaggia, and Trocmé, 2004) found that the South Asian immigrant parents in their sample did not differ significantly from other populations in their judgment of appropriate parenting approaches; that is, persistent and excessive use of physical discipline was considered to be inappropriate, behaviors of parents that may have negative emotional consequences for children were recognized as inappropriate, and lack of proper supervision of children was seen as a concern. As noted earlier, studies have identified the struggles of immigrant parents that may be missed in child welfare (Maiter et al., 2009).

Unaccompanied Minors

Ali, Tarabin, and Gill (2003) note that with respect to separated children seeking asylum, very little systematic data collection or research has been done. Information and knowledge on the experiences of unaccompanied children and of those who are trying to meet their needs, on institutional strategies and practices, and on governmental policies and their impact is very scant.

The office of Citizenship and Immigration Canada and the Immigration and Refugee Board considers children under the age of 18 not accompanied by a member of the family class to be "unaccompanied." Although all major international protocols define a child as someone under the age of 18 with the United Nations High Commission on Refugees defining an unaccompanied child as one separated from both parents and not being cared for by an adult (UNHCR, 2000), the age range for child protection services in Canada varies from under

19 years in British Columbia to under 16 years in Ontario, unless they are in the care of the state. Thus child protection services do not extend to unaccompanied minors over 16 in Ontario while also continuing to be patchy even if unaccompanied minors fall within the appropriate age for these services. In British Columbia, the Ministry of Children and Family Development has set up a Migration Services Team that is responsible for protection and support services for children up to the age of 19. The situation in Ontario, the province receiving the largest numbers of unaccompanied minors, is considered to be the worst. Unlike the situation in Quebec and British Columbia, there is no agreement between the Immigration and Refugee Board and the Children's Aid Society or the Catholic Children's Aid Society, the two organizations providing child protection service to children under 16.

Although the numbers for unaccompanied minors is relatively small in Canada, they have been increasing, as can be noted in the data: In 1999 there were 368; in 2000, 673; in 2001, 817; and in 2002, 1830. As noted previously, in Ontario, children in the 16- to 17-year-old age range do not qualify for the services provided by the child protection system, yet, because of their age, they are also the ones most likely to be exploited in the labor market and the sex industry. They are not required by law to attend school and do not qualify for student loans that would provide them access to postsecondary education, and it is unclear what publicly funded service, if any, can they continue to count on.

More recently, the Canadian Broadcasting Corporation reported that in 2011–2012, 289 migrant children of parents seeking asylum in Canada together with other deportees waiting to leave have been held in detention centers in Canada (CBC News, 2012). Mothers and children are in separate sections of the center, with children only being able to visit with their fathers during designated times. The report shows stunning pictures of barbed wire fences around these facilities. Sadly, while at the detention center, children do not attend school. The authorities note that the average length of stay is 6.6 days, but there have also been stays of up to 70 days.

Policy and Services

Child protection agencies in Canada respond to calls regarding concerns for the safety of children. Once calls are received, families are assessed and services provided either from the agency itself or through referrals to a range of relevant resources within the community. Services proceed from least intrusive, voluntary family services with children remaining in the home to seeking supervision orders to work with the family while the child/children remains in the home, to temporary placement with family, friends, or foster parents. Most agencies note that services are provided in ways that maintain connections with extended family and the culture of the child. Innovative services such as family group conferencing are used to help in seeking out solutions to keep children safe and, wherever possible, with family members.

Researchers, policymakers, and practitioners in Canada, as in other countries, have become more concerned about the need to develop social services to meet the needs of its increasingly diverse ethnoracial populations and newcomers to the country. This impetus has arisen from recognition of the harmful impact of traditional services for diverse ethnoracial, Aboriginal, and immigrant families. A number of different approaches to developing culturally relevant services have been suggested for social work practice generally and for child protection work specifically. These approaches range from what can be termed a "cultural competency" approach (Al-Krenawi and Graham, 2003) to an "antiracist/anti-oppression" approach (Maiter, 2009a). Problems identified with a cultural competency approach include the impossible task of becoming competent in a culture of another group, essentialization and generalizations of groups, a focus on culture that masks the social exclusion and marginalization of racialized and other minority groups, negative and positive stereotyping of groups, and lack of an understanding of contextual issues faced by particular groups (Maiter, 2009b). Bachelor's and master's of social work programs across the country offer a variety of courses that directly or indirectly relate to immigration and settlement and cultural, racial, and ethnic diversity. All schools of social work are required to include materials on these topics as required by the accreditation standards of the Canadian Association of Schools of Social Work. Its mission statement for their standards for accreditation notes that "Schools shall be expected to provide evidence of effective progress in attaining multicultural/multiracial diversity" (CASWE, June, 2013, 1.11) and this progress should be evident in curriculum, among other items. Each school then decides on how this material will be included. In examining course outlines, schools cover immigration and settlement-related matters in various ways in their curriculum either through stand-alone courses on racial and cultural diversity or embedded within theory, practice and policy courses, or specific courses on immigration.

Some suggested guidelines in child protection laws may indirectly relate to provision of services to immigrant families. The Child and Family Services Act of Ontario (2011), for example, notes that children's services should be provided in a manner that "(i) respects a child's need for continuity of care and for stable relationships within a family and cultural environment [and] (ii) takes into account physical, cultural, emotional, spiritual, mental, and developmental needs and differences among children. Additionally, services to families should also, wherever possible "be provided in a manner that respects cultural, religious and regional differences." Other jurisdictions have similar clauses in their statutes. The province of British Columbia notes in the principles of their protection act (2012) that "(e) kinship ties and a child's attachment to the extended family should be preserved if possible" and in their service principles that "(c) services should be planned and provided in ways that are sensitive to the needs and the cultural, racial and religious heritage of those receiving the services" and that "(e) the child's cultural, racial, linguistic and religious heritage should be considered when reference is made to the best interest of the child." Child protection organizations attempt to put these principles and guidelines into practice, but the workers' complex role of assessing risk and providing for the safety of the child trumps these considerations. Additionally, relevant resources are not always available to ensure the application of these principles.

Trends to understand and include material on cultural, racial, and ethnic diversity are also evident in child protection practice with these families. Although not set up as policy or law, child protection organizations across the country have made efforts to understand the cultural and contextual issues for families coming to their attention through the training of staff. Some examples include the efforts by the British Columbia Ministry of Social Services, as well as by the Ontario Association of Children's Aid Societies (Ontario Association of Children's Aid Societies, 2006). The OACAS's recent consultations regarding the transformation of child protection practice to a more strengths-based approach contains a section on delivering services to diverse ethno racial families that is relevant to their diverse situations. The Immigration and Refugee Staff Advisory Committee was also set up by the Children's Aid Society of Toronto and Catholic Children's Aid Society of Toronto (CCAS; the Refugee and Immigration Staff Advisory Committee, 2004) to address issues confronting the immigrant and refugee families served by these two very large organizations in the largest immigrant receiving city of Canada. The goal of this committee is: "to better understand the policies, procedures and problems, which immigrant/ refugee clients deal with in their attempts to settle in Canada. The Committee also explores ways to assist them in this process" (Refugee and Immigration Staff Advisory Committee, 2004: 4). Through this initiative, CCAS hired a Child Protection Immigration Specialist in 2007 to assist workers in addressing specific challenges of these immigrant children and families especially in terms of their legal situations in Canada. One major issue that had been identified was that children who were made permanent wards prior to their having Canadian citizenship would have no status once they reached the age of majority and were therefore at risk of being sent to their countries of origin once out of state care. Yet these children had been in Canada for long periods and, for some, most of their lives (Hare, 2007). CCAS, with the hiring of this worker, has had good success in obtaining citizenship for some of the permanent wards in their care who were vulnerable to being returned to the country from which they had come. It is not clear whether other child welfare organizations are making efforts to ensure that these children and youth have legal status in Canada once they reach the age of majority and are no longer in government care.

Children who come into state care while their parents' immigration status is still undecided are also in limbo. By virtue of being in care, these children gain "landed immigrant status," yet their parents don't have this status. Situations have arisen where parents are deported while the child is in care. At least in one instance, a youth was sent back with the parent, leaving the child welfare judge furious. These children are in care presumably because they are at risk of harm from their parent, and yet they are at risk of being put back in this harmful situation with their parent(s). On the other hand, if they are not returned with their parent then they risk losing the possibility of having family connections in Canada, as their parents have been deported. The lack of clarity between child welfare law—a provincial jurisdiction—and immigration law—a federal jurisdiction—can raise numerous dilemmas for workers, children, and families.

THE CANADIAN CONTEXT RELEVANT FOR IMMIGRANTS

There is considerable evidence that immigrant families often live in poverty or at risk of poverty as newcomers to Canada. Fleury (2007) found that one in five recent immigrants of working age lived in poverty in 2004 compared to fewer than one in 10 of their Canadian counterparts. They also encounter more difficulty finding employment, tend to earn less than the general population, and, compared to immigrants who arrived at a much earlier period (1970s–1980s compared to 1990s), possibly due to factors such as the change in source country resulting in greater numbers of racialized immigrants arriving, and decreased foreign credential recognition (Fleury, 2007). Interestingly, new immigrants are in the same category as lone parents, persons with disabilities, Indigenous persons, and single persons ages 45 to 64—all groups that are most likely to experience persistent poverty in Canada. Even with higher levels of education, more labor market experience, and not having a work-related disability, they continue to have struggles in gaining adequate work, leading researchers to suggest that race plays a role in immigrant poverty as "the vast majority of low-income recent immigrants were members of a visible minority (86%)" (Fleury, 2007: 25). Relevant for child welfare matters is that low-income recent immigrants tend to live in overcrowded (considered too small for the number of persons) and unaffordable housing (where housing costs account for more than 30% of income).

The 2004 report by United Way of Greater Toronto based on Census 1981 and 2001 for a 20-year comparison of residents' living conditions, workforce participation and income levels found that almost one in five families in 2001 was living in poverty, and while this rate had decreased for families across Canada since 1981, it appeared to have increased for families in Toronto. The report found that 30% of the total immigrant population in Toronto lives in poverty neighborhoods, accounting for two-thirds of the "poor" families living in these neighborhoods. Unemployment rates are higher in these neighborhoods; however, with 87% of people reporting that they were working, it appears that many were working very low-paying, precarious forms of employment rather than not having jobs.

Of concern is that immigrants within Toronto used to occupy 35% of the high income areas in 1971, but this number fell to 28% in 2005 (Hulchanski, 2007). Within the low income areas, immigrant families rose from 31% in 1971 to 61% in 2005. Additionally, immigrants are negatively impacted because of the movement of impoverished neighborhoods to the outskirts of the city borders where it is geographically less desirable because of less access to reliable, efficient transit and services needed by families. Although studies provide insights into the poverty faced by immigrant populations in Toronto—the largest settlement city for immigrants in Canada, one can expect similar situations across the country given the well-known challenges immigrant face in the labor market and in having professional credentials recognized. Immigrant families are also reluctant to move away from Toronto and the province, as living in these areas gives them benefits that other areas may not, such as better social support. There is also evidence that immigrants are moving in greater numbers to other Canadian cities to benefit from work available there. Nevertheless, the poverty identified by the aforementioned studies and the hardships in terms of obtaining adequate housing can have a detrimental impact on families and increase their vulnerability to child welfare intervention.

OVERVIEW OF IMMIGRANTS IN CANADA

Immigration over the past 40 years has increased substantially due to changes in Canada's immigration policy together with international events. Census 2006 reports that "foreign-born" persons represent one in five of the total population for a total of 6,186,950 persons (Statistics Canada, 2006). It appears to be the main driver for population growth, accounting for 69.3% of the growth from 2001 to 2006. Some argue that while this immigration rate is necessary for the nation's population growth and to drive the economy in terms of labor and capital, it may be changing the culture of Canada from a European origins (majority Caucasian) population to a racialized one (Bannerji, 2000). Driving this anxiety are the published statistics in the Census 2006 that the majority of recent immigrants from 2001 to 2006 were born in Asia and the Middle East (58.3%) with Central, South America, and the Caribbean providing 10.8% and Europe providing 16.1%—far less than racialized countries (Statistics Canada, 2011). Institutional and systemic racism at personal and individual levels has resulted in the term "immigrant" being used synonymously and sometimes derogatively to refer to racialized people, whether immigrant or not.

In July of 2010, the ruling conservative government in Canada enacted the far-reaching decision of replacing their "Longitudinal Survey of Immigrants to Canada" under an umbrella set of "Census of Population—Long Form" surveys, which have mandatory completion requirements of residents, to a shorter voluntary survey. The long form of the census survey was to be completed voluntarily, with the argument that this move would protect residents from the intrusion of a mandatory requirement to provide information. Thus the recent Census 2011 data collected by Statistics Canada did not include information on immigrants in Canada, and, at this time, Citizenship and Immigration Canada appears to be the most comprehensive source of data on immigrants in Canada. These data are limited as they are more focused on immigrants as newcomers to Canada and less on immigrants settled for longer periods. This shift will have drastic effects on the ongoing information that will be available about immigrants in Canada, and one can speculate about the government's reasons for this change.

Interesting changes have taken place in terms of source country where immigrants originate. Table 9.1 shows the changes from 2001 to 2010 of the top source countries from which immigrants (permanent residents who have as yet not obtained citizenship) arrived (www.cic.gc.ca/english/resources/statistics/facts2010/permanent/10.asp).

These changes can be surmised to an extent as reflective of the economic drive for labor and capital brought in by immigrants of these source countries and specific programs targeting them such as the Live-In Caregiver program, which brings in the majority of labor from the Philippines; however, other political issues also play into these decisions. Pakistan's drastic drop can be reflective of other global events such as the 9/11 terrorist attacks in the United States and the ensuing covert institutionalization of Islamphobia as part of the widespread antiterrorism measures (see Mountz, 2010, for discussion).

Some information on the place of birth of immigrant children under 15 years of age is available in Statistics Canada 2006 data and is shown in Table 9.2. The figures in Table 9.2 show the large number of immigrant children in Canada. Some of these children together with their families will come to the attention of the child welfare system.

Using Statistic Canada's Census 2006, figures in Table 9.3 show the number of different ethnic persons by age and urban residence. These figures highlight the immense ethnic diversity of the Canadian population.

Table 9.1. Changes in source countries of immigrants

Permanent residents by top five source countries				
Source country	2001	2010	% Increase	% Decrease
Philippines	12,928	36,578	183	
India	27,901	30,252	8	
China	40,365	30,197		25
United Kingdom	5,359	9,499	77	
Pakistan	15,353	6,213		60
United States	5,909	9,243	56	

Table 9.2. Immigrant children under age 15 and source countries, 2006

Source country	Number of children
China	39,315
United States	29,015
India	25,175
Philippines	20,780
Total Number of children born outside Canada	345,705

Source: Statistics Canada, 2006.

Table 9.3. Ethnic persons by age and urban residence

	Top ethnic groups under age 15			
	Montreal	Toronto	Calgary	Vancouver
Chinese	15,300	80,535	12,180	59,970
South Asian	17,585	169,215	14,085	47,435
Black	44,990	93,990	6,305	5,985
Filipino	4,580	36,355	5,810	17,050
Latin American	15,760	18,960	2,475	3,835
Southeast Asian	9,470	16,130	3,475	7,655
Arab	25,435	12,780	3,840	1,890
West Asian	2,845	14,875	1,400	4,125
Korean	1,090	9,165	1,605	8,905
Japanese	590	3,070	995	4,140

The diversity of the child population in Canada is also evident within statistics Canada. For example, the percentage of all children (ages zero to 14) who speak a mother tongue other than English or French ("Refers to the first language learned at home in childhood and still understood by the individual at the time of the census"; Statistics Canada, 2006) is as follows: Canada—14.7%, Calgary—17.3%, Montreal—17.8%, Toronto—30.5%, and Vancouver—31.7%.

SOCIAL WORK PRACTICE WITH IMMIGRANT FAMILIES: SURVEY FINDINGS

A total of 33 child welfare workers from the Toronto and surrounding area took part in an online survey. All reported experience working with immigrant families. Many workers themselves (45%, $n = 15$) were foreign born while

67% (*n* = 22) descended from foreign-born parents. Half the workers reported speaking the language of one of the immigrant groups with whom they worked, but it is not possible to assess whether they were fully fluent in the language and would be able to provide service in the language of their client. At the time of the survey, most of the workers reported having immigrant families on their caseload; however, the number of immigrants on their caseload was reported as being low—between one and three. This low number is likely the result of the survey being conducted in an area of Toronto that does not have a very high number of immigrant populations settled and would possibly change if the survey was completed by workers from areas with dense immigrant settlement. Predominant immigrant groups workers reported being on their caseloads include those from Asia, the Caribbean, and Africa, with a sizable number from South America and the Middle East and a small number from Eastern Europe followed by Western Europe.

The online survey comprised two case vignettes that required the respondents to identify the level of risk and make a decision on the type and nature of likely service provision they would offer. Vignette 1 concerned a marginalized unemployed immigrant family with a newborn baby (see appendix for vignette). Most workers reported that they would consider the risk in this family to be between moderate to very high. This risk is presented in the framework of prevention with 82% (*n* = 27), reporting that they would allow the child to remain in the parents' care and provide ongoing services. This speaks to the focus in the system on family preservation and unity and providing support services for families. Qualitative responses for reasons identifying level of risk included "age of child, family isolation, the lack of necessary amenities, being immigrants, and being young parents with a newborn." The small number who identified the risk as being low still raised concerns for the well-being of the child but identified strengths/positives in the family while showing concern for the safety of the child. Some comments made were "baby is healthy, mother is recovering well, poor housing condition, lack basic amenities, parents appear eager for positive change, motivated as they left country for a 'better' future." When given option of types of services that families would be referred to, some reported (*n* = 8) that they would assist the parents in becoming employed, while most reported that this was not an option in their system. This service may be one of those "soft" services where families are given information on connecting with employment agencies, a service that is voluntarily provided by workers. All reported that they would connect the family with welfare services to improve their financial situation as well as other community services. Sixteen of the 22 who responded reported that they would assist the family in finding housing with better amenities, with the rest reporting that this was not an option—perhaps a more accurate response given how busy child welfare workers are and the limited time to provide services. All except one reported providing access to other formal (public or statutory) services, suggesting a high level of concern for the child and a way to remain involved with the family even if the child would not be removed from the parents. Close to half of the workers responding ($n = 9/18$) indicated that they envisioned the family to be from a particular ethnic/cultural background, suggesting that workers may have some preconceived ideas about particular families.

When provided with a possibly value-laden option to encourage the family to return to their country of origin, 16 of 19 participants reported that they would not, while three reported that this was not an option in their system. When asked about the role of child welfare in situations of undocumented children, interestingly, although many workers recognized that an undocumented child was the responsibility of the child welfare authorities, 27% ($n = 9/33$) said that they were not and 21% ($n = 7/33$) responded that they did not know. Most reported that the interest of the child would supersede immigration concerns, while a small percentage noted that they did not know. Most workers responded that immigration concerns would not require resolution before child welfare concerns could be addressed, while a small number noted that they did not know. These mixed responses indicate a need for further training on legal matters relating to immigration and child welfare responsibilities as also noted earlier in the chapter.

In Vignette 2, we tested to see whether parental occupation status would alter social worker assessment. Two competing survey versions, 1 and 2 (employed versus unemployed parents, respectively) were issued of this vignette to different respondents. For both versions, the vast majority of social workers identified "moderate" to "high risk." A small difference was noted in responses where parents were employed versus unemployed: 5 of the 15 (33%) respondents for the vignette where parents were *unemployed* assessed the risk as "very high" compared to 3 of the 18 (17%) of the respondents choosing this option where parents were employed. Furthermore, 33% ($n = 5/15$) of respondents for the unemployed version of the survey compared to 11% ($n = 2/18$) for the employed parents also reported greater willingness to remove the 10-year-old from her family and start out-of-home placement plans. These findings need further exploration as it would appear that unemployment can result in a slightly higher level of risk being assessed and can perhaps lead to greater consideration of removal of a child from the caregiver's home.

All participants who responded to the survey had more than two years of experience working in the child welfare field with 39% ($n = 12$) having worked between three to seven years, 42% ($n = 13$) had 8 to 16 years, and 19% ($n = 6$) had 17 to 25 years. The vast majority of workers reported a university education in social work. In our survey, we asked about perceived competence in working with immigrant and nonimmigrant groups. Notably, 33% ($n = 11$) responded that they had not received training to work with immigrant populations—a surprising finding given the emphasis in social work and continuing education on competence in cultural and ethnic diversity related issues. Furthermore,

37% ($n = 12$) of respondents feel less competent working with immigrant families compared to nonimmigrant families, and 42% ($n = 14$) reported finding the work more challenging. Moreover, a large number of participants (79%; $n = 26$) highlighted that there were "more barriers" in working with immigrant families.

The sample size ($n = 33$) for the study was small, thus the findings must be viewed with caution and only as exploratory. However, the findings do begin to provide some insights into the struggles of child welfare workers in working with immigrant families. Surprisingly, some workers noted that they did not have training in working with immigrant families while a good number reported greater barriers when working with these families and thus found the work to be more challenging. Some difference between worker responses between employed families and unemployed families was also noted, suggesting a further examination of this issue. Knowledge and training on working with immigrant families and undocumented children is indicated from these findings, while studies with larger numbers would also be useful in providing better insights into these issues.

The topic of immigration and immigrants in Canada is laden. This, however, is not the case for all immigrants but for immigrants arriving from racialized countries. Earlier blatant racist immigration policies have been replaced by policies that are not overtly racist but continue to attempt to limit the arrival of immigrants from source countries that are seen as unfavorable but are essentially racialized countries, as can be seen in the earlier discussion of the changes in source countries from which immigrants are accepted. Racialized immigrants also continue to experience marginalization, exclusion, higher levels of poverty, and discrimination even into the second generation (Nakahie, 2006). Responding to criticism of inadequate services or a complete lack of services for families from diverse ethnoracial backgrounds, social service providers have been examining their responses to immigrant populations generally and to racialized immigrants specifically. Changes in practice approaches have taken place, resulting in a shift from earlier assimilation approaches to ethnic diversity to a multicultural perspective that embraces cultural sensitivity and cultural competency. Yet this approach also continues to have the potential to overlook the struggles experienced by individuals and families. Focusing on culture can lead to stereotyping and further blame on cultures for structural problems experienced by families. Disproportionate levels of poverty and settlement struggles, together with bias in reporting and substantiating maltreatment, can increase disproportionate representation of immigrant families on child welfare caseloads. Still, this should not be a sweeping indicator of differential approaches to parenting, as other structural issues also contribute to these numbers, as noted by researchers (Euser et al., 2011; Maiter et al., 2004, 2009).

Child welfare organizations have also taken the initiative to examine services to their racialized and immigrant families. The impact of these initiatives, however, remains unclear and needs further exploration. The child welfare service survey conducted as part of this study shows that the vast majority of workers reported experiencing "more barriers" when working with immigrant families; more than one-third feel less competent working with immigrant families compared to nonimmigrant families, and half find the work more challenging. While workers were cognizant of structural factors affecting the immigrant families on their caseloads, responses also indicate a need to improve knowledge on immigration-related matters.

NOTE

1 Statistics Canada (http://www.statcan.gc.ca/concepts/definitions/minority 01-minorite01a-eng.htm) in referring to the term "visible minority" notes: "This category includes persons who are non-Caucasian in race or non-white in colour and who do not report being Aboriginal," including black, Chinese, Latin American, Filipino, Korean, Arabic, South Asian, Southeast Asian, and Japanese.

REFERENCES

Ali, M.A., Taraban, S., & Gill, J.K. (2003). Unaccompanied/Separated Children Seeking Refugee Status in Ontario: A Review of Documented Policies and Practices. CERIS Working Paper 27. Toronto: CERIS.

Al-Krenawi, A., & Graham, J. (2003). *Cross-Cultural Social Work Practice with Diverse Ethno- Racial Communities in Canada*. Toronto: Oxford University Press.

Bannerji, H. (2000). *The Dark Side of the Nation: Essays on Multiculturalism, Nationalism and Gender*. Toronto: Canadian Scholars' Press.

Blackstock, C., Trocmé, N. & Bennett, M. (2004). Child welfare response to Aboriginal and non-Aboriginal child in Canada: A comparative analysis. *Violence Against Women*, 10(8), 901–906.

British Columbia Ministry of Children and Family Development. (2012). Protecting Children. Vancouver: Ministry of Children and Family Development. Retrieved December 18, 2012, from, http://www.mcf.gov. bc.ca/child_protection/index.htm

Canada and the World. (2011). *Canada's Racist Immigration Policies of the Past*. June. Retrieved July 20, 2012, from http://www.canadaandtheworld.com/ canadasracistimmigrationpolicies.html

CASWE-ACFTS Accreditation Standards—June 2013. Retrieved August 26/2014 from http://caswe-acfts.ca/commission-on-accreditation/coa-standards/

CBC News. (2012). Detention Centres No Place for Migrant Children, Critics Argue. Canada out of Step with Push to Keep Migrant Children out of

Detention Centres. Retrieved December 20, 2012, from http://www.cbc.ca/news/canada/story/2012/12/13/detention-children-canada.html

Chau, S., Fitzpatrick, A., Hulchanski, D., Leslie, B., & Schatia, D. (2001). *One in Five… Housing as a Factor in the Admission of Children to Care: New Survey of Children's Aid Society of Toronto Update 1992 Study*. Toronto: University of Toronto, Centre for Urban and Community Studies.

Dettlaff, A., & Rycraft, J. (2010). Factors contributing to disproportionality in the child welfare system: Views from the legal community. *A Journal of the Nation Association of Social Workers*, 55(3), 213–224.

Euser, E., IJzendoorn, M., Prinzie, P., & Bakermans-Kranenburg, M. (2011). Elevated child maltreatment rates in immigrant families and the role of socioeconomic differences. *Child Maltreatment*, 16(1), 63–73.

Fleury, D. (2007). A Study of Poverty and Working Poverty among Recent Immigrants to Canada. Catalogue no. SP-680-05-07E. Ottawa: Human Resources and Social Development Canada.

Hare, F.G. (2007). Transition without status: The experience of youth leaving care without Canadian citizenship. *New Directions for Youth Development*, 113, 77–88.

Hicks, S. (2009). *Social Work in Canada: An Introduction*. (3rd ed.) Toronto: Thompson Educational Publishing.

Hulchanski, J. (2007). *The Three Cities within Toronto: Income Polarization among Toronto's Neighbourhoods, 1970–2005*. Research Bulletin 41. Toronto: University of Toronto.

Lavergne, C., Dufour, S., Sarmiento, J., & Descoteaux, M.-E. (2009). La reponse du systeme de protection de la jeunesse montrealais aux enfants issus des minorities visibles (Response of Quebec's child protection system to visible minorities). J. Cookson & K. Montin (Trans.) *Intervention*, 131, 233–241. Retrieved December, 18, 2012 from http://www.centrejeunessedemontreal.qc.ca/recherche/PDF/Memento/5_EN_Lavergne_2011-08.pdf

Lavergne, C., Dufour, S., Trocmé, N., & Larrivée, M.-C. (2008). Visible minority, Aboriginal, and Caucasian children investigated by Canadian protective services. *Child Welfare*, 87(2), 23–86.

Leschied, A., Chiodo, D., Whitehead, P., & Hurley, D. (2003). *The Association of Poverty with Child Welfare Service and Child and Family Clinical Outcomes*. London: University of Western Ontario.

Leslie, B. (2005). Housing influences on child welfare: A practice response with service and policy implications. In J. Scott and H. Ward (Eds.), *Safeguarding and Promoting the Well-Being of Children, Families and Communities*, 36–59. London: Kingsley.

MacLaurin, B., Fallon, B., & Trocmé, N. (2003). Characteristics of investigated children and families referred for out-of-home placement. In K. Kufeldt & B. McKenzie (Eds.), *Child Welfare: Connecting Research, Policy and Practice*, 27–40. Waterloo, ON: Wilfrid Laurier University Press.

Maiter, S. (2009a). Social justice not assimilation or cultural competence. In J. Carrier & S. Strega (Eds.), *Walking this Path Together: Anti-Racist and Anti-Oppressive Practice in Child Welfare*. Halifax: Fernwood.

———. (2009b). Using an anti-racist framework for assessment and intervention in clinical practice. *Clinical Social Work*, 37, 267–276.

Maiter, S., Alaggia, R., & Trocmé, N. (2004). Perceptions of child maltreatment by parents from the Indian subcontinent: Challenging myths about culturally based abusive parenting practices. *Child Maltreatment*, 9(3), 309–324.

Maiter, S., Stalker, C., & Alaggia, R. (2009). The experiences of minority immigrant families receiving child welfare services: Seeking to understand how to reduce risk and increase protective factors. *Families in Society: The Journal of Contemporary Social Services*, 90(1), 28–36.

Matas, D. (1985). Racism in Canadian immigration policy. *Refugee*, 5(2), 8–9.

Mountz, A. (2010). *Seeking Asylum: Human Smuggling and Bureaucracy at the Border*. Minneapolis: University of Minnesota Press.

Nakhaie, R. (2006). A comparison of the earnings of the Canadian native-born and immigrants, 2001. *Canadian Ethnic Studies*, 38(2), 19–46.

Ontario Association of Children's Aid Societies (OACAS). (2006). Child Welfare in Ontario: Developing a Collaborative Intervention Model. Excerpts from a Position Paper submitted by the Provincial Project Committee on Enhancing Positive Worker Interventions with Children and their Families in Protection Services: Best Practices and Required Skills. Toronto: Ontario Association of Children's Aid Societies.

Pratt, A., & Valverde, M. (2002). From deserving victims to "masters of confusion": Redefining refugees in the 1990s. *The Canadian Journal of Sociology*, 27(2), 135–161.

Refugee and Immigration Staff Advisory Committee. (2004). Best Practices Guidelines for Serving Immigrant and Refugee Children, Youth and Families. Hamilton, ON: Catholic Children's Aid Society.

Statistics Canada. (2006). *Canada's Ethnocultural Mosaic, 2006 Census*. Catalogue no. 97-562-X. Ottawa. Retrieved May 25, 2012, from http://www12.statcan.ca/census-recensement/2006/as-sa/97-562/pdf/97-562-XIE2006001.pdf

———. (2011). *Population Growth in Canada: From 1851 to 2061, 2011 Census*. Catalogue no. 98-310-X2011003. Ottawa. Retrieved June 2, 2012, from http://www12.statcan.gc.ca/census-recensement/2011/as-sa/98-310-x/98-310-x2011003_1-eng.pdf

Swift, K. (2011). Canadian child welfare: Child protection and the status quo. In N. Gilbert, N. Parton, & M. Skivenes (Eds.), *Child Protection Systems: International Trends and Orientations*, 36–59. New York: Oxford University Press.

Thoburn, J. (2007). *Globalization and Child Welfare: Some Lessons from a Cross-National Study of Children in Out-of-Home Care*. Norwich: School of Social Work and Psychosocial Sciences, University of East Anglia.

Trocmé, M., Fallon, B., MacLaurin, B., Daciuk, J., Felstiner, C., Black, T., Tonmyr, L., Blackstock, C., Barter, K., Turcotte, D., & Cloutier. R. (2005). *Canadian Incidence Study of Reported Child Abuse and Neglect—2003: Major Findings.* Ottawa: Public Health Agency of Canada.

Trocmé, N., MacLaurin, B., Fallon, B., Daciuk, J., Tourigny, M., & Billingsley, D. (2001). The Canadian Incidence Study of Reported Child Abuse and Neglect: Methodology. *Canadian Journal of Public Health*, 92(4), 259–263.

United Nations High Commissioner for Refugees. (2000). *Refugee Children and Adolescents: A Progress Report.* Geneva: United Nations High Commissioner for Refugees. Retrieved December 8, 2012, from http://www.unhcr.org/cgi-bin/texis/vtx/home/opendocPDFViewer.html?docid=3bb3192da&query=Refugee

United Way of Greater Toronto. (2004). *Poverty by Postal Code: A Geography of Poverty 1981—2001.* Toronto: United Way of Greater Toronto.

Zapf, M. (2004). Concluding thoughts from social work. In N. Bala, M. Zapf, R. Williams, R. Vogl, & J. Hornick (Eds.), *Canadian Child Welfare Law: Children, Families and the State* (2d ed.), 409–419. Toronto: Thompson Educational Publishing.

10

CHILD WELFARE AND MIGRANT FAMILIES AND CHILDREN

A CASE STUDY OF ENGLAND

Ravinder Barn and Derek Kirton

INTRODUCTION

This chapter explores child welfare policy, practice, and provision in relation to migrant families and children in England. It is perhaps useful to offer a comment on our use of the term "migrant" here, not least as in an English context, "immigrant" is an overwhelmingly ethnicized, often racialized, and almost always highly politicized term. Many who migrated in the latter part of the twentieth century have established large and readily identifiable minority ethnic communities, while there is also a significant and growing number of "small communities" (Modood, 2007). It is also important to acknowledge the wide range of legal status, from citizenship and those with rights of refuge, settlement, or residence through to those who have an "irregular" status arising from refused asylum, overstaying, or illegal entry. The amalgam of temporal and legal variation creates an extremely diverse group of migrants, and we have chosen to consider the situations both of established minority ethnic groups and more recent migrants for two main reasons. The first is that there is considerable shared experience, as well as differences. A second and more pragmatic reason is that official and research data do not typically distinguish according to length of settlement or countries of origin. Where separate data are available or policy measures clearly apply to particular groups of migrants, this is made clear. Depending on the circumstances of arrival, settlement and subsequent life events, children's experiences of migration may be closely tied to those of their families or sharply separated.

Principally, five major areas are the subjects of consideration in this chapter—namely the English demographic context, law and policy, organization of child welfare systems, representation of migrant families and children in child welfare services, and social work practice. The latter includes findings from an online survey of child welfare social workers.

DEMOGRAPHICS

Since the Second World War, England has witnessed significant waves of immigration—from the Caribbean and the Indian subcontinent since the 1950s and other parts of the globe, including Africa, the Middle East, Bangladesh, and Sri Lanka, in the past few decades. Importantly, whilst scholars have documented that racial and cultural diversity has been a feature of England since the days of colonialism and slavery, and indeed there is evidence to suggest that black soldiers served in the Roman army over 2,000 years ago (Fryer, 1984), it is the recent concentration of migrant groups that is considered to be worthy of attention by law and policymakers and practitioners in the field of child welfare. Crucially, modern child welfare systems themselves are a relatively recent phenomena, pointing to the contextual and temporal nature of childhood, children's rights, and child welfare.

Patterns and Outcomes of Migration

The postwar period resulted in a crippled economy and a shortage of labor. Britain called upon its colonies and former colonies to help rebuild the mother country. The colonies and ex-colonies have been described by critics as places that were underdeveloped as a consequence of the harsh realities of slavery and colonialism (Sivanandan, 1976). Postwar migration led to the rebuilding project, but it also witnessed overt and covert racial discrimination in a range of areas from housing and employment to education and social services. Concentration of migrant families in rundown, poor neighborhoods was a direct consequence of employment opportunities, experiences of racism in housing and employment, poverty, and the desire to live among one's compatriots for reasons of safety and security and family and friends networks (Modood, Berthoud, and Nazroo, 1997). Today, migrant families are largely found in major urban conurbations such as London, the Midlands, Merseyside, and Bristol—places where there have been employment opportunities for newly arrived migrants.

Since legislation passed in the early 1970s (see section on law and policy) virtually ended all primary migration from the former colonies, continual migration from these areas has been largely a result of family reunion, labor migration, and refugee and asylum seeker arrivals. Attempts to end such family reunion migration by making migrant family forms and practices seem deviant appear to have been the concern of successive governments. An array of human rights abuses from the 'virginity tests' of the 1970s to the pathologization of migrant families as culturally dubious has been the state modus operandi to curb migration. It has been argued that immigration controls from the 1970s onward have encouraged other means of migration such as irregular migration and human trafficking (Boswell, 2005). Despite this controlling policy framework, however, family (re)unions based on the arrival of spouses, children, and other relatives remains a significant source of migration (Crawley, 2009).

Table 10.1 displays census data showing both the current ethnic profile of the population in England and the way this has changed in the early twenty-first century. The data reveal a broadly static white British and Irish population alongside significant growth in almost all minority groups. For a number of these groups—notably white other, black African, Asian other, Indian, Chinese, and other ethnic groups—the increase could largely be attributed to net migration. Conversely, for the mixed groups, the rise overwhelmingly reflects natural increase, while for groups such as Pakistani and Bangladeshi, there has been a relatively even split between the two factors (Office for National Statistics, 2011).

Table 10.1. Population by ethnic group: England and Wales, 2001–2011

Ethnic group	Population 2001	Population 2011	% Increase 2001–2011
White British	42,747,136	42,279,236	–1.1
White Irish	624,115	517,001	–17.2
White Other	1,308,110	2,484,905	90.0
Mixed White/Black Caribbean	231,424	415,616	79.6
Mixed White/Black African	76,498	161,550	111.2
Mixed White/Asian	184,014	332,708	80.8
Mixed other	151,437	283,005	86.9
Asian/British Asian: Indian	1,028,546	1,395,702	35.7
Asian/British Asian: Pakistani	706,539	1,112,282	57.4
Asian/British Asian: Bangladeshi	275,394	436,514	58.5
Asian/British Asian: Chinese	220,681	379,503	72.0
Asian/British Asian: Other	237,810	819,402	224.6
Black African	475,938	977,741	105.4
Black Caribbean	561,246	591,016	5.3
Black Other	95,324	277,857	191.5
Other groups	214,619	548,418	155.5
All ethnic groups	49,138,831	53,012,456	7.9

Source: Office for National Statistics, Neighbourhood Statistics Tables UV09 and QS201EW, 2012.

Varied data reveal that despite some fairly restrictive policies, there was a substantial rise in immigration during the new millennium. For example, average annual net migration to the United Kingdom (UK) was 195,000 between 2000 and 2011, compared to 65,000 in the 1990s (Vargas-Silva, 2013), while trends of settlement (permission to live in the UK without being subject to immigration control) were broadly similar (Blinder, 2012). Similarly, the Office for National Statistics (2012) indicates that from 2001 to 2011 the population in England and Wales born outside the UK rose from 4.6 million to 7.5 million (9%), though regionally, the figures range from 37% in London to 5% in the northeast of England. Rising immigration stemmed from a combination of increased asylum seeking, the effects of a globalized labor market, and, perhaps most dramatically, the enlargement of the European Union, although study remains the most common reason (Vargas-Silva, 2013). According to the Annual Population Survey, there were over 2 million European Union citizens living in the UK in the year to March 2011, while almost 40% of overseas workers obtaining National Insurance Numbers between 2004 and 2010 came from the eight Eastern European accession states (Sumption and Somerville, 2010). Increased migration from Europe, the rapid growth of mixed ethnicity groups, and diversification of countries of origin (including for asylum claims) have led to what some authors have referred to as "superdiversity" (Vertovec, 2007). In this context, it is also important to acknowledge the phenomenon of "irregular" migration, an umbrella term used to describe various situations in which migrants are living in England without authorization (e.g., overstaying on a visa, having asylum refused, or having entered illegally, including through trafficking). Inevitably, this is a somewhat "hidden" population but has been estimated for the UK at over 600,000, including 120,000 children, over half of them born in the country (Sigona and Hughes, 2012). Although their circumstances vary widely, irregular migrant children and families face obvious vulnerabilities in terms of access to services and for many the pressures of evading detection and possible deportation. Access to compulsory education has been found to be relatively straightforward but pre- and postcompulsory education more problematic, while access to health services is largely limited to primary and emergency care (Sigona and Hughes, 2012).

Data on ethnicity and age from the 2011 Census confirm that since migrants tend to be generally young and healthy, it is not surprising to find that the birth rate among migrant families is high. As a consequence, some black and minority ethnic communities are relatively young; for instance, almost two-fifths of the population within the Pakistani and Bangladeshi groups are between the ages of zero and 17, whilst the figure is even higher among those of mixed ethnicity at 49% (Office for National Statistics, 2013). These figures reflect the dominant tendency to collate official data in terms of ethnicity rather than migration. However, Crawley (2009) reports analysis of the 2001 Census that showed that around one in six children were in immigrant families (defined as having at least one parent born outside the UK), of whom a fifth had also been born outside the UK. Although no updated figures are available from the 2011 Census, it appears almost certain that these figures will have risen in the intervening decade.

Migration to Britain from within Europe and from non-Organisation for Economic Co-operation and Development countries presents a challenge in a number of ways, from concerns about pressures on public services to a shared national identity and social cohesion. Such concerns are shared with other European neighbors as Europe as a region now surpasses North America in its migrant population. According to the International Organisation on Migration (2003), there were 56.1 million migrants in Europe compared to 40.8 million in North America. It would appear that although European countries need migrant labor, they continue to manifest an ambivalence about migrants from some parts of the globe, particularly those coming from non-Organisation for Economic Co-operation and Development (non-OECD) countries. Boswell (2005: 5) reports that "anti-immigrant sentiment has manifested itself in public support for restrictive immigration and asylum policies, negative reporting on immigrants and asylum-seekers in the popular press, discrimination against resident ethnic minority groups, and racist or anti-immigrant harassment and violence."

LAW AND POLICY

In addition to laws and policy that restrict immigration and keep a check on eligibility for British citizenship, Britain has an array of legislation in the areas of nondiscrimination. This section outlines law and policy as it applies to migrant families.

A brief historical sketch is that whilst the 1948 Nationality Act afforded British citizenship to all residing in British colonies and provided work opportunities for others in ex-colonies to help postwar reconstruction (noted previously), there has been a catalogue of restrictive immigration laws since that period. Given the British self-image of being a fair and tolerant nation, Britain passed antidiscrimination laws during the 1960s and 1970s whilst simultaneously introducing restrictive immigration legislation. Such a twin approach was captured in Labour Minister Roy Hattersley's aphorism in 1965—"without integration, limitation is inexcusable; without limitation, integration is impossible." Law and policy in relation to integration has been hampered by a number of key factors, including lack of clarity about the meaning of integration, economic factors, and the ongoing appetite for politicians to exploit immigration as a populist electoral issue. Whilst antidiscrimination laws since the 1960s have existed to combat overt and covert acts of racial discrimination, in 2010 a new act was passed that reflects the need to address discrimination on different levels in a more holistic fashion. The Equality Act 2010 incorporates nine previous pieces of legislation in the areas of race, sex, age, religion, disability, and sexual orientation, seeking to strengthen previous legislation in protecting individuals from unfair treatment whilst promoting equality in society.

In the area of child welfare, British law has recognized multiculturality since the passing of the 1989 Children Act s22(5)(c), which stipulates that when making decisions in respect of children, an authority "shall give due consideration...to the child's religious persuasion, racial origin and cultural and linguistic background." This principle was adhered to in subsequent legislation for some time. However, in a bid to increase adoption rates for minority ethnic children in state care, the government, in England, in spite of oppostition from child welfare experts, has now repealed the relevant sub-section of the Adoption and Children Act 2002 which gave 'due consideration to...religious persuasion, racial origin and cultural and linguistic background'. Thus, the importance of ethnicity is now diminished in the new Children and Families Act 2014. (For a discussion of these plans and their weak evidence base, see Barn and Kirton, 2012).

Working with Refugee and Asylum-Seeking Children and Young People

Whilst some minority ethnic groups continue to experience multiple social and economic problems, including social exclusion, poverty, unemployment, poor-quality housing, discrimination, and problematic access to public services, this situation is particularly exacerbated for refugees and asylum seekers. Over the past two decades, the lives of child asylum seekers have been profoundly shaped by a wider climate of hostility, reflecting successive governments' priorities to minimize the number of people granted refugee status and deter requests for asylum. A succession of laws has progressively tightened the conditions for application, reduced and removed entitlement to social benefits and housing, prevented asylum seekers from working, and restricted rights of appeal (Sales, 2007). Under the Asylum and Immigration Act 1999, a policy of dispersal has been practiced in order to ease financial burdens on key geographical areas (typically near points of entry to the UK) with high numbers of asylum seekers. However, as Beirens, Mason, Spicer, Hughes, and Hek (2006) argue, the dispersal policy has fostered isolation among refugee and asylum-seeking families, housing them in neighborhoods with previously small minority ethnic populations. It is argued that services in those areas are often not aware of, nor geared to address, the variety of different needs of these groups.

The treatment of children depends crucially on whether they are seeking asylum as part of a family or alone. However, in both instances, there are deep tensions between the workings of immigration law and the legal framework for child welfare. In the case of children with their families, two key issues have arisen. The first is that families have often been held in detention centers, sometimes on initial reception but also pending possible deportation. A report on behalf of the Children's Commissioner found that roughly 2,000 children were subject to detention each year (11 Million, 2009). Conditions for children in such centers and poor provision in areas such as education have been severely criticized by both prison inspectors and children's rights organizations along with their experiences of arrest and locked transportation. Rights activists reject the principle of administrative detention and contend that the UK is in breach of the United Nations Convention on the Rights of the Child by failing to use detention as a "last resort" (11 Million, 2009; Children's Rights Alliance, 2011). In response to campaigning, the coalition government has pledged to phase out the use of detention for children but has yet to do so.

Second, such was the strength of UK governments' prioritization of immigration matters that for many years this was a "reserved" area (in effect an opt out) of their compliance with the United Nations Convention on the Rights of the Child, although this reservation was formally lifted in 2008. The prioritization of deterrence over child welfare was equally apparent in Section 9 of the Asylum and Immigration (Treatment of Claimants) Act 2002, which prohibited child social care agencies from offering help to families seeking asylum, instead offering only for the child(ren) to be received into state care if their needs could not be met. The thrust of the policy—namely that intact families will not be supported to stay within the UK—is clear but equally clearly in contravention of duties under the Children Act 1989 to keep families together wherever possible (Cunningham and Tomlinson, 2005). Once again, however, campaigners have enjoyed some success in challenging this prioritization, notably through Section 55 of the Borders, Citizenship and Immigration Act 2009, which imposes a legal duty on the UK Border Agency to safeguard and promote the welfare of children in carrying out its work.

In certain respects, unaccompanied children and young people seeking asylum may fare better in terms of services under the Children Act 1989 but nonetheless often face significant difficulties in addition to those emotional and psychological challenges arising from their experiences in countries of origin, the migration process, or life in the UK (Kohli, 2007; Chase, Knight, and Statham, 2008). Moreover, policy remains crucially framed by wider immigration and asylum concerns, emphasizing dispersal and preparation for return to the country of origin (Border and Immigration Agency, 2008). Whether due to deterrence or not, a recent written Parliamentary answer indicates a sharp fall in new unaccompanied asylum seeking children (UASC) applications, from 4,285 in 2008 to 1,717 in 2010 (WA325 1.2.12). Gateways to services crucially depend on age determination and legal status. Typically young asylum seekers do not bring proof of age with them, and hence this has to be gauged through processes often including extensive interviewing and medical examination. Needless to say, this is a difficult process and while there are undoubtedly some over the age of 18 who are treated as children, the reverse is also true (Lane and Tribe, 2006).

UASC may receive help by one of two routes. The first, under Section 20 of the Children Act 1989, involves them being accommodated, typically for younger children in either foster or residential care, with bed and breakfast or hostel accommodation often used for those ages 16 and 17. In March 2012, there were 2,150 unaccompanied asylum seekers within the looked after children population. Nearly 90% of these were male and 75% ages 16 or 17 (Department for Education, 2012b). Looked-after status should guarantee access to leaving care services, but UASC often reach 18 without having their asylum claims accepted, which, apart from them facing the threat of deportation, has the effect of making it very difficult to pursue further or higher education routes (Lane and Tribe, 2006). Prior to 2003, 16- and 17-year-olds often received help under Section 17 of the Children Act 1989, in effect giving them fewer entitlements, but a judicial review known as the Hillingdon judgment (*R [Beher and others] v Hillingdon Borough Council* [2003] EWHC 2075 [Admin]) directed that they too should be dealt with under Section 20 or receive equivalent services. However, cost pressures on local authorities mean that they are sometimes keen to divest themselves of responsibilities for UASC at the earliest opportunity. Nonetheless, the Hillingdon judgment has had a significant impact in increasing the availability of accommodation and leaving care services for UASC (Wade, Sirriyeh, Kohli, and Simmonds, 2012).

Yet despite some positive moves, the pressures facing young asylum seekers approaching 18 may be acute. In addition to potential loss of support from local authorities, many face continuing uncertainty regarding their claims for asylum, prompting some to go "missing" from care or leaving care services. As Pinter (2012) charts, these developments have led to increasing experiences of destitution on the part of young migrants and associated vulnerabilities to homelessness and/or exploitation. Such experiences may be equally if not more common for irregular migrants or those in private fostering placements (which include many unaccompanied migrant children) if family support is lacking (Shaw et al., 2010; Sigona and Hughes, 2012). In some situations, this can lead to children becoming stateless (Adesina, 2012).

ORGANIZATION OF CHILD WELFARE SYSTEM

In Britain, Children's Departments were founded in 1948 as a consequence of the death of 13-year-old Dennis O'Neill who was killed in 1945 at the hands of his foster carers. With the introduction of the 1948 Children Act, local authorities were under a duty to "receive the child into care" in cases of abuse and neglect. Subsequent legislation enhanced local authority powers to investigate neglect and take preventive action to support families. Over the years, the distinctions between children who were abused, neglected, and deprived from others who were considered to be in "moral danger" and "young offenders" have been somewhat blurred. A key piece of legislation was the 1989 Children Act, which sought to balance and strengthen support for families and children in need. The notion of "significant harm" was a central feature of this act. This refers to "ill-treatment or the impairment of health or development" or if the child or young person is considered to be "beyond parental control."

Following its implementation, there have been consistent tensions between the Children Act's emphasis on supporting (birth)families and protecting children by removing them from the family if necessary. High-profile deaths of children both before the act and since have tended to stress this protective role but, according to critics, have also prompted a defensive, proceduralized practice on the part of professionals. A consistent theme has been to improve communication and coordination between agencies, including health, education, police, and social care services. The death of eight-year-old Victoria Climbié (herself a migrant child brought to England by an aunt who, with her partner, went on to kill her) in 2000 was followed by the Laming inquiry and the Labour government's *Every Child Matters* Green Paper (Chief Secretary to the Treasury, 2003). This initiative again emphasized interagency coordination, to be aided by shared communication and a national database (later withdrawn by the coalition government) allowing all children to be tracked and concerns about them recorded. Specific reference was made in the Green Paper regarding UASC, although the emphasis on support and coordination with immigration services also included promotion of a de facto "dispersal" policy. Moreover, the overall framework, which models itself on the public health approach, has been criticized for its acontextual treatment of risk factors (France and Utting, 2005).

Another high-profile child death, that of Peter Connelly in 2008, prompted a potentially more radical review of child protection work by Professor Eileen Munro. Her recommendations are designed to help shift the child protection system from being "over-bureaucratised and concerned with compliance to one that keeps a focus on whether children are being effectively helped and protected" (Munro, 2011: 6). However, implementation to date has been patchy, and it remains to be seen how far the promised refocusing will be achieved. What is now evident is that Baby Peter's death sparked a steady rise in referrals, child protection plans, and children being taken into public care, as can be seen in Table 10.2.

While is it difficult to attribute such an increase entirely to the Baby Peter tragedy, the figures do reveal a problematic and point to a picture of insecurity, uncertainty, fear, and risk where allocation of blame has become individualized when systems of governmentality fail. The trend of increased child protection referrals and plans can also be seen to enjoy government support, evident in a recent speech by Secretary for Education Michael Gove (2012) in which he called for more decisive action to remove children from neglectful environments (Rogowski, 2012).

Table 10.2. Referrals, child protection plans, and children looked after, year ending March 2008–2012

Year	2008	2009	2010	2011	2012
Number of referrals	538,500	547,000	603,700	615,000	605,100
Number of child protection plans	34,000	37,900	39,100	42,700	42,900
Number of children looked after	59,400	60,900	64,400	65,520	67,050

Source: Department for Education, 2012b.

It should be noted that the reach and gaze of the child welfare system has extended over the past two decades, often in response to campaigning on the part of children's organizations. A pertinent example relating to migration is the recognition given to the trafficking of children into the UK (Beddoe, 2007), although a recent report on modern slavery has highlighted continuing shortcomings in the identification and treatment of those trafficked, who are often treated with suspicion or criminalized (Slavery Working Group, 2013).

For a detailed description of the organization of child welfare systems in England, see the comprehensive account provided by Nigel Parton and David Berridge in the book *Child Protection Systems* (Gilbert, Parton, and Skivenes, 2011).

REPRESENTATION OF MIGRANT BACKGROUND CHILDREN IN THE CHILD WELFARE SYSTEM

In England, research and government statistical evidence has consistently pointed to the disproportionate representation of some minority ethnic children in the child welfare system. It is useful to point out that with the exception of UASC, the word "migrant" or "immigrant" is not employed to refer to these children. Instead, along with other descriptive characteristics, children's ethnic background is recorded by local authorities, and this data is made available at a local and national level.

Children in Need

Under the 1989 Children Act, local authorities are under a duty to provide services to children considered to be in need in their areas to promote child safety and well-being. Although under the Children (Leaving Care) Act 2000, the duties of local authorities have been extended to young people over the age of 18, in general terms those between the ages of zero and 18 are considered children. Local authorities are required to identify the extent of need in their areas and to make decisions about level of services to be provided to help achieve or maintain a reasonable standard of health or development, to prevent significant or further harm to health or development, and to provide for children who are disabled.

In March 2012, a total of 369,410 children were considered to be in need in England. Of these, 73% were white, 6.9% were black or black British, 6.7% were mixed, 5.4% were Asian or British Asian, and 2.2% were of other ethnicity. The ethnicity of 5.6% ($n = 21,460$) of the children was not known (Department for Education, 2012a). Compared to their figures in the total child population (which is 4.9% black/black British and 5.2% mixed ethnicity), children of black/black British and mixed parentage are more likely to be among the "in need" statistics, although this ratio has fallen in recent years. Research has suggested that black and minority ethnic families often receive poorer "preventive" services than their white counterparts or face ethnocentric provision (Barn, 1993; Thoburn, Chand, and Procter, 2004). Little is known about the experiences of recent migrants. Within official data collection, reporting categories are based purely on ethnicity and are very broad-brush (e.g., white, black, Asian). It is highly likely, however, that children from migrant families may be underrepresented in relation to their levels of need, either due to lack of awareness of services or (especially in the case of irregular migrants) a desire to avoid contact with "the authorities." As was noted earlier, asylum seekers were specifically excluded from receiving support *as families* under the Children Act 1989 Section 17.

Child Protection

British literature on child protection and ethnicity over the past two decades has seen a steady growth (see Thoburn et al., 2004, for a summary). Both research studies and official data have indicated patterns of overrepresentation among child protection cases of children from mixed and black/black British backgrounds and typically underrepresentation from their (British) Asian peers (Barn, Sinclair, and Ferdinand, 1997). Government statistics reveal a similar profile, showing that in March 2012, of the 42,850 children who had a child protection plan, 75.9% were white, 7.9% were of mixed background, 5.4% were Asian or Asian British, 4.9% were black or black British, and 1.2% were of "other" ethnicity. In 4.6% of the cases, ethnicity was not known (Department for Education, 2012a). However, official statistics on ethnicity must be treated with caution as they are decontextualized in terms of social class, religion, and length of stay in the UK. Moreover, there has been significant debate as to the reasons for this pattern. For instance, some studies have found that minority ethnic children are more likely to suffer physical abuse due to harsh punishment (sometimes involving the use of implements), but a wider nonclinical population study found no significant differences in physical punishment between different groups (Barn, Ladino, and Rogers, 2006). Similarly, set alongside a strongly ethnicized official data, wider population studies have found relatively few such differences in self-reported maltreatment (Cawson, 2002).

Such apparent discrepancies have raised questions about the operation of the child protection system. Evidence on this remains fairly limited, although it is known that there are instances both of ethnocentric application of "white" norms and cultural relativism that may lead to over- and underinvolvement, respectively (Channer and Parton, 1990). For example, the inquiry into the death of Victoria Climbié heard allegations that her fearful demeanor in the presence of her aunt was (mis)interpreted "culturally" as respect. Some minority ethnic communities may be less willing to report cases of abuse due to concerns with family honor, ostracization, or fear of racist treatment (Bernard and Gupta, 2008), but research by Brophy, Jhutti-Johal, and Owen (2003) found that, once involved, minority ethnic families were often drawn more deeply into the child protection system than their white counterparts. In a context when the workings of ethnicity and cultural difference in and upon families are highly contested (Modood et al., 1997), Barn et al. (1997) found that in general, white practitioners and managers emphasized culture as the key concern, while minority ethnic professionals deemphasized culture and placed greater stress on issues of race, racism, and Euro-centric thinking.

Relatively little is known about the treatment of (recent) migrants in the child protection system and the significant "hidden" population, including children in private fostering and irregular migrants, which gives rise to concerns that maltreatment may go unrecognized. The system itself has undergone important changes, for example framing female genital mutilation as a form of child abuse rather than as an acceptable "traditional" practice (London Safeguarding Children Board, 2009) and attempting to address abuse linked to faith groups and beliefs in witchcraft (Department for Education, 2012c). However, the continuing prioritization of immigration control has led critics to argue that important child protection concerns are often neglected when immigration claims are being dealt with (Crawley, 2012).

Children Looked After

Since 1954, when the National Children's Home published a study titled *The Problem of the Coloured Child*, there has been concern about the situation of minority ethnic children in the child welfare system. Over the years, a plethora of research evidence, albeit based on localized studies, has consistently pointed to the high rates of entry of some minority ethnic children into the care system (Bebbington and Miles, 1989; Barn, 1993). With the current availaibility of government statistical data, pertaining to children "in need," on the child protection register, and those looked after, Owen and Statham (2009) confirmed previous findings in documenting the disproportionality of black/black British and mixed-parentage children

Table 10.3 shows the numbers of children looked after by ethnicity from 2008 to 2013 compared to their representation in the general child population.

Table 10.3. Looked-after status by ethnicity and year (%)

	2009	2010	2011	2012	2013	General child population (2011)
	Looked after children (%)					
White	76	76	77	78	78	78.5
Mixed	9	9	9	9	9	5.2
Asian or Asian British	5	5	5	4	4	9.5
Black or Black British	7	7	7	7	7	4.9
Other ethnic group	2	2	2	2	2	1.8

Source: Department for Education, 2012a.

A comparison of figures from the general child population and the looked-after population by ethnicity shows that children of mixed and black or black British background are disproportionately represented in the care system. For example, children of mixed-ethnicity background comprise 5% of the child population, yet they represent 9% of those who are looked after.

Government figures reveal that there were 2,150 UASC who were looked after as of March 31, 2012, a fall of 45% since 2009. The vast majority of the looked-after UASC are over 16 years of age, and most are male (87% in 2012). With respect to ethnicity, the main categories were "other Asian background" (40%) and "other ethnic group" (30%). Sixteen percent were of black African origin, a decrease from 31% in 2007. Such fluctuations point to global and geographical instability, which results in the movement of people. Crucial issues facing UASC are those of securing high-quality, culturally appropriate placements and, given the dominant age profile, effective transition planning.

SOCIAL WORK PRACTICE WITH MIGRANT FAMILIES—SURVEY FINDINGS

A total of 72 child welfare social workers contributed to data collection via an online survey from in and around London. The vast majority of the workers reported "working experience" with migrant families and children—predominantly with migrants from Africa, Asia, or Eastern Europe. Given the move toward the professionalization of social work in England over the past couple of decades, we were not surprised to learn that almost all of the social workers were qualified with the relevant social work qualification, that is, a bachelor's or master's in social work. Moreover, three-quarters of the sample reported that they had more than five years of relevant child welfare experience.

Almost 2 out of 10 workers described themselves as "foreign-born immigrants," while a quarter reported that their parents were foreign born. About a fifth reported a shared language with at least one of the immigrants groups with whom they worked. Crucially, 8 out of 10 workers did not speak the same language as the migrant family. Social work literature in the UK emphasizes the importance of good communication between practitioners and service users. The role of interpretation and translation services is well recognized in social care; however, increasing diversity presents its own challenges (Chand, 2005).

The online survey comprised two case vignettes that required respondents to identify the level of risk and make a decision on the type and nature of likely service provision they would offer. These vignettes are described in detail in the methodological appendix.

In assessing risk in Vignette 1 involving a small baby and her immigrant parents, the majority of the respondents identified "moderate" to "high" and "very high risk". Interestingly, this risk is presented in the paradigm of prevention, and almost all respondents demonstrate their decision making within a framework of family unity and integrity and the need for in-home service provision. Thus the vast majority expressed a preference in allowing the baby to continue to stay with the parents, and less than 10% reported that they would remove the baby from the parents. With regard to the immigration status of the family, it is instructive to note that the majority of the practitioners prioritized the interests of the newborn child over immigration issues. There is some confusion among the rest, however, where practitioners express ignorance and 15% also report that they would "encourage the family to return to their home country." Similarly, in response to a question about education and undocumented children, 86% of the practitioners stressed that an undocumented child not attending school would indeed be the responsibility of their child welfare system, but a small minority (12%) reported ignorance on this issue. The findings of confusion over immigration laws support a recent parliamentary committee that reported the disparate response from local authorities where some local authorities were "letting UKBA's desire for immigration control trump the welfare needs of children" (Solomon 2012: 9).

In Vignette 2, we tested to see whether parental employment status would alter social worker assessment. Two competing survey versions (employed vs. unemployed parents) were issued of this case to a different set of respondents. Interestingly, whilst the vast majority of social workers identified "moderate" to "high risk," the group to whom the parents were presented as "unemployed" reported greater willingness to remove the 10-year-old from her family and start out-of-home preparations for a substitute family placement. In other words, almost half of the sample where the parents were described as "unemployed" reported that they would remove the girl from her parents immediately or initiate preparations to remove her from her family compared to less than a third of the sample where the parents were presented as "employed." The impact of intersectionality, that is, the ways in which diverse axes of disadvantage and discrimination may militate against the best interests of individuals and groups, may be relevant here. Given the small size of this sample, however, it is not possible to view this difference in any conclusive way regarding parental employment status. More research is needed of this kind to determine the impact of parental involvement in the labor market and child welfare decision making.

An ongoing concern amidst the British social work profession is around the competency framework. This entails competency in assessing risk, knowledge of theories and models, and an understanding of broader structural disadvantage and discrimination along various social divisions in society, including social class, ethnicity, gender, disability, religion, and sexual orientation. In our survey, we asked about competence in working with immigrant and nonimmigrant groups. Interestingly, only half of the sample reported that they had received relevant training in relation to working with immigrants. A similar proportion stated that they felt "less competent" in working with immigrant families, whilst almost a third of the sample reported working with such groups as more challenging than nonimmigrant families. Moreover, an overwhelming proportion, almost 8 out of 10, workers highlighted that there were "more barriers" in working with immigrant families. Notably, the term "immigrant" is conceptually limited, temporal, contextual, and contested, and it is difficult to know how the respondents understood this category. It is surprising to learn, nevertheless, that a significant proportion of the sample reported a lack of training in working with immigrant groups, particularly given the historical focus on racial and cultural diversity in British social work education and training since the 1980s.

CONCLUSION

In conclusion, this chapter shows that over the past 60 years or so, England has become a society that comprises significant numbers of diverse ethnic groups. This diversity, which is a consequence of England's historical legacy in slavery and colonialism, is now accompanied by modern and increasing globalization, "rich north/poor south divide," and ongoing international wars and conflict.

Whilst England prides itself on its self-perceived values of fairness and tolerance, we can see that the experience of the vulnerable migrant family and child does not speak to this. Some migrant families are overrepresented as service users of child welfare services as a consequence of poverty, unemployment, poor housing, and the impact of these vulnerabilities on family functioning. The disproportionality of some migrant children in child welfare institutions and foster care has been witnessed as a consistent and growing trend for the past 60 years.

Arguably, English child welfare policy and practice has, over time, attempted to tackle disadvantage and discrimination. This is manifest in key pieces of legislation such as the Children Act 1989 s22(5)(c), which gives credence to a child's "religious, cultural, racial, and linguistic background" and advises practitioners to take these into consideration in their decision making. Since the 1980s, there has been recognition of the impact of racial discrimination and the importance of cultural sensitivity in social work education and training (de Waal & Shergill, 2004; Thompson, 2012). With the shift toward deracialization (see the Children and Families Act 2014), and increasing anti-immigrant and restrictive laws, however, a new landscape is taking shape (Williams & Johnson, 2010). The focus on racial and ethnic diversity in social work education has become significantly minimal as practitioners struggle to make sense of the tensions that exist between immigration and child welfare laws.

Our own survey findings show that half of our sample reported lack of relevant training to work with migrant groups and that they felt "less competent" in working with such groups. Moreover, we found that 8 out of 10 practitioners did not have a shared language with their migrant service users. Whilst the use of interpreters and translators in English social work practice is well known, it is also important to understand that the appropriateness and ready availability of skilled interpreters remain key concerns.

Allied to findings on training, this highlights the need for significant improvements in this area of work, with confusion over the interrelationship between immigration controls and child welfare amply highlighted in our survey. In relation to immigration and asylum, the ensuing tensions have been exacerbated by working within a framework that is widely seen as oppressive, exclusionary, and prioritizing immigration control over the welfare of children. Researchers such as Dunkerley, Scourfield, Maegusuku-Hewett, and Smalley (2005) have been critical of much social work practice for its "complicity" with such discriminatory policies. While specialist knowledge and training can contribute to improving practice in this area (Grady, 2004), our survey findings suggest that this is not available on anything approaching the scale required. Responses to the second vignette of the survey also show how, even in the abstract, questions of ethnicity and migration intersect with those linked to material standards and implicitly to social class.

Although it is difficult to gauge effects precisely, it is also important to acknowledge the broader turn in the early twenty-first century against multiculturalism and back toward assimilation. Albeit incorporating a range of perspectives, the primary critique of multiculturalism is that it has promoted "separatism"—allegedly influential in a range of phenomena from educational underachievement to rioting and the rise of Islamic extremism—and weakened social cohesion. Although such views have been forcefully and persuasively countered (Modood, 2007; Finney and Simpson, 2009), this has had limited impact on policy. A partial switch of focus toward migration from Eastern Europe is another important development. On the one hand, this can be seen to have deracializing effects on perceptions of and attitudes toward immigrants. On the other hand, however, this shift has witnessed a rising xenophobia—built around a range of moral panics linked to welfare benefits, employment, and housing—which impacts on both recent and established migrants.

In the current climate, it is difficult to be sanguine regarding the prospects for policy and practice in relation to migrant and minority ethnic families. Political and public discourse has been progressively deracialized—for example, with a de-emphasis on interpretation and translation of public services in minority community languages and with the removal of "ethnicity" as a consideration in adoption legislation—yet it is difficult to argue that this reflects a corresponding decline in racism. Instead, it can better be understood as manifesting a resurgence of assimilationist "color blindness," despite the latter's discredited past. For recent migrants, the environment is harsher—anti-immigrant policy and sentiment have become respectable, even "common sense" in ways that no longer apply to racism. This situation poses great challenges for social workers working with migrant and minority ethnic families, and their response remains to be seen.

REFERENCES

Adesina, Z. (2012). Children "with no state" in UK. BBC News, November 5. Retrieved March 16, 2013, from http://www.bbc.co.uk/news/uk-england-london-20186588.

Barn, R., & Kirton, D. (2012). Transracial adoption in Britain: Politics, ideology and reality. *Adoption and Fostering, 36*(2), 25–37.

Barn, R., Ladino, C., & Rogers, B. (2006). *Parenting in Multi-Racial Britain.* London: National Children's Bureau.

Barn, R., Sinclair, R., & Ferdinand D. (1997). *Acting on Principle: An Examination of Race and Ethnicity in Social Services Provision for Children and Families.* London: British Agencies for Adoption and Fostering.

Barn, R. (1993). *Black children in the public care system.* London: BT Batsford Limited.

Bebbington, A., & Miles, J. (1989). The background of children who enter local authority care. *British Journal of Social Work, 19*(1), 349–368.

Beddoe, C. (2007). *Missing Out: A Study of Child Trafficking in the North-West, North-East and West Midlands.* London: ECPAT UK.

Beirens, H., Mason, P., Spicer, N., Hughes, N., & Hek, R. (2006). *Preventive Services for Asylum Seeking Children.* Birmingham, UK: University of Birmingham.

Bernard, C., & Gupta, A. (2008). Black African children and the child protection system. *British Journal of Social Work*, 38(3), 476–492.

Blinder, S. (2012). *Settlement in the UK*. Oxford: Migration Observatory Briefings.

Border and Immigration Agency. (2008). *Better Outcomes: The Way Forward—Improving the Care of Unaccompanied Asylum Seeking Children*. London: Border and Immigration Agency.

Boswell, C. (2005). *Migration in Europe*. Hamburg: Hamburg Institute of International Economics.

Brophy, J., Jhutti-Johal, J., & Owen, C. (2003). *Significant Harm: Child Protection Litigation in a Multi-Cultural Setting*, London: Department for Constitutional Affairs.

Cawson, P. (2002). *Child Maltreatment in the Family: The Experiences of a National Sample of Young People*. London: National Society for the Prevention of Cruelty to Children.

Chand, A. (2005). Do you speak English? Language barriers in child protection social work with minority ethnic families, *British Journal of Social Work*, 35(6), 807–821.

Channer, Y., & Parton, N. (1990). Racism, cultural relativism and child protection. In Violence Against Children Study Group (Ed.), *Taking Child Abuse Seriously: Contemporary Issues in Child Protection Theory and Practice*, 104–120. London: Unwin Hyman.

Chase, E., Knight, A., & Statham, J. (2008). *The Emotional Well-Being of Unaccompanied Young People Seeking Asylum in the UK*. London: British Association for Adoption and Fostering.

Children's Rights Alliance England. (2011). *The State of Children's Rights in England 2011: Review of Government Action on United Nations' Recommendations for Strengthening Children's Rights in the UK*. London: Children's Rights Alliance for England.

Crawley, H. (2009). *The Situation of Children in Immigrant Families in the United Kingdom*. Florence: UNICEF.

———. (2012). *Working with Children and Young People Subject to Immigration Control Guidelines for Best Practice*. London: Immigration Law Practitioners' Association.

Cunningham, S., & Tomlinson, J. (2005). "Starve them out": Does every child really matter? A commentary on Section 9 of the Asylum and Immigration (Treatment of Claimants, etc.) Act, 2004. *Critical Social Policy*, 25(2), 253–275.

Department for Education. (2012a). *Characteristics of Children in Need in England*, 2011–12. London: Department for Education.

———. (2012b). *Children Looked After by Local Authorities in England (Including Adoption and Care Leavers)—Year Ending 31 March 2011*. London: Department for Education.

———. (2012c). *National Action Plan to Tackle Child Abuse Linked to Faith or Belief*. London: Department for Education.

de Waal, M., & Shergill, S. (2004). Recognising and celebrating children's cultural heritage. In V. White and J. Harris (Eds.), *Developing Good Practice in Children's Services*, 124–136. London: Jessica Kingsley.

Dunkerley, D., Scourfield, J., Maegusuku-Hewett, T., & Smalley, N. (2005). The experiences of frontline staff working with children seeking asylum. *Social Policy and Administration*, 39(6), 640–652.

11 Million. (2009). *The Children's Commissioner for England's Follow Up Report to the Arrest and Detention of Children Subject to Immigration Control*. London: 11 Million.

Finney, N., & Simpson, L. (2009). *"Sleepwalking to Segregation"? Challenging Myths about Race and Migration*. Bristol: Policy Press.

France, A., & Utting, D. (2005). The paradigm of "risk and protection-focused prevention" and its impact on services for children and families, *Children and Society*, 19(2), 77–90.

Fryer, P. (1984). *Staying Power: The History of Black People in Britain*. London: Pluto Press.

Gilbert, N., Parton, N., & Skivenes, M., eds. (2011). *Child Protection Systems: International Trends and Emerging Orientations*. New York: Oxford University Press.

Gove, M. (2012). The Failure of Child Protection and the Need for a Fresh Start. London: Department for Education. Retrieved November 20, 2012, from www.education.gov.uk/inthenews/speeches/a00217075/gove-speech-on-child-protection.

Grady, P. (2004). Social work responses to accompanied asylum-seeking children. In D. Hayes and B. Humphries (Eds.), *Social Work, Immigration and Asylum: Debates, Dilemmas and Ethical Debates for Social Work and Social Care Practice*, 132–150. London: Jessica Kingsley.

International Organization on Migration. (2003). *World Migration 2003, Managing Migration: Challenges and Responses for People On the Move*. Geneva: International Organization on Migration.

Kohli, R. (2007). *Social Work with Unaccompanied Asylum Seeking Children*. Basingstoke: Palgrave.

Laird, S. (2008). *Anti-Oppressive Social Work: A Guide for Developing Cultural Competence*. London: SAGE.

Lane, P., & Tribe, R. (2006). Unequal care: An introduction to understanding UK policy and the impact on asylum-seeking children. *International Journal of Migration, Health and Social Care*, 2(2), 7–14.

London Safeguarding Children Board. (2009). *London Female Genital Mutilation Resource Pack*. London: London Safeguarding Children Board.

Modood, T. (2007). *Multiculturalism: A Civic Idea*. Cambridge: Polity.

Modood, T., Berthoud, R., & Nazroo J. (1997). *Ethnic Minorities in Britain: Diversity and Disadvantage*. London: Policy Studies Institute.

Munro, E. (2011). *The Munro Review of Child Protection Final Report: A Child-Centred System*. (Cm8062). London: Department for Education.

Office for National Statistics. (2011). *Current Estimates, Population Estimates by Ethnic Group Mid-2009 (Experimental)*. London: Office for National Statistics. Retrieved September 23, 2012, from www.ons.gov.uk/ons/publica-tions/re-reference-tables.html?edition=tcm%3A77-50029.

———. (2012). *International Migrants in England and Wales, 2011*. London: Office for National Statistics.

———. (2013). *2011 Census: Ethnic Group by Sex by Age*. Retrieved August 23, 2013, from www.nomisweb.co.uk/census/2011/DC2101EW.

Owen, C., & Statham, J. (2009). *Disproportionality in Child Welfare: Prevalence of Black and Ethnic Minority Children within "Looked After" and "Children in Need" Populations and on Child Protection Registers in England*. London: Department for Children, Schools and Families.

Pinter, I. (2013). *"I Don't Feel Human": Experiences of Destitution among Young Refugees and Migrants*. London: Children's Society.

Rogowski, S. (2012). Social Work with Children and Families: Challenges and Possibilities in the Neo-Liberal World. *British Journal of Social Work*, 42(5), 921–940.

Sales, R. (2007). *Understanding Immigration and Refugee Policy: Contradictions and Continuities*. Bristol: Policy Press.

Shaw, C., Brodie, I., Ellis, A., Graham, B., Mainey, A., de Sousa, S., & Willmott, N. (2010). *Research into Private Fostering*. London: National Children's Bureau.

Sigona, N., & Hughes, V. (2012). *No Way Out, No Way In: Irregular Migrant Children and Families in the UK*. Oxford: Centre on Migration, Policy and Society.

Sivanandan, A. (1976). Race, class and the state: The black experience in Britain. *Race and Class*, 17(4), 347–368.

Slavery Working Group. (2013). *It Happens Here: Equipping the United Kingdom to Fight Modern Slavery*. London: Centre for Social Justice.

Solomon, E. (2012). Destitution among asylum-seeking and migrant children. Education Committee, Oral evidence, July 4. London: UK Parliament. Retrieved January 23, 2013, from http://www.publications.parliament.uk/pa/cm201213/cmselect/cmeduc/uc149-i/uc14901.pdf.

Sumption, M., & Somerville, W. (2010). *The UK's New Europeans: Progress and Challenges Five Years after Accession*. Policy Report. Manchester: Equality and Human Rights Commission.

Thoburn, J., Chand, A., & Procter, J. (2004). *Child Welfare Services for Minority Ethnic Families*. London: Jessica Kingsley.

Thompson, N. (2012). *Anti-Discriminatory Practice: Equality, Diversity and Social Justice*. Basingstoke: Palgrave.

Vargas-Silva, C. (2013). *Long-Term International Migration Flows to and from the UK*. Oxford: Migration Observatory Briefings.

Vertovec, S. (2007). Super-diversity and its implications. *Ethnic and Racial Studies*, 30(6), 1024–1054.

Wade, J., Sirriyeh, A., Kohli, R., & Simmonds, J. (2012). *Fostering Unaccompanied Asylum Seeking Children: Creating a Family Life across a "World of Difference."* London: British Association for Adoption and Fostering.

Williams, C., & Johnson, M. (2010). *Race and Ethnicity in a Welfare Society*. Maidenhead: Open University Press.

11

CHILD PROTECTION OF MIGRANTS IN AUSTRALIA

Ilan Katz

INTRODUCTION

Since its settlement, Australia has been a country that has attracted large numbers of migrants. As of June 30, 2011, 27% of the estimated resident population was born overseas, and half had at least one parent born overseas (ABS, 2012). The largest group of migrants was from the United Kingdom (UK) followed by New Zealand, China, India, and Vietnam. Australia has also become ethnically diverse, with migrants coming from virtually every country in the world. Although migrants make up a large proportion of the population, Australia has a history of suspicion and hostility toward migrant populations, especially those from non-English-speaking backgrounds. Migration, and especially the treatment of refugees and asylum seekers, has always been a difficult and contested area of policy in Australia.

The history of the child protection system (CPS) in Australia has also been complex and challenging and has been intertwined with the colonial history of the country itself. This is perhaps best illustrated by the fact that in recent years the Australian government has apologized to various groups of people who have been harmed by the CPS, including Indigenous Australian children forcibly removed from their families, "Forgotten Australians" who were brought to Australia from the UK as children, often under false pretences, the victims of forced adoptions, which were prevalent until the 1970s, and victims of abuse in institutions, particularly those run by churches. This history has had a profound effect on the CPS.

The CPS in Australia, as in most other English-speaking countries, is categorized as a "residual" or "child protection" system (Gilbert, Parton, and Skivenes, 2011; Hetherington, Cooper, Smith, and Wilford, 1997; Higgins and Katz, 2008). In essence this means that the system is primarily focused on identifying and assessing the risk of abuse to children and intervening to protect children, rather than addressing child protection as part of a broader spectrum of family support interventions. In this way Australia is similar to other English-speaking countries such as the United States, Canada, and the UK.

In this chapter I describe the CPS in Australia and how it operates. A particular focus of the chapter is the situation of Indigenous Australians in the system, because the system has been shaped to a large extent by its impact on Indigenous children and families. I then go on to briefly describe the history of migration in Australia and current migration policies before focusing specifically on the current state of knowledge about child protection with migrant families in Australia. Despite the large numbers of migrants in Australia, relatively little is known about migrant children in the CPS, and child protection of children from migrant families has not been a key focus of policy or research. The research that has been done indicates that child protection policies and practice does not address the needs of many migrant children, particularly those from refugee backgrounds.

LAW AND POLICY

Although Australia has a federal government structure, child protection is primarily a state-level responsibility. Each state therefore has its own CPS governed by separate laws and policies (Bromfield and Higgins, 2005). Nevertheless, there are similarities in all these systems and they share many common features. Historically the federal government did not engage with child protection policy or practice other than to provide annual statistics for all the states and territories. However, in the past five years the Australian government has been developing a national framework for child protection. This aims to better coordinate the work of the states and to move toward a "public health" approach to child protection focused on prevention rather than investigation and removal (COAG, 2009). Initiatives under this framework include the trialing of a common assessment approach across professions, common standards for the provision of out-of-home care (OOHC) services, a national research program, and information sharing across states about children at risk. It is worth noting that the concept of children's rights and the United Nations Convention on the Rights of the Child are not particularly influential in policy development on child welfare in Australia, although several Australian states have Children's Commissioners and the government has recently appointed a Federal Commissioner for Children.

State Child Protection Services

As mentioned, each Australian state has its own CPS. In general the role of the CPS (named differently in different states and territories) is to receive notifications of alleged child abuse and neglect, assess the risk to children, and investigate those notifications where children are in need of protection. If necessary children are removed and placed in OOHC or the family is referred to nongovernment organizations (NGOs) or other statutory services for support or counselling. CPS caseworkers seldom engage in ongoing work with families in the system, nor do they offer preventive services (except for some specific programs in some states). In some states, for example New South Wales, notifications are made to a central referral point or "helpline," which conducts an initial risk assessment before passing the case on to local child protection teams.

Family Support

Family support is generally provided by NGOs funded by state or federal governments, often supplemented by fundraising from the public. Many of the larger NGOs started off as faith-based organizations, and most are still aligned with one or other Christian denomination. NGOs tend to be located in one or perhaps two states, and there are few that provide services across the nation.

As a result of this arrangement, services for vulnerable children and families are fragmented and disparate. They differ considerably by state and are also variable in different geographic locations. Australia is a huge country, and service provision in remote areas is particularly challenging, often relying on "fly in fly out" practitioners and therefore involving constant changes of staffing, providing little continuity for clients. Clients living in remote areas sometimes have to travel hundreds of kilometers to access services. For example, many children taken into care from remote communities are accommodated in urban centers far from their families and communities.

Each jurisdiction has its own criteria for notifications and also slightly different criteria for who is mandated to report child abuse and neglect (Higgins, Bromfield, Richardson, Holzer, and Berlyn, 2010).

RECENT REFORMS

In response to the growing numbers of children referred to the CPS and rising numbers of children in care, most states have recently initiated reforms that attempt to increase the resources available for prevention, enhance interagency and interdisciplinary collaboration in child protection, and reduce the number of children in OOHC. Although the situation of migrant children is not directly addressed in most of these reform processes, they do have important implications for work with migrant and refugee families.

Risk Assessment

Interestingly, in tandem with the move toward a broader approach to child protection, most jurisdictions are moving toward "actuarial" models of risk assessment within the CPS such as structured decision making. Even those states that do not use these methods have fairly rigid criteria for assessing whether an investigation is required and timescales for investigation and assessment. In some states, CPS and police form joint investigation teams that undertake investigations of more serious cases, especially sexual abuse.

INDIGENOUS AUSTRALIANS

It is not possible to understand the Australian CPS and its relation to migrant families without understanding the history of Australian settlement and the interaction between white settlers and the first nations of Australia (Aboriginals and Torres Strait Islanders). Australia has a colonial history characterized by conflict, violence, and tension ever since the first settlement. Unlike New Zealand and Canada, both of which have signed treaties with their Indigenous populations, Australia does not recognize its first nations constitutionally.

Policy toward the Indigenous population has shifted between open hostility, paternalism, protection, integration, self-determination, "practical reconciliation," and, more recently, "tough love" (Sanders, 2010). All of these policy positions have had damaging effects on the Indigenous population who have, as a result, suffered "generational trauma."[1]

Indigenous Australians continue to be the most disadvantaged group in Australian society, with lower socioeconomic status, shorter life expectancy, higher rates of incarceration, and lower levels of education than the non-Indigenous population (ABS, 2010). Aboriginal and Torres Strait Islander children are hugely overrepresented in the CPS in every jurisdiction in Australia. Overall the rate of notifications for Indigenous children is around 10 times that for non-Indigenous children, and the rate of Indigenous children in OOHC is around nine times higher. This is an ongoing challenge for the Australian CPS, which, despite the best efforts of policymakers in every state and territory, has failed to decrease the overrepresentation of Indigenous children.

The Stolen Generations

One of the most traumatic chapters in the history of Aboriginal and Torres Strait Islander policy and practice is known as the "stolen generations." The term refers to the actions of the Australian government together with churches and NGOs in which Indigenous children, particularly those with white parents, were forcibly removed and placed in white institutions and families. This policy started out with the ultimate aim of "breeding out" the Indigenous population and later changed to rescuing "neglected" Indigenous children. These removals lasted from the early part of the twentieth century and finally ended in the 1960s. The traumatic stories of the victims of the stolen generations were made public in the *Bringing Them Home* report, which was published by the Australian Human Rights and Equal Opportunities Commission after an in-depth inquiry (HREOC, 1997).[2] This history continues to cast a long shadow over many Aboriginal and Torres Strait Islander individuals, families, and communities who are still suffering the consequences. These include dislocation from language, community, and country.[3] The stolen generations has had a profound effect on child protection practice in Australia over the past two decades.

One of the consequences of the stolen generations history is that, as a response to the previous practices, CPS in Australia developed what is known as Aboriginal Placement Principles. These principles state that, if possible, Aboriginal and Torres Strait Islander children should be kept in their own family and not removed and that if they are removed they should always be placed with a member of their extended family. If this is not possible, they should be placed within their community or the broader Indigenous community, and Aboriginal and Torres Strait Islander communities should be consulted around the placement of these children (SNAICC, 2013). For example, the Queensland Department of Communities, Child Safety and Disability Services' (2011) policy states that in making decisions about the placement of Aboriginal and Torres Strait Islander children, the order of priority is

(1) a member of the child or young person's family
(2) a member of the child or young person's community or language group
(3) another Aboriginal person or Torres Strait Islander who is familiar with the child or young person's community or language group
(4) another Aboriginal or Torres Strait Islander person

Although officially the Aboriginal Placement Principle applies only to care placements, the underlying philosophy has underpinned a range of initiatives to provide culturally appropriate services to Indigenous children and families.

It is very important to note that Indigenous Australians do not see themselves as a minority ethnic community or racial group within the wider Australian population. Rather their status is that of the first nations of Australia, and they therefore have a specific and historical relationship to the land and country. Policies and practices relating to Indigenous children and families cannot simply be extrapolated to other minority communities, even though there are similarities in terms of values and approaches relating to cultural competence and antiracist practice.

MIGRANT COMMUNITIES IN AUSTRALIA

Despite the unique position of Aboriginal and Torres Strait Islanders in Australia, it is within the context and history of child protection services to Indigenous Australians that services to children from migrant families need to be understood. Australia additionally has a complex history of migration and policy toward migrant communities that bears significantly on the experiences of migrant children and families in the CPS. Within the overall policy of migration, policies toward refugees and asylum seekers require specific attention as they differ somewhat from the broader migration policies, in particular in relation to child protection issues.

Migration Policy

Australia has had a complex and challenging migration policy history. The country has, since settlement, always relied on the influx of large numbers of migrants to remain economically viable. For many years the migration policy was governed by the maxim "populate or perish," and migration was encouraged. Nevertheless there is a shameful history of xenophobia and racism in Australia. For many years immigration was regulated by the "white Australia" policy framework. This policy began in the early years of the twentieth century and persisted until after World War Two. At that time, immigration was largely limited to British and Irish nationals. In the late 1940s, immigrants from southern Europe began to flow in as a result of acute labor shortages after the Second World War. It has been only since the 1970s that Asians and others not of European origin have been allowed to emigrate to Australia in any numbers (Jupp, 2007). Waves of refugee migration began with a large number of "boat people" from Vietnam who arrived in Australia in 1975, followed by refugees from the Lebanese war. Since then there have been successive migrations from Asia and the Pacific. In the 1970s Australia officially adopted "multiculturalism" as the policy framework for integrating migrant populations. Multiculturalism continued to be official government policy until the change of government in September 2013 but has been downplayed by successive governments (Jupp, 1997) and is not supported by the Coalition (conservative parties, now in government). Australia is now one of the most diverse countries in the world, with almost a third of the child population having a parent born overseas (Katz and Redmond, 2010). The main groups of migrants from non-English-speaking backgrounds are Lebanese, Vietnamese, Greek, Italian, and Chinese.

Reasons for migration to Australia include skilled migration, family reunification, and humanitarian migration. The majority of migrants come via the skilled migration program. Skilled migrants are strictly controlled and are subject to a points system whereby points are given for education, age, English proficiency, and need for a particular skill. Thus the majority of these migrants are well educated and have reasonable proficiency in English. It is partly because of this demographic profile that migrants in Australia tend to have relatively higher levels of well-being and settlement outcomes than in many other countries, despite the fact that they are subject to the same barriers and challenges (disruption of families, dislocation from community and language, racism, and discrimination) migrants face in all countries.

As in most countries, migrants in Australia tend to be housed in the major urban areas (Sydney, Melbourne, Brisbane, Adelaide, and Perth), although there are some communities in regional areas. There are areas with high proportions of migrants in all the major conurbations, and some suburbs have become associated with particular migrant groups. However, there are few "ghettos" in Australia, and migrants tend to be spread through the suburban areas of the major cities.

Refugees and Asylum Seekers

Migration is an important and highly charged political issue that often attracts adverse media attention, particularly with respect to Muslim migrants and how they integrate into Australian society and adopt "Australian" values (Mansouri and Marotta, 2012). Migration is also part of a broader discussion relating to the question of whether there should be a "Big Australia"—that is, whether policies should encourage population growth to ensure a dynamic economy or whether population growth should be curtailed to ensure environmental and social sustainability. However, by far the most charged political debate relates to policies toward asylum seekers who arrive by boat in Australian territory.

In Australia there is a very clear distinction made between two groups of refugees. "Humanitarian" refugees come to Australia via the United Nations High Commission for Refugees (UNHCR). These refugees have had their status approved by the UNHCR. Australia accepts a fixed number of these refugees each year (around 13,000 per year in recent years). Refugees in this category come from a range of different regions, including Somalia, Burma, and other parts of Asia. On arrival in Australia, refugees are given permanent residence and are provided with the full range of social and welfare services and benefits available to all permanent residents. However, the settlement support services are not very well developed, and families are provided with only six weeks of specific settlement support from NGOs before they are expected to fend for themselves.

Asylum seekers who arrive on Australian territory by boat are known as "irregular maritime arrivals" (IMAs) or, more recently, "illegal maritime arrivals." Australia has a policy of mandatory detention for IMAs, and every person who arrives by boat in Australia is taken for processing to Christmas Island[4] and is then sent to an immigration detention facility, either in Australia or elsewhere. This policy was implemented following a comprehensive review of the system for dealing with IMAs that recommended that people arriving by boat should not be at an advantage compared to people who "waited their turn" by going through the UNHCR (Houston, Aristotle, and L'Estrange, 2012). This policy includes children in families and unaccompanied minors (UAMs). Border protection (i.e., the policies and programs put into place to deter boat people and asylum seekers) has become one of the most charged political debates in Australia over the past two years. In the general election held in September 2013, the Coalition (center-right party), which had been in opposition, ran on a policy of "turning back the boats"—that is, refusing to let boats containing asylum seekers enter into Australia. The Labor government had already considerably tightened the policy by reinstating "offshore processing"—the policy of diverting asylum seekers to third countries to process their refugee claims and then ensuring that those countries, rather than Australia, became their country of refuge. Kevin Rudd, the previous prime minister, had stated that under the new policy, no person arriving by boat in Australia would be given refugee status in Australia. New refugee processing detention centers were established on Manus Island in Papua New Guinea and Nauru in early 2013 to accommodate these asylum seekers. There have been mixed reports about how UAMs would be processed under the new regime. At first it was stated that minors and families would be accommodated in these offshore centers on the grounds that if they were excluded, the "people smugglers" would exploit the situation by sending more young people and families. However, conditions in these camps were not suitable for young people, and few appear to have been sent there to date, with some who were having to return to detention in Australia.

After spending some time in detention, asylum seekers are either offered refugee status and settled in the community, sent to community detention (where they are under similar conditions to detention facilities but are housed in the community), or put on a "bridging visa," which gives them more freedom but less support than community detention. If their claim is rejected, they are returned to their country of origin if possible. Currently the majority of IMAs originate from Afghanistan, Sri Lanka, Iraq, and Iran.

There is enormous hostility in Australia toward IMAs and constant battles between the political parties about who has the toughest response toward them. The media gives constant attention to this issue.

UAMs are generally housed at first in alternative places of detention, detention facilities that are slightly less restrictive than those in which single adults are held. They are then generally moved into community detention, where they are housed with other minors. Although they have freedom of movement, they must live in a residence provided by the Department for Immigration and Border Protection, and they are not allowed to work. Children are required to attend schools, and families have access to a range of services. Children who are in immigration detention, either as part of a family or as UAMs, are the responsibility of the Department for Immigration and Border Protection, and state CPS do not have jurisdiction over them. However, adults in community detention who commit crimes, including child abuse related crimes such as sexual abuse or neglect, are subject to the state criminal justice system.

Once they are given protection visas (i.e., are recognized as legitimate refugees), UAMs become the responsibility of states and territories along with all permanent residents of Australia. If they are still under 18, they are placed in OOHC. Australia does not keep statistics on the numbers of UAMs in OOHC, and little is known of their numbers, location, or well-being (Barrie and Mendes, 2011). As indicated here, the policy on refugees and asylum seekers is constantly changing, and the protection of children in the refugee system remains a significant concern, but there is little empirical evidence to underpin practice in this area.

ORGANIZATION

There is very little information about the situation of migrant children and families in the CPS in Australia. Relatively little information is collected about these families.

The Australian Institute of Health and Welfare (AIHW) annual report does not report on migrant or culturally and linguistically diverse (CALD) families, nor do any of the states or territories. It is not known, for example, whether migrant children are over- or underrepresented in the CPS, and if so which groups are more represented than others. The *Framework for Protecting Australia's Children* contains a significant focus on the protection of Indigenous children but does not explicitly refer to migrant children. However, some effort has recently been made to address this issue in some states. The Queensland and New South Wales CPS agencies have developed guidance for practitioners on culturally sensitive practice (Community Services New South Wales, 2010; Queensland Department of Communities, Child Safety and Disability Services, 2010). Recent statistics indicate that over 50% of referrals to CPS in New South Wales are for children from CALD backgrounds (personal communication). While there are no reliable figures, it appears that certain migrant communities are overrepresented in the CPS whereas others are underrepresented. Of all the major inquiries and state reform activities, only the Cummins inquiry in Victoria (Cummins, Scott, and Scales, 2012) contains a chapter on migrant communities (Chapter 13: Meeting the Needs of Children and Young People from Culturally and Linguistically Diverse Communities, pp. 312–328). The chapter summarizes submissions from a number of organizations to the inquiry, and calls for a much higher priority to be placed on developing culturally sensitive service provision within the state. In particular, the inquiry notes that CALD families have limited access to preventive services and therefore are likely to be caught up in tertiary or statutory services when they encounter difficulties. A key recommendation of the inquiry is that data on language and ethnicity should be improved considerably so that the service response to CALD children and families can be monitored and improved.

How Indigenous Policy Has Influenced Child Protection of Migrant Children
The Language of Race, Migration, and Ethnicity
One example of how the history of settlement and colonization and the response to it has affected the conceptualization of migrant communities relates to the use of language in official documents and policies. Although the idea of a white Australia was historically a key component of the development of Australian national identity, the concept of race has deliberately been excluded from the official lexicon in Australia in recent years. When the white Australia policy was eventually abandoned, it was superseded by the official adoption of multiculturalism and, more recently, citizenship (Koleth, 2010). Terms such as "BME" (black and minority ethnic), "visible minority," or "minority ethnic" are not used in Australia, and migrant groups have been labelled, respectively "NESB" (non-English-speaking background), "LOTE" (language other than English [spoken in the home]), or, more commonly "CALD" but never "ethnic" or "racial." The opposite of CALD is "Anglo-Australian" or "Anglo-Celtic," not "white." CALD includes not only people of, for example, Chinese and Somalian heritage but also those of Polish and Italian origin. The term is therefore not even a good designation for people of color or visible minorities. Nevertheless, it is often used as a rather poor proxy for disadvantages and visible minority status (Sawrikar NS Katz, 2009). It should be noted that the term "migrant," although used here and in official statistics, is seldom used in the context of service delivery because a very high proportion of migrants are people from English-speaking countries (particularly the UK and New Zealand). These populations are not considered minority groups in the same sense as those from "developing" countries.[5]

Whilst CALD groups are often identified collectively, they are also classified with "Anglo" in contrast to Indigenous, and most official reports either ignore them altogether or still classify them by country of origin (e.g., families where at least one parent is born overseas) or language. All official categorizations in Australia are by cultural or religious affiliation or country of origin, and there is no official way of differentiating visible or racial minorities.

Another area in which the history of Aboriginal and Torres Strait Islanders has affected CPSs is that in Australia there is virtually no use of adoption or institutional care. In 2012–2013 there were a total of 339 adoptions in Australia, of which 54 (16%) were local adoptions (defined as "adoptions of children who were born or permanently residing in Australia before the adoption, who are legally able to be placed for adoption, but who generally have had no previous contact or relationship with the adoptive parent[s]"; AIHW, 2013: 2).One aspect of the decline in adoptions over time (9,798 in 1971–1972, 1,501 in 1988[6]) has been the reaction to the stolen generations. In recent years another group of children have been identified who were adversely affected by child protection policy: the so-called Forgotten Australians. These were children who had been brought to Australia from the UK as "orphans" and placed either in families or institutions. As a result of the work of the Child Migration Trust and others, it has now become known that most of these children were not orphans at all but were taken from single mothers and other disadvantaged families, and their experiences of adoption and institutionalization were often appalling. Prime Minister Kevin Rudd apologized to this group as well, in November 2009. Other recent apologies have included an apology by Prime Minister Julia Gillard in 2012 to mothers whose children had been taken from them at birth under false pretenses and placed for adoption This was common practice in Australia until the early 1970s. Adoption is thus a highly contested issue in Australia, despite the small numbers of people now involved.

The most recent significant development in policy in Australia has been the appointment of a Royal Commission to examine child sexual abuse in institutions.[7] The Royal Commission began hearing evidence in mid-2013 and is expected to sit for at least three years and to hear testimony from hundreds of victims, as well as alleged perpetrators and other stakeholders. The Royal Commission is also developing a large program of research into various aspects of child sexual abuse in institutions. This follows several years of revelations of child sexual abuse in institutions, particularly churches and schools run by religious organizations. There is no specific remit for the commission to examine abuse of migrant children.

These developments have been initiated by determined campaigners who have fought against significant odds to uncover the truth of the implications of past child protection policies and to change policy and practice. There has not been an equivalent group of people campaigning for the needs of migrant children, and consequently there is far less policy, practice, or research in Australia relating to migrant families than is the case for similar countries with high levels of migration such as the UK, the United States, and Canada. Nevertheless, the situation of migrant families is beginning to be recognized in policy in some states and also at the federal government level, and steps are being taken in some states to improve policies and practices, for example by paying more attention to accurate data collection about CALD families and ensuring that resources such as interpreters and translated information materials are made available.

Training

Training of child protection workers is a significant challenge in Australia. Perhaps uniquely among rich countries, child protection practitioners are not required to be social workers but in most jurisdictions can be drawn from a range of human services professions. Similarly, in the nongovernment sector workers tend to come from a range of backgrounds (Cortis and Meagher, 2012). Newly recruited practitioners are provided with training in assessment and working with families and with opportunities for further training. Some social work courses do contain modules on diversity, multiculturalism, or culturally sensitive practice, but this is not the case for all the professions involved in child protection. Practitioners are not required to undertake courses on working with migrant families, although this training is provided on an ad hoc basis in a number of jurisdictions (Kaur 2009). In some states such as New South Wales, practitioners have access to advice and support from a multicultural or diversity unit. Nevertheless, many practitioners in the statutory CPS do not feel adequately trained in culturally sensitive practice (Sawrikar and Katz, 2013).

Very few statutory or nongovernment agencies in Australia have made significant advances in the managerial or strategic domains, however. Work with migrant families is therefore still viewed primarily as a matter of training practitioners in culturally sensitive practice. In some organizations the protocols around Indigenous practice have been extended to migrant groups so that children from migrant communities are placed with foster carers from similar backgrounds if possible. However, it is only recently that specific programs have been developed to recruit and support foster carers from migrant communities by some NGOs, such as Settlement Services International (2013).

REPRESENTATION OF MIGRANT CHILDREN

Incidence of Child Protection

Annual statistical reports about the functioning of the system are produced by the AIHW (2011). Australia has a high rate of notifications and substantiations. According to the AIHW, the number of children subject to notification in 2010–2011 was 163,767, a decrease of 13% from 2009–2010 (AIHW, 2012). During the same period, the number of children subject to a substantiation of a notification remained relatively stable (increasing by less than 1%, from 31,295 to 31,527.

There is considerable variation between states in both the number of children in the CPS and the rates of children being notified, substantiated, and subject to orders. New South Wales has by far the highest rate of CPS activity and the largest number of children in the CPS, accounting for nearly a third of children subject to notifications in 2010–2011.

The rate of children in OOHC is similar to that of Sweden, although the demography of children in care differs between the two countries (Healy, Lundström, and Sallnäs, 2011). Overall the numbers of children in the CPS have been steadily rising for many years, more than doubling in the past 10 years. Unlike some other countries such as the UK, Australia does not collect statistics on "children in need" or children in the broader child welfare system. Although all child protection statistics are disaggregated by Indigenous status, official data are not provided for migrant children or other minority groups.

Research

There is a very limited research evidence base on this population (Kaur, 2012). Jatinder Kaur has undertaken the only comprehensive review of the empirical literature on CALD and refugee families in the CP system in Australia, and this review confirms the paucity of research. Most of the research that has been undertaken provides relatively consistent findings. With regard to the representation of migrant groups, the review found that there appear to be broadly representative proportions of migrant children as a whole in the CPS but over- and underrepresentation of particular groups.

It is particularly challenging to gauge the representativeness of migrant families in the CPS in Australia. First, figures differ considerably according to the specific definition of "migrant" that is used. The most widely accepted definition in Australia—having one parent who is born overseas—is very broad and includes a high proportion of the population but excludes some who would consider themselves from minority communities. Migrant families are no more likely to have contact with child protection than Australian-born families. However, it does appear that certain groups are overrepresented, including families with a refugee background, as well as Pacific Islanders and Maoris. These are migrant families who tend to be in the lower socioeconomic brackets and to live in disadvantaged areas. Second, there is a lack of accurate information about migrant families because the information itself is not collected systematically. Although many states include a field for "CALD" or "language spoken in the home" in their administrative information systems, this is not a mandatory field in the data and therefore is seldom accurately completed by practitioners, leading to significant underreporting of CALD status in child protection statistics. Although there have been similar concerns expressed about Aboriginal and Torres Strait Islander identification, most states have worked hard to improve the accuracy of reporting on these children and families and have made the reporting of Indigeneity mandatory.

Type of Abuse Reported

Kaur (2012) found that there appeared to be higher levels of physical abuse and neglect reported for migrant families than for the overall population. It is difficult to disaggregate the extent to which cases of physical abuse and neglect are caused by stressors to parents in migrant families who are struggling with issues such as cultural shock, as well as the loss of support from extended families and communities. Research in Australia attests to the difficulty many parents experience when coming to a new country with different expectations of parenting and also where their own support systems are lacking (Lewig, Arney, and Salveron, 2010; Renzaho and Vignjevic, 2011). On the other hand, at least some of the involvement of these families is likely to be due to cultural misunderstandings on the part of child protection workers (Kaur, 2009).

One of the consistent findings across research projects has been the relative lack of understanding by migrant families of the Australian CPS, accompanied by fear of children being removed and concern that their own culturally appropriate parenting behavior will be construed as being neglectful or abusive.

A number of research projects have found that many migrant families, especially those from countries without well-developed CPSs, are very anxious and suspicious of the Australian child protection authorities. For example Pe-Pua and colleagues (2010) found that, for many Muslim parents, fear of the child protection services was one of the most significant causes of stress, in some ways greater than racism and discrimination. These parents felt that Australian expectations about parenting, especially the requirement not to physically chastise children, undermined their authority as parents. They also felt that if their children did misbehave or acted in antisocial ways, the parents were held responsible and blamed for not disciplining children adequately. In many cases these beliefs were further exacerbated by their suspicion of statutory authority due to experiences in their country of origin and also by rumors within the community relating to children who had been "unjustly" removed from parents who had being parenting in culturally appropriate ways. Renzaho and Vignjevic (2011) found very similar reactions among African parents and also found that parents were often confused about the specific requirements and expectations of Australian laws relating to child protection. In response to these findings in the research literature, the second three-year plan of the *Framework for Protecting Australia's Children* contains an action to develop culturally appropriate information for migrant and refugee families about Australian norms and laws relating to parenting (FaHCSIA, 2012).

One of the reasons that some migrant groups appear to be overrepresented in the CPS is that it is much more difficult for migrant and refugee families to access preventive and early intervention services. This is first because the services themselves are often not designed in a culturally appropriate manner. This can be for a number of reasons, including that they do not provide information in different languages, do not employ workers from migrant communities, provide services in a culturally insensitive manner (e.g., they do not separate men and women), or because they are physically less accessible to migrant and refugee families (Sawrikar and Katz, 2007). Families themselves may also be reluctant to access services, partly because of their general suspicion of authority but also because for some, the concept of a "service" may be alien to their experience. These families would be far more comfortable accessing community elders or religious leaders than formal services.

The consequence of this for child welfare is that families may only become "visible" to services when they reach such a point of crisis, when they are forced to go for help outside the community, or when a professional such as a teacher or general practitioner recognizes that there is a difficulty. Even in these situations, families may only minimally engage with preventive services.

Many groups of migrants face a range of challenges, including economic adversity, racism, isolation, cultural disorientation, intergenerational conflict, posttraumatic distress, domestic violence, and social exclusion. Refugee families in particular face challenges over and above other migrant families. The difference between refugees and other migrants is particularly significant in Australia, because most migrants other than refugees are relatively highly educated and have reasonably good English skills. Refugees, on the other hand, tend to be poorly educated and lack proficiency in English. In addition, their own traumatic experiences in their country of origin and the hazardous journey to Australia often takes a toll on families, and children from refugee families are a particularly vulnerable group who are ill-served by mainstream services (McFarlane, Kaplan, and Lawrence, 2011).

For child protection workers, it is often very challenging to understand the contribution of cultural differences and the effects of migration, pre-migration experiences, trauma, poverty, unemployment, and discrimination in Australia. All these factors can affect the parenting practices of refugees, and it is difficult to disaggregate the effects of these different processes (Sawrikar, 2009).

Practitioners Committed to Cultural Competency But Lacking Training and Confidence

Most practitioners in child protection services in Australia are sympathetic to the principles of cultural competency. Cultural competency is a fundamental component of practice with both Indigenous and migrant families. Nevertheless, practice itself often falls short of cultural competence. Practitioners feel unsupported and lacking in confidence about working in a culturally competent manner (Kaur, 2009). More important, however, services lack the management and policy frameworks that facilitate the provision of culturally appropriate practice (Cummins et al., 2012; Sawrikar and Katz, 2007). Despite the child protection workforce's overall commitment to cultural sensitivity, research has found it is still fundamentally Euro-centric in its orientation (Walter, Taylor, and Habibis, 2011), and CALD practitioners often feel challenged to work in culturally appropriate ways, even with families from similar cultural backgrounds (Sawrikar, 2013). Many of these issues are, of course, not confined to Australia and are found in research on migrant families internationally (Korbin, 2002).

Other examples of research in Australia include that of Bourke and Paxman (2008) who undertook a small-scale audit of files of children in OOHC. They found that workers are sensitive to cultural issues but that there were a number of barriers to placing children in culturally appropriate placements. In a much larger study that involved file audits, in-depth interviews with caseworkers, families, and other stakeholders, and examination of administrative data, Sawrikar found that practice was variable and that many families from CALD

backgrounds felt disempowered and misunderstood, whilst many practitioners were aware of cultural issues but were less aware of racism as an issue
for these families; they also felt that there were a lack of appropriate resources
(Sawrikar, 2009).

In a later part of her research, Sawrikar (2011: 22–23) identified three types
of issues that affect the interactions between migrant families and CPS:

Cultural: physical abuse, inadequate supervision, traditional cultural
practices, culture difference in "child-centered" family functioning,
academic pressure, and exposure to trauma;

Migration-related: lack of awareness about child protection laws and
agencies, lack of extended family support, and generational difference
in migration and language issues; and

Generalist: homelessness, poverty, mental health issues, domestic violence, and alcohol or drug issues.

This finding points toward the fact that cultural differences are only one area
of concern for migrant families, and, as pointed out previously, refugees face
additional challenges. These families face a number of adversities that need to
be addressed in order to secure the well-being of children and parents, and culturally sensitive practice on its own is unlikely to make a significant difference
to the multitude of issues faced by these families. According to Sawrikar and
Katz (2007), in order to provide an effective service, the needs of migrant families need to be addressed at three levels:

Practice
Managerial/organizational
Strategic

At the practice level, the priority is to help practitioners develop awareness
of cultural differences in child rearing and also of issues such as institutional
racism and intergenerational issues related to migration and culture shock.
However, this is not sufficient. Frontline practice needs to be carried out within
a managerial context that provides the resources and supports for practitioners
engaged in cross-cultural work. This means, for example, providing interpreters
where necessary, making available cultural consultants, specifically targeting
migrants for recruitment as practitioners and managers, and making premises accessible to migrant families, for example by providing separate areas for
women. At the more strategic level, policies and programs must acknowledge
the specific needs of migrant families and put in place mechanisms for ensuring that their needs are appropriately met—for example, ensuring that cultural
competence is included in professional training for the relevant professional
groups, including background in data collection and reporting, and developing

specific programs aimed at supporting migrant families to access preventive services. Additionally, services need to acknowledge the structural barriers for many of these families to engage in mainstream society, particularly to find secure employment and housing.

CONCLUSION

Australia's fragmented, reactive, and risk-focused CPS provides a particularly difficult context for undertaking effective work with migrant families. Although most states now provide some cultural awareness training for staff, there are systemic barriers to offering a responsive and holistic service to these clients. In particular, agencies have not addressed the question of migrant children and families strategically. The great diversity of migrant communities means that there are few locations in Australia where there is a predominance of any one migrant community, further complicating service delivery in areas where there are high concentrations of migrants and refugees. Overall, therefore, there is a significant need for research, policy development, and practice enhancement to better protect and safeguard the needs of migrant children in Australia.

Australia's child protection history has been profoundly influenced by the history of settlement and the colonization of the Indigenous population. Although as first nations of Australia, Aboriginal and Torres Strait Islander people have a specific status within the society, there are a number of lessons that can be learned from work with Indigenous families that could support improved policy and practice with CALD families.

Although there is increasing recognition that the needs of particular groups of migrant children, particularly those from refugee and asylum-seeking backgrounds, are not well met by the child welfare and CPS, there is still a significant dearth of research, policy, and practice development in this area, and therefore there is still much to be learned about the best way forward for addressing these issues in the Australian context.

NOTES

1 A good summary of the history of Indigenous policy and its effect on Indigenous families is available from the Australian Human Rights Commission http://www.hreoc.gov.au/bth/taken/track_the_history.html

2 The inquiry was set up under the Keating Labor Government but reported when the new Liberal (conservative) government came into power, and their response was to contest the accuracy of the report's findings and to reject the need for apology. Ten years later when Kevin Rudd was elected, he did finally

apologize to the Aboriginal community for the stolen generations in his first act on becoming prime minister of Australia in November 2007.

3   A fundamental aspect of Aboriginal and Torres Strait Islander culture involves connection to country (i.e., to the specific area inhabited by each community). Culture, language, and country are all inextricably bound together, and the removal of children from communities has disrupted this fundamental connection, leaving both individuals and communities bereft and disrupted.

4   Christmas Island is situated relatively near the coast of Indonesia but is Australian territory.

5   Migrants' country of origin is not always a good indicator of their social status. In Australia some migrants from relatively poor countries are themselves relatively advantaged; Australia recruits large numbers of skilled workers including professionals from many Asian countries. In addition, there are other anomalies, including a relatively large proportion of "African" migrants being white South Africans (Katz and Redmond, 2010).

6   However, there is a strong push toward increasing the numbers of adopted children in Australia. In December 2013 the prime minister, Tony Abbott, announced a high-profile task force to make adoption easier for Australians (Morton, 2013).

7   http://www.childabuseroyalcommission.gov.au/

REFERENCES

Australian Bureau of Statistics (ABS). (2010). The Health and Welfare of Australia's Aboriginal and Torres Strait Islander Peoples, 2010. Retrieved on September 8, 2014, from http://www.abs.gov.au/ausstats/abs@.nsf/mf/4704.0.

———. (2012). Migration, Australia, 2010–11. Retrieved on September 8, 2014, from http://www.abs.gov.au/ausstats/abs@.nsf/Products/84074889D69E738 CCA257A5A00120A69?opendocument.

Australian Institute of Health and Welfare (AIHW). (2011). Child protection Australia 2009–10. Child Welfare Series No. 51. Cat. no. CWS 39. Canberra: AIHW.

———. (2012). Child Protection Australia 2010–11. Canberra: AIHW.

———. (2013). Adoptions Australia 2012–2013. Canberra: AIHW.

Barrie, L., & Mendes, P. (2011). The experiences of unaccompanied asylum-seeking children in and leaving the out-of-home care system in the UK and Australia: A critical review of the literature. International Social Work, 54(4), 485–503. doi: 10.1177/0020872810389318

Bromfield, L., & Higgins, D. (2005). National comparison of child protection systems: Child Abuse Prevention Issues 22. Melbourne: National Child Protection Clearinghouse.

Burke, S., & Paxman, M. (2008). Children and Young People from Non-English Speaking Backgrounds in Out-of-Home Care in NSW. Sydney: NSW Department of Community Services.

Community Services New South Wales. (2010). Culturally Appropriate Service Provision for Children and Families in the NSW Child Protection System. Sydney: NSW Community Services.

Cortis, N., & Meagher, G. (2012). Social work education as preparation for practice: Evidence from a survey of the New South Wales community sector. *Australian Social Work*, 65(3), 295–310. doi: 10.1080/0312407X.2012.707666

Council of Australian Governments (COAG). (2009). *Protecting Children is Everyone's Business: National Framework for Protecting Australia's Children 2009–2020*. Canberra: COAG.

Cummins, P., Scott, D., & Scales, B. (2012). *Report of the Protecting Victoria's Vulnerable Children Inquiry*, Vol. 2. Melbourne: State Government of Victoria.

Department of Families, Housing, Community Services and Indigenous Affairs (FaHCSIA). (2012). Protecting Children Is Everyone's Business: National Framework for Protecting Australia's Children 2009–2020: Second Three-Year Action Plan, 2012–2015. Canberra: FaHCSIA.

Gilbert, N., Parton, N., & Skivenes, M., eds. (2011). *Child Protection Systems: International Trends and Orientations*. New York: Oxtord University Press.

Healy, K., Lundström, T., & Sallnäs, M. (2011). Worlds apart? A comparison of out-of-home care for children and young people in Australia and Sweden. *Australian Social Work*, 64(4), 416–431.

Hetherington, R., Cooper, A., Smith, P., & Wilford, G. (1997). *Protecting Children: Messages from Europe*. Lyme Regis: Russell House Publishing.

Higgins, D., Bromfield, L., Richardson, N., Holzer, P., & Berlyn, C. (2010). Mandatory Reporting of Child Abuse: National Child Protection Clearinghouse Resource Sheet. Melbourne: Australian Institute of Family Studies. Retrieved April 30, 2012, from http://www.aifs.gov.au/nch/pubs/sheets/rs3/rs3.html.

Higgins, D., & Katz, I. (2008). Enhancing service systems for protecting children: Promoting child wellbeing and child protection reform in Australia. *Family Matters*, 80, 43–50.

Houston, A., Aristotle, P., & L'Estrange, M. (2012). *Report of the Expert Panel on Asylum Seekers*. Canberra: Australian Government.

Human Rights and Equal Opportunities Commission (HREOC). (1997). *Bringing Them Home: Report of the National Inquiry into the Separation of Aboriginal and Torres Strait Islander Children from Their Families*. Canberra: HREOC.

Jupp, J. (1997). Immigration and national identity: Multiculturalism. In G. Stokes (Ed.), *The Politics of Identity in Australia*, 132–157. Melbourne: Cambridge University Press.

———. (2007). *From White Australia to Woomera: The Story of Australian Immigration*. Sydney: Cambridge University Press.

Katz, I., & Redmond, G. (2010). Review of the circumstances among children in immigrant families in Australia. *Child Indicators Research*, 3(4), 439–458.

Kaur, J. (2009). Developing "culturally sensitive" practice when working with CALD communities in child protection—An Australian exploratory study. *Developing Practice*, 23, 22–35.

———. (2012). *Cultural Diversity and Child Protection: Australian Research Review on the Needs of Culturally and Linguistically Diverse (CALD) and Refugee Children and Families*. Queensland: JK Diversity Consultants.

Koleth, E. (2010). Multiculturalism: A review of australian policy statements and recent debates in Australia and overseas. Research Paper No. 6, 2010–11. Canberra: Parliament of Australia.

Korbin, J.E. (2002). Culture and child maltreatment: Cultural competence and beyond. *Child Abuse & Neglect*, 26(6–7), 637–644. doi: http://dx.doi.org/10.1016/S0145-2134(02)00338-1

Lewig, K., Arney, F., & Salveron, M. (2010). Challenges to parenting in a new culture: Implications for child and family welfare. *Evaluation and Program Planning*, 33(3), 324–332.

Mansouri, F., & Marotta, V. (2012). *Muslims in the West and the Challenges of Belonging*. Melbourne: Melbourne University Press.

McFarlane, C., Kaplan, I., & Lawrence, J. (2011). Psychosocial indicators of wellbeing for resettled refugee children and youth: Conceptual and developmental directions. *Child Indicators Research*, 4(4), 647–677. doi: 10.1007/s12187-010-9100-4

Morton, R. (2013). Tony Abbott announces adoption taskforce, backed by Furness, Jackman. *The Australian*, December 19. Retrieved on December 14, 2013, from http://www.theaustralian.com.au/national-affairs/tony-abbott-announces-adoption-taskforce-backed-by-furness-jackman/story-fn59niix-1226786541811

Pe-Pua, R., Gendera, S., Katz, I., & O'Connor, A. (2010). *Meeting the Needs of Australian Muslim Families: Exploring Marginalisation, Family Issues and "Best Practice" in Service Provision*. Report Prepared for the Australian Government Department of Immigration and Citizenship. Sydney: Social Policy Research Centre, University of New South Wales.

Queensland Department of Communities, Child Safety and Disability Services. (2010). *Working with People from Culturally and Linguistically Diverse Backgrounds. Brisbane*. South Brisbane: Queensland Department of Child Safety.

———. (2011). Child Placement Principle. Retrieved April 30, 2012, from http://www.communities.qld.gov.au/childsafety/foster-care/aboriginal-and-torres-strait-islanders/child-placement-principle.

Renzaho, A., & Vignjevic, S. (2011). The impact of a parenting intervention in Australia among migrants and refugees from Liberia, Sierra Leone, Congo, and Burundi: Results from the African Migrant Parenting Program. *Journal of Family Studies*, 17(1), 71–79.

Sanders, W. (2010). Ideology, evidence and competing principles in Australian Indigenous affairs: From Brough to Rudd via Pearson and the NTER. *Australian Journal of Social Issues*, 45(3), 307–331.

Sawrikar, P. (2009). *Culturally Appropriate Service Provision for Culturally and Linguistically Diverse (CALD) Children and Families in the New South Wales (NSW) Child Protection System (CPS)*. Sydney: Social Policy Research Centre, University of New South Wales.

———. (2011). *Culturally Appropriate Service Delivery for Culturally and Linguistically Diverse (CALD) Children and Families in the NSW Child Protection System (CPS): Final Report*. Sydney: Department of Human Services, NSW.

———. (2013). A qualitative study on the pros and cons of ethnically matching culturally and linguistically diverse (CALD) client families and child protection caseworkers. *Children and Youth Services Review*, 35(2), 321–331. doi: http://dx.doi.org/10.1016/j.childyouth.2012.11.012

Sawrikar, P., & Katz, I. (2007). *Enhancing Family and Relationship Service Accessibility and Delivery to Culturally and Linguistically Diverse (CALD) Families in Australia*. Melbourne: Australian Family Relationships Clearinghouse.

———. (2009). How Useful is the Term "Culturally and Linguistically Diverse" (CALD) in Australian Research, Practice, and Policy Discourse? Paper presented at the Australian Social Policy Conference, Sydney. http://www.sprc.unsw.edu.au/media/File/Paper276.pdf

———. (2013). "Normalizing the novel": How is culture addressed in child protection work with ethnic-minority families in Australia? *Journal of Social Service Research*, 39(5), 39–61. doi: 10.1080/01488376.2013.845126

Secretariat of National Aboriginal and Islander Child Care (SNAICC). (2013). Aboriginal and Torres Strait Islander Child Placement Principle. North Fitzroy: SNAICC. Retrieved on September 8, 2014, from http://www.snaicc.org.au/policy-advocacy/dsp-landing-policyarea.cfm?loadref=36&txnid=12&txnctype=post&txncstype=

Settlement Services International. (2013). Multicultural Foster Care Service. Ashfield, NSW: Settlement Services International. Retrieved December 12, 2013, from http://www.ssi.org.au/services/child-and-family-services/multicultural-foster-care-service

Walter, M., Taylor, S., & Habibis, D. (2011). How white is social work in Australia? *Australian Social Work*, 64(1), 6–19. doi: 10.1080/0312407x.2010.510892

12

IMMIGRANT CHILDREN AND FAMILIES IN THE ESTONIAN CHILD PROTECTION SYSTEM

Merle Linno and Judit Strömpl

INTRODUCTION

In September 1991, soon after the emancipation from the Soviet Union, the young independent Republic of Estonia adopted its first international law: the United Nations Convention on the Rights of the Child. The first law accepted by the Estonian Parliament was the Child Protection Act (CPA; 1992, entered into force in on January 1, 1993). Children seemed to be the first priority of the emancipated Estonian Republic. Unfortunately, these first efforts to act in the best interests of children were not so easy to follow. The duties connected with the United Nations Convention on the Rights of the Child were executed with difficulties.[1]

In the process of "restoring" (a term used at that time) the independent national state, other priorities became more important. Nation-state and ethnicity have essential importance in the Estonian context. This is the reason ethnic origin is more important than immigrant background of the population in Estonia.[2] In fact, the categorization of people is done on the basis of their ethnic belonging (Estonians vs non-Estonians); however, behind ethnic belonging, people's immigrant past is emphasized. Thus we use the terms interchangeably in this chapter.

In the early 1990s, one of the most important situations Estonia had to deal with was the demographic situation, which was the result of the Soviet colonization policy. One-third of population formed a group of people who had entered Estonia during the time of the Soviet regime. Estonia had to both integrate and protect itself from these people, who were considered a potential danger to the Estonian culture and state independency. One tool to deal with these problems was the Estonian citizenship policy, the aim of which was to verify the loyalty toward the Estonian Republic and respect toward the Estonian culture through the mastery of the Estonian language. As a result of citizenship and language policies, the separation of two groups (Estonians and Russophones) deepened. The integration process was and still is rather complicated. All of this has had an important impact on the immigration policy and the situation of the immigrants today. However, recent immigrants differ from those who entered during the time of the Soviet regime. The Organisation for Economic Co-operation and Development (2013) data about the Estonian population show two important figures that should be interpreted to understand the situation: first, 16.7% of the population are marked as foreign-born people, but among them are also people who entered Estonia during the Soviet period, and these are not identified by Estonian people as immigrants but as an ethnic minority. People belonging to this group do not identify themselves as immigrants either, because they did not cross the official state border of the USSR. The other number indicates 17.6% of the Estonian population are foreigners, but this figure may include third- and fourth-generation immigrants who officially do not belong to the category of immigrants but have chosen Russian citizenship (7.3%), or have citizenship in a former Soviet Union country, or are people with undetermined citizenship (7.3% of the Estonian population; UNHCR, 2011).

In this chapter we describe the particular demographic situation in Estonia and use historical arguments to create a context necessary to understand the response of the Estonian child protection system to the needs of migrant children and families. We give a short overview of recent migration, including the situation of the asylum seekers and refugees, while concentrating on children's and adolescents' situations. Then we analyze the Estonian citizenship regulation and its impact on the process of integration and development of national identity of children and young people with an immigrant background and especially stateless children. Next, the Estonian child protection system specifics are presented with the emphasis on the rights to services of immigrant children and families. All this provides the Estonian context to the cross-country survey data analysis and interpretation. (For more information, see the appendix – survey method overview.)

LAW AND POLICY

Overview of Migration and Current Demographic Situation

The Estonian demographic situation changed dramatically during and after the Second World War. During WWII, Estonia lost almost 25% of its population, going from 1,133,917 in 1939 to 830,000 in 1945 (Parming, 1978: 34; in Kallas and Kaldur, 2010: 82). Emigration was connected with both German and Soviet occupations during WWII. After the incorporation of Estonia into the USSR in 1945, an intensive immigration process started, the results of which are still significant. The immigrant population increased from approximately 12% ethnic minorities in 1934 to 38.5% in 1989 (Kallas and Kaldur, 2010: 83). The majority of immigrants were ethnic Russians (30.3%), Ukrainians (3.0%), and Byelorussians (1.8%). Other ethnic minorities (hundreds of different ethnic groups) formed 3.4% of the population. During these years a large so-called Russophone part of population emerged, which was segregated from the Estonian population because of the language and regional location. Immigrants were settled intently in north and northeast cities and towns.[3] The official explanation of immigration was connected with industrial development: factories and laborers were taken to Estonia by the Soviet power (Kallas and Kaldur, 2010: 83; Misiunas and Taagepera, 1993).

Immigration stopped in 1991 when the independent Estonian Republic was restored. Between the years 1990 and 1997, some 4.6 million former Soviet Union citizens migrated from the former occupied territories back to Russia (Okólski, 2004: 38; cited in Järv, 2009: 43). Among them were Russophone people who returned to Russia with the Soviet Army. As a result of the emigration process, the percentage of Estonian people in the total population increased from 61.5% in 1989 to 68.7% in 2008. In 2000 and 2008, the percentage of Russians was 25.6%. At the beginning of 2012, the general population in Estonia was 1,339,662 persons (Statistics Estonia, 2013). This number is 5.5% lower than that of the last population census in 2000. During the time between the two censuses, the percentage of children ages zero to 15 decreased from 18% in 2000 to 15.6% in 2012.

Migration Trends after 1991: Recent Migrants, Asylum Seekers, and Refugees in Estonia

The first reliable data on external migration is obtainable since 2000. According to these data between 2000 and 2007, 10,326 persons came to Estonia, and 26,518 persons (2% of the Estonian population) left Estonia. Migration events became more vivid after the country joined the European Union (EU) in 2004. Despite the small numbers, immigration has been a growing trend over the years. Most immigrants came from Finland (3,145 persons, or 31% of all immigrants) and Russia (2,467 persons, or 24% of all immigrants). According to Anniste (2009: 64), 45% of immigrants were Estonian citizens, former emigrants who returned to Estonia within a few years. Fifteen percent of immigrants were people with Russian citizenship, 11% with Finnish, and 5% with Ukrainian (Anniste, 2009: 64). Because the statistics on immigrant population in Estonia are not very clear, we can only guess at some tendencies in this category of the population. Table 12.1 represents information about countries of

Table 12.1. Immigrants by year of migration and country of birth (all age groups and sexes)

	Estonia	Russia	Finland	Other country	Country unknown	Total
2004	250	144	233	284	186	1,097
2005	355	169	311	412	189	1,436
2006	611	209	494	647	273	2,234
2007	1,296	273	820	948	404	3,741
2008	1,184	675	316	1,416	80	3,671
2009	1,250	672	317	1,595	50	3,884
2010	1,188	534	167	881	40	2,810
2011	1,539	1,085	56	991	38	3,709
2012	2,133	923	69	1,093	26	4,244

Source: Statistics Estonia, 2013.

Table 12.2. Immigrants by year of migration, age group zero to 19 and country of birth (all sexes)

Year	Estonia	Russia	Finland	Other country	Country unknown	Total
2004	56	14	32	41	13	156
2005	63	17	42	56	23	201
2006	121	27	71	85	32	336
2007	327	46	111	169	56	709
2008	155	128	54	294	6	634
2009	119	168	48	288	1	624
2010	107	115	22	222	1	467
2011	144	256	41	246	1	688
2012	233	201	47	343	40	824

Source: Statistics Estonia, 2013.

birth of people who immigrated to Estonia during the years after joining the EU in 2004. Statistics show that joining the EU inspired Estonian-born people to return to their home country.

Table 12.2 shows the number of young immigrants to Estonia between 2004 and 2011.

Here we use the term "immigrant" to mean people from the former USSR states and Finns (i.e., representatives of neighboring cultures). We can only guess that people born in Estonia who emigrated and then immigrated back to Estonia are not identified by child protection workers as immigrants.

After Estonia joined the EU it became a country of transition from third-world countries to the EU. Most asylum seekers used Estonia as a gateway to some other EU country (Anniste, 2009; Strömpl, 2011).

The number of recently arrived immigrants from distant countries and asylum seekers is not large. Since 1997, when Estonia joined the United Nations Convention of Asylum Seekers and the Refugee Act was adopted, until July 2013, 415 applications were submitted (see Police and Border Guard Board statistics) and 83 persons received the refugee status (Estonian Refugee Council, 2013). In 2011, the number of applications has doubled comparing to 2010 (Toodo, 2012: 139). In 2012, there were 75 applications submitted, which is more than in earlier years but still the smallest number in Europe. In the same year, 10 persons received refugee status, then received humanitarian help; only five received subsidiary protection (Eurostat Commission, 2013). Among both asylum seekers and refugees, the number of children and adolescences is very small. Until January 1, 2011, the number was up to 10. By their citizenship, the asylum seekers are mainly people from Iraq, Russia, Turkey, Belarus, Georgia, Pakistan, and Afghanistan (Citizenship and Migration Bureau 2009; Kallas and Kaldur, 2010: 89).

Citizenship and Other Relations with the State

Before Estonia regained independence, all residents living in Estonia had USSR citizenship. After 1991, the Citizenship Act of 1938 was reintroduced. Accordingly, only those who had been citizens before 1940 and their descendants were automatically granted Estonian citizenship. Immigrants during the Soviet period had to go through the process of naturalization, which required two years of residence before applying, the loyalty oath, and the required knowledge of the Estonian language. According to the Estonian Citizenship Act, double citizenship is not allowed. The immigrant population had to choose among three options to formalize their relations with the independent state: naturalized Estonian citizens, citizens of independent Russian Federation or other country of their origin, or [remain] citizens of the extinct Soviet Union. The later group became people with undetermined citizenship or stateless people who had to apply for a residence permit (Kallas and Kaldur, 2010: 84).

Children are granted citizenship according to their parents' citizenship. Problems arise with having no information about parents' citizenship. According to the law, if one of the parents has Russian citizenship and the other is a person with undetermined citizenship with a resident permit, the child is identified as a Russian citizen.[4]

There is ongoing discussion about the modification of Estonian Citizenship Act. In the early 1990s the aim of the single citizenship was a kind of test of loyalty toward independent Estonia. Today people choose citizenship based on economic considerations. Living in Estonia and having Russian citizenship or being an undetermined citizen and having a permanent resident permit gives people more possibilities to travel without visas both in Europe and in Russia and other countries of the former Soviet Union. But undetermined citizenship affects people's identity, which is especially important for children and their national identity development. As Jacqueline Bhabha (2011: xiii) writes: "children need to have a demonstrable legal identity to flourish. Without it, they are in effect stateless, and their claims to citizenship, belonging, protection, and inclusion in the community in which they live are compromised."

The current citizenship policy demonstrates the state's excluding attitude toward the descendants of the so-called Soviet-time immigrants and grounds their status, which is more like an immigrant's status than the status of a native resident. Such a state attitude generates certain reactions in people, and they demonstrate their passiveness in applying for the Estonian citizenship. However, the situation is improving. At the beginning of 1992, one-third of the population was stateless. However, "On December 31 in 2009, there were 104,813 persons with undetermined citizenship in Estonia, including 2,153 children under 15 years of age who held long-term residence permit and whose both parents had undetermined citizenship" (Vetik, 2011: 162). This is approximately 1% of all children of the same age. After 20 years of independence, in January 2012, the number of stateless people was 97,749 (UNHCR, 2012), or 7.3% of the total population. The data show that many adult residents, although they do not so for themselves, apply for Estonian citizenship for their children.

In 2005 a new Act on Granting International Protection to Aliens was ratified by the Parliament to harmonize EU norms and international obligations of Estonia. This act entered into force on July 1, 2006 (Roots, 2007). This new act has some shortages compared with EU laws. Lehte Roots and Kristina Kallas (2011) in their comparative analysis of the European Council directive from January 27, 2003, and the Estonian Act from 2006 find that, among other important differences, the Estonian act does not define the notion of asylum seekers with special needs sufficiently enough. Only unaccompanied minor aliens are mentioned in the Estonian act, and there is not a word about children and adolescents who enter Estonia with their families or elderly people and disabled people. Because of this insufficient definition, the meaning of the special living conditions is not clear in the Estonian act.

Since 2000, asylum seekers can live in the Reception Centre for Asylum Seekers in Illuka. Qualitative research (Kadur and Kallas, 2011) carried out among asylum seekers living in Illuka Centre shows that especially families with small children are not satisfied with the living conditions. Children have no other space for playing besides the bedroom of the family. Families with children have to ask specially for the opportunity to visit a family doctor when the child is ill, but routine medical control for children is not organized by the center. However, it is common for Estonian medical systems in general to give the responsibility of the regular medical observation of children to the parents, so one can argue that the idea is in harmony with the general Estonian health care policy. However, newcomers, especially refugees or victims of trafficking, do not know anything about the Estonian system, and there is little attention paid to providing newcomers with sufficient information.

During this research, two confusing cases were mentioned. The first is the case of a young woman who came to Illuka with a three-week-old baby and who did not have postnatal care, because no one offered her this opportunity and she did not know that she had to ask for it. Another is the case of a 16-year-old boy with posttraumatic stress disorder who had to wait nine months before he could get psychiatric help. There are also problems with getting adequate education (Strömpl, Kaldur, & Markina, 2012). Because the Illuka Centre is very far from any large towns, there are no schools in the nearest neighborhood. Organizing school attendance for children requires a special effort. These cases illustrate the communication problems between the service providers and the users. When the head of the Illuka Centre takes the floor about the situation in Illuka, he, as a rule, blames the asylum seekers for their passiveness about organizing their life and for an expectant attitude toward the center staff.

In conclusion, although the number of asylum seekers and refugees is small, state and local governments do practically nothing to help these people to integrate into the Estonian society (see the letter of the chancellor of justice to the minister of social affairs, Kaldur and Kallas, 2011).

Child Protection Policy in Estonia

The CPA, mentioned earlier, defines the rights and obligations of children and parents and regulates child protection, which is first of all connected with possible harm and abuse of children in a family. The CPA was later much criticized because of its declarative character and low functional capacity. The implementation of the act became entangled in the lack of supportive regulations (Henberg, 2003). A new CPA is currently in the works. This new act was prepared as several documents (e.g., the Child Welfare Concept in 2005). On October 20, 2011, the government approved the *Strategy for Children and Families for 2012–2020* (Ministry of Social Affairs, 2011; hereafter Strategy), which, compared with the previous strategic documents, pays more attention to simultaneously improving the skills of the parents and developing the systems for noticing and helping the children in need. The Strategy emphasizes the importance of ensuring secure and friendly living environments for all families living in Estonia regardless of their nationality, religion, language, or place of residence. The Strategy does not mention immigrant families specifically but pays special attention to unaccompanied and trafficked children and emphasizes the development of services designed for them.

The everyday work in social work practice is regulated besides the CPA, as well as the Social Welfare Act (1995), the National Family Support Act (2002), the Parental Benefit Act (2004), and the Family Act (2010). Every family living in Estonia with legal status (citizenship, residence permit, asylum-seeking or refugee status) has an equal right to receive universal child support benefits stated in the National Family Support Act (2002) and the Parental Benefit Act (2004). Universal benefits are paid on the state level. The National Family Support Act states several types of family benefits paid to parents for every child until the age of 16 (see Family Benefit Act, Section 3). Children enrolled in basic or secondary schools or vocational education institutions operating on the basis of primary education have the right to receive family benefits until the age of 19 (Social Insurance Board, 2014a). The Parental Benefit Act is designed to contribute to the successful intertwining of parents' work and family life. The benefit itself provides parents with their average salary from the preceding calendar year for the time that they temporarily take off work to care for their children; unemployed parents receive parental benefits in the sum of a minimum amount (in 2013 it was 290 Euros). Any parent, adoptive parent, stepparent, guardian, or foster parent who is rearing a child and who is a permanent resident of Estonia or a foreigner living in Estonia on the basis of a temporary residence permit has the right to receive the parental benefit (Social Insurance Board, 2014b). State support of families in rearing their children is limited to the listed financial benefits.

The Estonian Ministry of Social Affairs was appointed as the National Contact Point for Unaccompanied and Trafficked Children already in 2004, but special regulations, services, preparation, and so on were missing until the spring of 2013. In April 2013, Parliament passed the specifications to the victim support services regulation and included unaccompanied and trafficked children in the target group. According to these changes, the Estonian National Insurance Board will hold the responsibility for organizing services and help such children at the moment public procurement for finding substitute home and health services providers is in progress.

ORGANIZATION

There are three levels in the organization of child protection work in Estonia: the state, the county, and the local government level. Service provision to people in need is incumbent on local governments. At the state level, the coordinator of national child protection work is the Ministry of Social Affairs. The Ministry's responsibility is to work out suitable legislation and elaborate strategies and developmental plans for providing services and benefits, to develop child protection professions, and to organize supervision and evaluation of services. The state is responsible for ensuring the supplies for children in care and organizing intercountry adoption (Ministry of Social Affairs).

Estonia is divided into 15 counties, and it is the county governments that are responsible for adoption, evaluation, and supervision of social services provided by local authorities and consulting local governments in child protection. There are 215 local municipalities in Estonia. They vary by size and number of inhabitants, from 99 persons in Piirissaare to 419,707 persons in Tallinn, the capital city of Estonia (as of January 1, 2013, Ministry of Internal Affairs). Regardless of differences, all local municipalities hold the same responsibility of helping people and ensuring their welfare. The coordination of child welfare work of cities and rural municipalities and also direct assistance of those in need is performed by child protection workers, but the task can also be entrusted to social workers, youth workers, or education specialists. This indicates that in Estonia there is no uniform perception of child welfare work by local governments yet. According to the annual reports of the Ministry of Social Affairs and to the recent audit carried out by the National Audit Office, only 38% of local governments employ a child welfare official. One-fifth of children in Estonia live in local government units that do not employ a child protection worker (National Audit Office of Estonia, 2013). Although according to the Child Welfare Concept prepared in 2005 there should be one child welfare official for every 1,000 children (Ministry of Social Affairs, 2005), there were approximately 1,491 children for every child welfare official in Estonia in 2010 (Poopuu, 2011: 23).

Services for children and families are provided mainly through institutions in municipal ownership or nonprofit organizations, whereas local governments are often more in the role of service buyers than providers. Services are divided into in-home and out-of-home services. The aim of the in-home services is to enhance families' capability to take care of their children and to avoid placement into substitute care. Some in-home services are assigned to the parents, for example, support-person services, different educational programs for raising parental capability, counseling services, participation in family center activities to avoid exclusion from community life, and so on. Some of the in-home services are aimed at the children, such as day care centers, counseling, rehabilitation, and so forth. As usual, services are selected according to the problems the families face; preventive services are lacking. Despite the possibilities that local governments have, the help does not reach children at the right time (i.e., in the early stages of problem). Usually local governments predominantly provide assistance in cases where a problem has become so serious that the parent or guardian has decided to ask for help from the system (National Audit Office of Estonia, 2013). Other studies (e.g., Linno, 2012) indicate also the child protection workers' tendency rather to wait for clients' initiative than to act themselves actively toward people in need. Such kind of waiting for clients' activeness in seeking help demonstrates that prevention and early intervention is not the issue of local government child protection practice, which also means that many of the children in need can be left without any help while their guardians are not active in seeking help. One reason why immigrant families are left out of child protection practice could be that they are not active seekers of help due to insufficient language skill and lack of appropriate and understandable information.

Local governments' child protection officials' activity first of all focuses on protecting children from abusive parents (see also Toros, 2011). They have the power and jurisdiction to separate a child from parents if the circumstances at home are dangerous to the life and health of the child. Child protection workers are required to present an application for the decision concerning child's separation in court of law. The child protection worker has to find a placement for the child among available opportunities. There is a well-organized institutional care system in Estonia. A foster family system also exists, but the number of children who are placed into the foster families has diminished over the years (National Audit Office of Estonia, 2009). Besides that, local government's child protection workers have to continue working with the family to assure child's and parents' reunification. However, recent studies (see, e.g., Julle, 2010) have shown that child protection workers are skeptical toward such kind of work. They lack motivation to make the reunification happen and consider placement as the final solution mainly because they do not believe in parents' ability to change their behavior.

Information about children and families—service users of child welfare—is insufficient. For years the national statistics registered only children taken into out-of-home care (i.e., separated from parents). Children taken into in-home care have been registered only since 2006. The number of children taken into out-of-home care are presented in Table 12.3.

TRAINING

There is no statistical data on the preparation and level of the education of the child welfare officials, but, according to the results of the 2004 survey by the Ministry of Social Affairs, the average child protection worker was 46 to 55 years old and had been working in the field for at least five years; approximately two-thirds of the participants in the survey had acquired higher education, but only one-third had acquired professional (i.e., social work) higher education (Luik, Reinomägi, Tomberg, Riisalo, Kurves, and Sõmer, 2004). Twenty-eight percent of the participants were child protection workers, and 72% were social workers fulfilling the duties of child protection workers. In 2010 Kati Kütt also conducted a survey among child protection workers. According to her results, the average age of child protection workers was 40, and 82% of them had higher social work education (Kütt, 2011: 24–25). According to the latest study carried out by the Estonian Social Work Association (2012), approximately 51% of all social workers working in local governments have higher social work education.

It is evident that, compared with all social workers working in local governments, the child protection workers are professionally more educated. But, as mentioned previously, only 38% of local governments employ child protection workers, and in the majority of local governments, the task of child protection is entrusted to the social workers, who quite often do not have professional education.

Table 12.3. Children first registered and taken into out-of-home care, 1998–2012[a]

Year	Registered children in the beginning of the year[b]	First registered/ taken into care[c]	Institutionalized[d]	Children in care at the end of the year[e]
1998	362	1,671	1,595	440
1999	440	1,752	1,749	443
2000	443	1,227	1,305	365
2001	364	1,255	1,288	331
2002	331	1,249	1,301	279
2003	281	1,276	1,326	231
2004	230	1,092	1,073	249
2005	249	858	979	128
2006	822	1,680	645	1,848
2007	1,319	1,529	543	2,305
2008	1,984	1,738	585	2,430
2009	2,738	2,184	664	3,334
2010	3,334	2,054	460	3,904
2011	3,904	2,574	454	4,611
2012	4,751	2,808	410	5,213

[a] Since 2006, in addition to the children without parental care and orphans, other children in need were also included in statistics.

[b] Clients of child protection at the beginning of the year.

[c] Children who became child protection users during the year.

[d] Children who were separated from parents during the year.

[e] Children whose separation process was still in progress at the end of the year or who received supportive services to avoid placement.

Source: Ministry of Social Affairs.

The Social Welfare Act states that social workers have to have higher education and adequate professional preparation, but it does not specify the need for social work higher education. However, higher education doesn't mean that social workers are trained to work with different cultural and religious groups, especially the distant ones.

Social work curricula at two Estonian universities include special modules of social work with children, youth, and their families, providing competence for child protection workers on bachelor's and master's levels. The Institute of Social Work at the University of Tallinn offers, for example, a two-year master's program in Social Pedagogy and Child Protection (120 credits). However, even this curriculum has no subjects on working with immigrant children or multicultural/intercultural social work. In spring 2013 a new course on asylum seekers and refugees was taught at Tallinn and Tartu Universities. The course was initiated by the Centre for Human Rights and was prepared by lecturers and specialists working with the topic theoretically and practically. This course gives some basic knowledge for social workers working with immigrant people from distant cultures. Also, social work students work during their study practice and as volunteers with asylum seekers and refugees in Estonian Refugee Council. During some courses, it is possible to conduct research with immigrants or representatives of different cultures.

REPRESENTATION OF MIGRANT CHILDREN

When talking about the experiences of working with children and families with immigrant backgrounds, it should be kept in mind that there are at least three categories of families who might be categorized as immigrants:

(1) Formally immigrant but factually Estonian remigrant families, who spent some years abroad and returned to Estonia. These people can have some problems with the reintegration into the Estonian society, but they are hardly defined as immigrants by the social workers.

(2) Russophone families, who are formally not defined as immigrants because they can be people of a third or even fourth generation of immigrants, but they still have integration problems. Among these people may be also stateless people; however, they are rather defined by the social workers as ethnic minorities. Child protection work with this group is precise because of the specific problems of Russophone people, especially those who live in the northeastern part of Estonia. Because of economic backwardness of this part of Estonia, there are many unemployed people with several problems, such as drug abuse and poverty, which in turn result in many cases of child neglect (Linno, Soo, and Strömpl, 2011). Statistics about children with an immigrant background connected with social care systems are nonexistent. Until 2006 there were available data in the national statistics about children with temporary residence permit taken into care, but not anymore. However, on the basis of statistics provided by the local governments, one can see that the children from Ida-Virumaa (the northeastern part of Estonia with a high concentration of Russophone people, people with undetermined citizenship, and a high level of unemployment) are much more often registered as service users and placed into out-of-home care compared with children living in other counties.

(3) Recent immigrants who entered Estonia after 1991 (in Estonian: uusimmigrandid), including asylum seekers and refugees. This group of immigrants is so small that the system is just starting to recognize it as a specific category of clients. The term "immigrant" or "newcomer" is not mentioned in legal acts connected with child protection.

PRACTICE

To assess the real practice with immigrant children, a cross-country survey was carried out in the summer of 2012. We invited all the frontline child protection officials working in municipalities at that time. According to the Ministry of Social Affairs, there were 176 child protection officials working in municipalities and 12 child protection officials working in county governments. Child protection officials working in county governments were not included in sampling; because their duties are more general, they do not meet service users directly. As the survey had two versions, we created an alphabetical database of local municipalities and selected every first person on the list to receive the survey version 1 and every second person to receive the survey version 2. The first and second versions were distributed equally to 88 people each. We monitored every municipality employing more than one child protection worker to participate in the survey with both versions.

In sum, 176 persons were invited to participate in survey, which is 100% of all social workers of local municipalities dealing with child protection all over Estonia. Eighty-one (46%) of invited persons opened the questionnaire and answered the first question (see information about cross- country survey in the appendix), but only 22 respondents (27%) reported some working experience with immigrant children and their families. Also, the working number of respondents proved very low: most respondents working with immigrant families spend only 5% to 10% of their time and only two social workers spend 40% to 60% of their time helping immigrant families. One can assume that these were those social workers who were invited to participate in the study later who work not in a local municipality but in some special nongovernnmental organization for asylum seekers and refugees.

It is also remarkable that none of respondents were immigrant and only two respondents' parents were foreign-born people. This fact let us conclude that child protection workers from Ida-Virumaa (northeast part of Estonia) did not participate in this survey. The reason of nonparticipation may be explained by the fact that the survey was distributed only in the Estonian language and Russophone social workers had problems filling in the questionnaire. We did not translate the survey into Russian, because Estonian is obligatory to know for every state and municipality officials.

The Estonian survey data shows that 18 out of 22 respondents had higher social work education, but only 3 of 22 social workers working with immigrant families had received some special training.

The Estonian data of cross-country survey indicate that respondents specified the children and families from Russia, other former Soviet Union countries (Moldova, Latvia, Lithuania), and Finland more frequently as the immigrant clients of the child protection system. Nevertheless, single clients from Asia,

Africa, and Western countries (e.g., Spain, Portugal, Italy) were also mentioned by respondents.

One of the most interesting results of the survey was identifying parents' unemployment status as one of the high risk factors. We argue this result to be characteristic of Estonian child protection work and to be in accordance with findings from recent studies (Julle, 2010; Toros, 2011), concluding the material well-being as one of the most important aspects during the assessment of the family as suitable for the child. Child protection workers who participated in survey reacted to problems more strictly when the parents were described as unemployed people. The respondents were asked to assess the level of risk and offer action to a case of battered 10-year-old girl—daughter of an immigrant family (the second vignette of the survey). There were two versions of same case. In one version both parents were employed and worked long hours, while in other they were unemployed. In the second version the risk for the child was assessed as high (37%) and very high (62%), and the reaction of child protection workers was stricter: most social workers would ponder separation of the child from the family (two of eight were ready to do this immediately and three of eight would start proceedings for out-of-home placement). The other three of eight would have left the child in the family and provided the parents with in-home services. In the case where the parents were employed, half of respondents would have offered the family in-home services, 5 respondents of 14 would have separated the girl immediately or started separation and 2 would have chosen some other solving procedure; unfortunately we don't know what exactly this would have been.

It was especially interesting to read the explanations added by respondents. Two more frequent explanations emphasized when the parents were unemployed were the following: first, coping problems of parents who had not found a job during five years of living in Estonia ("The parents have lived in Estonia for five years already and they have not been able to find job, they still live from social benefits"), and second, cultural differences and parents' inability to change their values ("The parents still live according to their cultural traditions and are not able to change their values"). In the case when the parents had long working hours some respondents guessed that the problem was in child neglect ("The girl is unattended by parents"); relationship problems between parents and the child ("Disturbance in relations between parents and the girl"; "Parents cannot understand a 10-year-old girl"), and cultural differences ("Parents don't understand that they do something wrong, they approach from the point of view of their cultural traditions, which are in contradiction with the Estonian law"). According to these explanations the social workers were going to advise parents to change their values. Separation in this case means temporary separation and the placement of the girl in a shelter. Among the explanations for the social worker's activity the best interest of the child and Estonian laws that prohibit children's corporal punishment were mentioned.

Among the ethnicity of parents—in case of the cultural difference—Russian, Roma, and Muslim/Arabic or Asian background was marked. In case vignette 1 Africa, some other Southern countries were marked as the immigrants' home country and also Roma ethnicity was mentioned. Thus in both vignettes some exotic culture or country of far distance was mentioned. In the case of comparing Estonian and Russian cultures the differences in values seems to be important to emphasize. Because of the small number of respondents, we cannot make any wide generalisations; however, the tendency that unemployed parents receive less trust from social workers compared with employed parents seems to be evident.

Until now the Estonian child protection work was first of all focused on saving the children and less on helping the family. However, some recent studies (Linno et al., 2011; Soo, Ilves, and Strömpl, 2009) on daily work with child maltreatment and domestic violence show that child protection workers try to help first the mothers of the children in need if and as long as it is possible. The latest developments (see the Strategy mentioned before and the new CPA in progress) indicate that parents and family should be supported to better cope with child rearing. The Estonian survey data also show that most social workers (20 out of 22) chose in the first vignette—describing a young immigrant family with a small baby living in very poor conditions—to help the family, while the risk for the baby was assessed by them as high or very high. This vignette, however, deals with material support of a newcomer family, and it seems that the services available in Estonian child protection have the potential to provide the family with the necessary material resources.

The small number of respondents who filled out the survey could be explained as a sign of some uncertainty of child protection workers' awareness about their service users' origin. This situation could be explained, on the one hand, by the people with an immigrant background not having specific problems that force them to turn to the child protection system. On the other hand, one can argue that the child protection workers' decision to participate in the survey depended on the fact that they had worked with a recently migrated family that maybe became service users specifically because of their immigrant status. Here asylum seekers and refugees form a specific group, and this may be the reason why many social workers who in fact work with immigrant families did not define them as immigrants because they were not refugees.

CONCLUSION

Immigrant children in the Estonian child protection system are invisible. This is explainable by the specifics of the Estonian migration process and factual and formal definitions of immigrant groups. Estonian citizens are mobile people and use the opportunities offered to them by the EU membership, and many of them return to Estonia after some years of living abroad. Children belonging to this group are not defined by the child protection system as immigrants; however, officially they are fixed in immigration statistics. On the other hand, there is a large group of children and families who stay in Estonia for a long time and who have an immigrant background and are marked in official statistics as foreign born, but for the Estonian people they are identified first of all as an ethnic minority (Russian or Russophone), not immigrants. They have problems with integration into the Estonian society, but in fact all they have the same access to services and benefits that the state offers all residents. The universalistic character of benefits does not obligate the social workers to delve into families' backgrounds; it is enough to have the information that the family has the legal right to live in Estonia. The situation is a bit different with children living in Estonia illegally (i.e., whose parents are not registered in the population register). These children are not included in child protection system either. The classically understood immigrants' group (e.g., foreign people coming to Estonia after 1991) is still very small, and they are hardly seen in the Estonian child protection system. Another group of children are the children of the refugee people or asylum seekers. This group is also very small, and our data show that they are not even recognized by child protection workers; it is nonprofit organizations that work with this contingent. However, the last Estonian integration program for 2008–2013 promises that recent immigrants will be welcomed with good integration regulations and programs.

NOTES

1 Estonia produced its first annual report regarding the obligations of the Convention in 2001, after an eight-year delay. The second, third, and fourth country reports were to be presented in 2008 but have not been presented as yet. The position of children's ombudsman was established 10 years after the signing of the Convention, in 2011 (Hallimäe, 2012: 147–151).

2 There is detailed information about ethnic composition of the population in official Estonian statistics, but information about immigrant population is represented only through the number of annual migrations, the foreign-born population, and the foreign population. The ethnic origin and immigrant background partly overlap.

3 Soviet military were placed everywhere in the country, but the largest bases were in South Estonia, in the northwest, and on the islands.

4 According to Citizenship Act of Russian Federation (section 11, a) children of Russian citizens who live on the territory of Russia or former Soviet Union and have no other citizenship, are granted Russian citizenship by birth. (see http://www.fms.gov.ru/documents/grazhdanstvo/Pdf/62-fz.pdf)

REFERENCES

Act on Granting International Protection to Aliens [Estonia]. (2005). Retrieved September 1, 2012, from https://www.riigiteataja.ee/en/eli/530102013009/consolide.

Anniste, K. (2009). External migration of Estonia in 2000–2007. In A. Tammur & H. Rannala (Eds.), *Ränne. Migration*, 50–66. Tallinn: Statistics Estonia.

Bhabha, J. (2011). Preface. In J. Bhabha (Ed.), *Children Without a State: A Global Human Rights Challenge*, xiii–xvi. Cambridge, MA: MIT Press.

Estonian Refugee Council. (2013). http://www.pagulasabi.ee.

Estonian Social Work Association. (2012). *Kohalike omavalitsuste sotsiaaltöötajate haridus* (Education of Local Governments' Social Workers). Tallinn: Estonian Social Work Association. Retrieved October 20, 2012, from http://eswa.ee/index.php?picfile=875.

Hallimäe, M. (2012). Rights of the Child. In *Human Rights in Estonia 2011: Annual Report of the Estonian Human Rights Centre*, 147–156. Tallinn: Foundation of Estonian Human Rights Centre. Retrieved March 1, 2013, from http://humanrights.ee/wp-content/uploads/2011/09/EIKaruanne2011.eng_.pdf.

Henberg, A. (2003). *Lastekaitse seaduse alusanalüüs* (Basic Analysis of Child Protection Act). Tallinn: Sotsiaalministeerium (Ministry of Social Affairs). Retrieved February 4, 2013, from http://lapsedjapered.sm.ee/fileadmin/Sisu_laadimine/Lapsed_ja_pered/Alusdokumendid/Lastekaitse_seaduse_alusanal-ueues.pdf.

Julle, A. (2010). *Perekondade taasühendamine—tühimik Eesti sotsiaaltöö maastikul* (Family Reunification—Gap in Estonian Social Work). Unpublished master's thesis, University of Tartu.

Järv, K. (2009). Recent migrant in Estonia. In E. Saar (Ed.), *Immigrant Population in Estonia*, 43–57. Tallinn: Statistics Estonia. Retrieved July 15, 2012, from http://www.stat.ee/publication-download-pdf?publication_id=18391

Kaldur, K., & Kallas, K. (2011). *Satisfaction Expectations by Asylum Seekers Towards Living Conditions and Offered Services*. Tartu: Institute of Baltic Studies.

Kallas, K., & Kaldur, K. (2010). Estonia: A post-Soviet predicamen. In K. Fangen, K. Fossan, and F.A. Mohn (Eds.), *Inclusion and Exclusion of Young Adult Migrants in Europe: Barriers and Bridges*, 81–108. London: Ashgate.

———. (2011). *Eestis rahvusvahelise kaitse saanud isikute hetkeolukord ning integreeritus Eesti ühiskonda* (The Current Situation of Refugees and their Integration into Estonian Society). Tartu: Institute of Baltic Studies.

Kütt, K. (2011). Eesti lastekaitsetöö sisu ja dünaamika 2001–2010 (The content and dynamics of Estonian child protection work). *Sotsiaaltöö* (Social Work), 4, 24–28.

Linno, M. (2012). Eriala esitamine lastekaitsetöötajate lugudes laste vastu suunatud vägivallast (The presentation of profession in child protection workers' stories about child abuse). In J. Strömpl, M. Selg, and M. Linno (Eds.), *Narratiivne lähenemine sotsiaaltööuurimuses: Laste väärkohtlemise lood* (Narrative Approach in Social Work Research: Stories about Child Abuse), 120–165. Tartu: Tartu University Press.

Linno, M., Soo, K., & Strömpl, J. (2011). *Perevägivalla levikut soodustavad riskid ja perevägivalla ulatus praktikute hinnangutes* (Risks of Distribution of Domestic Violence in Opinion of Practitioners). Tallinn: Justiitsministeerium (Ministry of Justice).

Luik, M., Reinomägi, A., Tomberg, M., Riisalo, S., Kurves, T., & Sõmer, S. (2004). *Lastekaitsetöö tegijad ning nende hinnangud valdkonna korralduse ja seadusandluse kohta: Küsitlus lastekaitsetöö tegijate seas* (Child Protection Workers and their Evaluation of Regulation and Legislation of the Field: Survey among Child Portection Workers). Tallinn: Ministry of Social Affairs. Retrieved May 10, 2012, from http://www.sm.ee/fileadmin/meedia/ Dokumendid/Sotsiaalvaldkond/lapsed/lastekaitse/Lastekaitsetoeoetajate_ kuesitlus.pdf.

Ministry of Social Affairs. (2004). *Lastekaitse kontseptsioon* (Child Welfare Concept) Tallinn: Sotsiaalministeerium (Ministry of Social Affairs). Retrieved October 20, 2012, from http://lapsedjapered.sm.ee/fileadmin/Sisu_laadimine/ Lapsed_ja_pered/Alusdokumendid/Lastekaitse_seaduse_alusanalueues.pdf.

———. (2011). *Laste ja perede arengukava 2012–2020* (Strategy for Children and Families for 2012–2020). Tallinn: Sotsiaalminsteerium (Ministry of Social Affairs). Retrieved August 21, 2012, from http://www.sm.ee/ fileadmin/meedia/Dokumendid/Sotsiaalvaldkond/kogumik/Laste_ ja_perede_arengukava_2012_-_2020.pdf.

Misiunas, R., & Taagepera, R. (1993). *The Baltic States: Years of Dependence, 1940–1990.* London: Hurst.

National Audit Office of Estonia. (2009). Activities of the State in Organising State Welfare Services for Children. Tallinn: National Audit Office of Estonia. Retrieved September 1, 2012, from http://www.riigikontroll.ee/ Riigikontrollipublikatsioonid/Auditiaruanded/tabid/206/Audit/2105/lan-guage/et-EE/Default.aspx.

———. (2013). Organisation of Child Welfare in Municipalities, Towns and Cities. Tallinn: National Audit Office. Retrieved August 20, 2012, from http://www.riigikontroll.ee/Suhtedavalikkusega/Pressiteated/tabid/168/ ItemId/664/View/Docs/amid/557/language/et-EE/Default.aspx.

Organisation for Economic Co-operation and Development. (2013). Country statistical profile: Estonia. *Country Statistical Profiles: Key Tables from OECD.* OECD iLibrary. Retrieved November 22, 2013, from http://dx.doi. org/10.1787/csp-est-table-2013-2-en.

Parming, T. (1978). *Population Changes and Processes: A Case Study of a Soviet Republic: The Estonian SSR.* Boulder, CO: Westview Press.

Poopuu, T. (2011). Eesti lastekaitsesüsteem vajab laiapõhjalist arendamist (Estonian child protection system needs a comprehensive development). *Sotsiaaltöö* (Social Work), 4, 22–23.

Roots, L. (2007). *National Report Done by the Odysseus Network for the European Commission on the Implementation of the Directive on Reception Conditions for Asylum Seekers in Estonia.* Academic Network for Legal Studies on Immigration and Asylum in Europe. Retrieved May 10, 2012, from http://ec.europa.eu/home-affairs/doc_centre/asylum/docs/estonia_2007_en.pdf.

Roots, L., & Kallas, K. (2011). *Välismaalasele rahvusvahelise kaitse andmise seaduse ja Euroopa Nõukogu direktiivi 2003/9/EÜ, 27.jaanuar 003 võrdlev analüüs erivajadustega isikute vastuvõtutingimuste osas* (Comparative Overview of the Implementation of the Directive 2003/9 of 27 January 2003 Laying Down Minimum Standards for the Reception of Asylum Seekers with Special Needs in the EU Member States and the Estonian Act on Granting International Protection to Aliens). Tartu: Institute of Baltic Studies.

Social Insurance Board. (2014a). Family Benefits. Social Insurance Board. Retreived September 2, 2014, from http://www.sotsiaalkindlustusamet.ee/family-benefits/.

Social Insurance Board. (2014b). Parental Benefit. Social Insurance Board. Retreived September 2, 2014, from http://www.sotsiaalkindlustusamet.ee/parental-benefit/.

Soo, K., Ilves, K., & Strömpl, J. (2009). *Laste väärkohtlemise juhtumitest teavitamine ja võrgustikutöö* (Notification of Cases of Child Maltreatment and Network). Tallinn: Ministry of Social Affairs.

Statistics Estonia. (2013). http://www.stat.ee/statistics.

Strömpl, J. (2011). *Asylum Seekers—Challenges for Estonia in a Post-Modern Europe. Illustrative cases.* Oslo: EUMARGINS. Retrieved November 27, 2013, from http://www.sv.uio.no/iss/english/research/projects/eumargins/illustrative-cases/documents/estonia-illustrative-case-illuka-final.pdf.

Strömpl, J., Kaldur, K., & Markina, A. (2012). Pathways in education. In K. Fangen, T. Johanson, & N. Hammarén (Eds.), *Young Migrants: Exclusion and Belonging in Europe*, 87–116. New York: Palgrave Macmillan.

Toodo, K. (2012). Rights of the refugees and asylum seekers. In *Human Rights in Estonia 2011: Annual Report of the Estonian Human Rights Centre*, 137–146. Tallinn: Foundation of Estonian Human Rights Centre. Retrieved March 1, 2013, from http://humanrights.ee/wp-content/uploads/2011/09/EIKaruanne2011.eng_.pdf.

Toros, K. (2011). *Assessment of Child Well-Being: Child Protection Practice in Estonia.* Dissertations on Social Sciences. Tallinn: Tallinn University.

United Nations High Commissioner for Refugees (UNHCR). (2011). *Asylum Levels and Trends in Industriallized Countries: Statistical Overview of Asylum Applications Lodged in Europe and Selected Non-European Countries.*

Geneva: UNHCR. Retrieved November 27, 2013, from http://www.unhcr.
org/4e9beaa19.html.

——. (2012). *2011 Statistical Yearbook*, 11th ed. Geneva: UNHCR. Retrieved
November 27, 2013, from http://www.unhcr.org/51628f589.html.

Vetik, R. (2011). Statelessness, citizenship and belonging in Estonia. In B.K.
Blitz & M. Lynch (Eds.), *Statelessness and Citizenship: A Comparative Study
on the Benefits of Nationality*, 160–171. Northampton, MA: Edward Elgar.

PART IV

CONCLUDING REMARKS

13

MIGRANT CHILDREN AND CHILD WELFARE SYSTEMS

A CONTESTED CHALLENGE

Ravinder Barn, Katrin Križ, Tarja Pösö, and Marit Skivenes

Children are in the midst of migration processes that are occurring due to economic crises, military conflicts, and natural disasters in many countries (UNICEF, 2009; Williamson, 2006). However, research rarely focuses on the challenges and problems that children may experience during migration, in the process of starting a new life, and after they and their families have settled in another society. This book explores how the child welfare systems of different countries in the global north perceive migrant children who are vulnerable, that is, at risk of abuse or neglect, and how they interact with these children. The chapters discuss children who migrate with their parents, as well as those who migrate alone, and children of parents who migrated. The aim of this book is to shed light on the situation of these children and compare the types of interventions and supports that child welfare systems provide for them. We explore the ideologies, policies, and responsibilities of child welfare systems in 11 countries as they work with migrant children who are in need of assistance or protection from harm. At the outset of this project, we identified five key themes in which we expected to find significant information about the book's areas of interest: (1) law and policy, (2) organization, (3) training, (4) representation of migrant children, and (5) practice. In this concluding chapter, we focus on three areas. First, we present the main tendencies and the ways in which the disparate child welfare systems carry out their roles and responsibilities. Second, given the diversity in this book, we delineate the differing findings to arrive at some meaningful conclusions. Finally, we identify areas for possible future research.

TENDENCIES

Law and Policy

The chapters in this book analyze the types of legal and policy platforms that countries create for the well-being of migrant children in general and the role of the child welfare system in particular. We asked to what degree migrant children are a focus of governmental policies and how laws and policies define problems and solutions. We saw that, on one hand, the platforms that countries and child welfare systems offer migrant children at risk are very similar overall, because all countries' child welfare systems assume the responsibility for all children who are at risk. However, if we think that migrant children are in an especially disadvantaged situation compared to other children, due to a higher poverty risk and their families' lack of social networks, lack of language proficiency, and knowledge of society and welfare systems when they arrive in the destination society, for example, then we see that very few countries report explicit legislation or guidelines to handle this group of children. Overall, the country reports on migration policies hardly mention children at all, which leads us to believe that children are not a central concern of migration policies; further, these policies may even be at odds with the interests of migrant children. Even Norway, a country that is highly focused on children, does not report a comprehensive legal and political platform that is specifically oriented toward migrant children. The schism between child welfare and migration policies is reflected at the organizational level as well in that child welfare and migration systems are separate systems with their own specific sets of goals and tasks.

Organization

When we examined how different child welfare systems work with migrant children from an organizational standpoint, three themes emerged. These themes echo the findings of Gilbert, Parton, and Skivenes (2011) with regard to the organizational aspects of child welfare systems in different Organisation for Economic Co-opertion and Development countries. First, recent organizational changes have taken place in some of the child welfare systems, reflecting the fact that this is a public sector that is constantly under scrutiny for reform. Second, several country authors discuss the decentralization and fragmentation of public child welfare services. They point to the fragmented aspect of the overall child welfare system, which may lead to variation in the types of services available to migrant families and their children, depending on where in a country they reside. In the countries under study, we also detected some evidence of the twin processes of supranationalization (such as European Union enlargement) and devolution of public services to the local level.

We found that in several of the countries, the statutory child welfare agencies themselves are not involved in providing services that are targeted specifically at migrant children and migrant families and their children: in countries that subscribe to residual or liberal welfare regimes (Esping-Andersen, 1990), including Australia, Estonia, Canada, England, and the United States, child welfare services themselves tend to focus on intervention rather than prevention or ongoing service provision (cf. also Gilbert et al., 2011). Intervention can be culturally sensitive or specific where child welfare workers have received cultural competency or diversity training, are hired for their ethnic and cultural background (as in so-called bilingual units in the United States), and/or where there are specific practice guidelines in working with migrant families (as in some local authorities in England). In countries such as Finland and Norway, both "family service" systems (Gilbert et al., 2011), child welfare services are embedded in a welfare state that provides universal public services, regardless of whether or not a person is a migrant. There are, however, also public services specifically targeted at migrant children to secure social inclusion and education. In Australia, Canada, and the United States, whose child welfare systems are protection-focused (Gilbert et al., 2011), the public child welfare system is not primarily involved in providing preventive or ongoing services. Similarly to England, these child welfare systems (as well as other parts of the state) work with "community service providers" that provide services targeted at migrant children and their families as well as other (not child welfare–specific) statutory services. In Austria, too, statutory child welfare services themselves do not offer public services specifically targeting migrants; migrant families are supported by civil society organizations and nongovernmental organizations. Italy drew up a 2012 national plan for developing public services available specifically to migrant families at the local level, but this plan has yet to be implemented. Further, some countries report using actuarial risk assessment tools, and it is noteworthy that most of these countries also subscribe to a protection-focused child welfare practice. Future research will need to explore in what ways these tools take into account the specific challenges faced by migrant children and their families, as well as examine how the needs of migrant children and families of different migrant statuses are met. The comparatively high poverty levels of migrant children and families are also emphasized by several country chapters. Future research will need to examine to what extent fiscal policies, such as child benefits and benefits through the tax system aimed at parents to prevent poverty among children, affect migrant children and their families differently from nonmigrant children and families.

Training

How are frontline child welfare workers who are employed by public child welfare agencies trained in working with migrant service users? What do training curricula look like? Although it is widely acknowledged that social work education is at the forefront of introducing new, relevant practices and tools for the profession, almost all of the chapters in this book report training that insufficiently prepares workers to practice with migrant children and families. We can see this tendency in the workers' responses to the survey as well. When child welfare workers were asked whether they had received training relevant to working with migrant children and families, almost half (45%) reported insufficient training. However, more workers in the United States reported receiving relevant training as compared to their colleagues in other countries: 83% of US respondents, most of whom practiced in California, reported relevant training. The lowest figures were in Finland (21%) and Estonia (14%). This is not surprising, given that these countries have recent migration histories and low levels of migration overall. These levels of experience with training relevant to migrant children specifically are also reflected in the survey responses about workers' ratings of their competency level in working with migrant children and families compared to working with nonmigrant families. A total of 40% of the practitioners reported feeling less competent when working with migrant than with nonmigrant families; however, only 19% of US respondents felt that they were less competent—the lowest percentage among all the countries that participated in the survey. Again, the Finnish and Estonian survey respondents were most likely to express that they felt less competent working with migrant children and families. However, this also means that 60% of the practitioners surveyed reported that they felt equally or more competent working with migrant families compared to other families.

We found that *multiculturalism* and *cultural competency* approaches are the two main paradigms embraced by child protection systems when addressing migration issues in child protection systems. Teaching about cultural competencies differs among countries, but we do see a strong emphasis on cultural dimensions. This is, of course, very relevant for child welfare work with migrant families, but other migration-related and antidiscrimination issues could be considered as well, such as issues related to migrants' legal status and residency or citizenship and other issues related to different types of migration and social problems stemming from disadvantage, discrimination, and migration histories. The impact of such experiences on migrant children should be included in training curricula. In particular, the complex issues related to undocumented families and unaccompanied children may require a wide and flexible mix of rights-based, culturally competent, and antidiscriminatory practice skills. However, the individual chapters do not provide ample evidence suggesting that training curricula address these important issues.

Jim Ife (2001), emeritus professor at the Centre for Human Rights Education at Curtin University of Technology in Perth, Australia, draws a distinction between "deductive" and "inductive" approaches to human rights practice. According to Ife, the deductive approach considers legislation and policy documents as the starting point for human rights practice, whereas the inductive approach "does the reverse, starting rather with the grounded and real world of practice, identifying issues, needs or problems, and then seeing what human rights issues lie behind them" (Ife, 2001: 137). This distinction could be a helpful theoretical backdrop to looking at the steps that social work education needs to take to meet the needs of migrant children and families. We suggest that, following the deductive approach, the declarations and politics of human—and especially children's—rights should serve as an essential starting point for social work education. The tensions between children's and human rights and migration policy should be considered as well, among other related issues. From the point of view of the inductive approach to human rights practice, social work training should be equally sensitive to the experiences of different migrant children and families and teach practitioners to consider the problems these families experience socially, culturally, and economically in their everyday lives.

With the exceptions of Australia and the Netherlands, surveys with child welfare professionals were gathered in all of the countries represented in this book. Given that the survey showed that in Austria, England, Finland, and Norway between 80% and 93% of the workers reported that they did not speak the same language as any of the immigrant groups with whom they work, it is surprising that the issues of language played only a weak role in the practice analysis. The use of interpreters, in general, tends to be a neglected issue in social work practice even though the lack of shared language between children, families, and practitioners fundamentally challenges social work practice and its ethics; indeed, it is also an issue of human rights. Križ and Skivenes (2010), for example, demonstrate that social workers encounter several challenges when using interpreters in their work with minority ethnic families as they lose information, time, and trust (also see, e.g., Chand, 2005, and Humphreys, Atkar, and Baldwin, 1999). Accurate information, in their own language, about their position as service-users and newcomers in the country is, however, essential for migrant children and families. Yet the use of interpreters is not a key issue in many of the child welfare systems studied here, and most of the chapter contributors do not present it as a major issue. This could be a sign that the countries have managed to cope with the challenge of linguistic differences, but is it not clear how this is achieved. On the other hand, it may signal that there is not enough sensitivity in the field of social work to recognize the challenges that the use of interpreters or the lack of shared language entail. If it is the latter, it is a serious challenge that social work training needs to address.

Representation of Migrant Children

We analyzed to what extent migrant children are represented in the child welfare system and explored their characteristics. Are they overrepresented or underrepresented compared to nonmigrant children? Who exactly are the migrant children represented in the child welfare system (i.e., in terms of ethnicity, religion, language, country of origin, first- or second-generation status)? What are the types of risks and problems of the migrant children who have entered the child welfare system?

It is striking that there is a lack of recording of such data at official levels in the majority of the participating countries. These include Austria, Australia, Canada, Estonia, Finland, Italy, and Spain. In spite of a lack of availability of official data on migrant children's representation in child welfare, there is evidence that academic research is beginning to document the plight of such children in relation to child welfare services. In Britain, for instance, isolated and localized research studies have for many decades reported the overrepresentation of some migrant children in the child welfare system (Barn, 1993, 2007). The drive from such studies and specific key recommendations to central government to recognize the importance of collating such data led to the introduction of the policy of ethnic monitoring by the New Labour government in 2000 (Barn, Sinclair, and Ferdinand, 1997).

Interestingly, in some countries where such information is available, there appears to be a disproportionate representation of some migrant children in in-home and out-of-home services. We can see noteworthy and potentially helpful patterns for policymakers and practitioners. For example, in Texas, Latin American immigrant children and children of Latin American immigrants were found to be underrepresented among children in care, whereas Latino children of native parents are overrepresented (Vericker, Kuehn, and Capps, 2007). Research into these differences reveals important trends in parenting and family life and the implications of these for children and families. In Norway, where detailed data exist into some aspects of the representation of migrant children in child welfare statistics, it is possible to document a clear sense of over- and underrepresentation. For example, data show that migrant children are not only overrepresented among those in receipt of in-home services, but the number represented in this category has grown exponentially over the years. In Norway, data on children on care orders and out-of-home placements show a small underrepresentation of migrant children. However, there is a concern that "voluntary" placements, which are not captured in the official data and which do not require a court order but may have an element of force, could be on the rise. We would suggest that there is an urgent need for this kind of information to understand the nature and extent of such "voluntary" placements.

It is important to systematically gather data on migrant children if one is interested in knowing whether child welfare systems are hands-off or hands-on

(Skytte, 2002) when it comes to initial interactions with migrant children, and if one wants to know how migrant children fare compared to other children once they are in contact with the child welfare system. The country reports suggest that information about the origin of the country of migration is not sufficient because of the importance of migrant status. There are, however, obvious challenges and pitfalls when gathering information about the sensitive issues related to migrant status, especially legal status. The position of undocumented children and children of undocumented parents as potential (non-) receivers of child welfare services is especially challenging for data gathering and national statistics.

Practice

One important aim of this book was to gather comparative data about what frontline practice with migrant families looks like in different countries. How do child welfare workers actually practice with migrant children and their families in different child welfare systems? We were able to answer this question with the help of an identical survey that was answered by child welfare workers in nine of the 11 countries ($n = 838$). In each country, we used the same questions and presented child welfare workers with two case vignettes. Workers were asked about their perceptions of the risk in the case and what action they would take. Further, we asked workers about their experiences when interacting with service users that have a migrant background. The details and methodology for this cross-country survey can be found in the book's methodological appendix.

In the survey, we presented respondents with a case involving physical discipline, as we know that there are clear differences in countries' legislation and norms around using physical discipline as means for raising children (Global Initiative to End All Corporal Punishment of Children, 2012). Thus we expected that a case about a child being beaten by her parents would be assessed differently by workers across countries. With the same case, we also analyzed whether child welfare workers were influenced by parents' connection to the labor market when they assessed risk in a child welfare case. We anticipated that workers would be inclined to think that children whose parents are employed, able to support themselves, and contributing to society would be less at risk than children whose parents are not working and live on welfare support. To examine whether employment matters in workers' assessment, we randomly presented half of the sample in each country with a vignette in which parents were employed; the other half received an identical vignette in which the child's unemployed parents received financial support through welfare services. The survey results showed that there are only few differences within countries, indicating that, overall, child welfare workers do not put particular weight on parents' connections to the labor market when considering risk for a child. Of course, the fact that this is a case involving physical violence may overshadow the differences in parents' characteristics between the two vignettes.

Even though we were not able to verify our hypothesis that employment status matters to this sample of workers, we did find significant cross-country differences in risk assessment of the case and in workers' suggested decisions. Most workers assessed the case to be a high or very high risk situation, with the United States at the low risk end of the spectrum. Further, when asked about what their decision would be in the case, we found a very interesting split in workers' suggestions. About half would start care order proceedings or undertake an out-of-home placement; the other half would provide in-home services. Italy was the exception, with about 75% of the workers in the sample suggesting out-of-home placement. We grouped countries together based on welfare state model, child welfare system, and ranking on child welfare indices to see whether these dimensions resulted in similar outcomes. We did not find any significant results.

We also asked workers to respond to a vignette involving a young couple who are labor migrants. They have a newborn baby and are living in harsh conditions. We anticipated that, given the different country contexts, welfare state models, and child welfare systems, we would find significantly different assessments of the risk for the baby. When we examined country differences in terms of workers' assessments of risk level, we were surprised to find that cross-country differences were few. More workers assessed the risk to be high or very high (59%) than moderate (33%), and few (8%) assessed the case to be no or low risk. The only country in which workers assessed the risk to be significantly lower was the United States, and, on the other end of the spectrum, Estonia, which assessed the risk to be very high. This is interesting because these countries are both considered liberal welfare states. However, there were only 22 respondents from Estonia. The results also showed that most workers (95%) would provide in-home services. Very few would suggest an out-of-home placement or, on the other end, would take no action, and there were no significant cross-country differences.

All respondents who suggested that in-home services should be provided for the young couple and the baby (n = 730) were asked whether they would help parents become employed, link them to financial welfare services, find them better housing, encourage them to return to their home country, link them with other formal services, or link them with informal services. We thought that the responses to this question would provide information about workers' attitudes and how they view their abilities and responsibilities within their systems when they work with vulnerable families. The results show that workers in all countries would provide services that help the family's financial situation. They would also provide other statutory services, as well as link the family to community services. However, the results look different when it comes to housing and employment. Workers in three countries (Estonia, Italy, and Spain) indicated that they would help parents become employed. In Canada, England, and the United States, the country samples are split, with about half of respondents stating that they would help parents become employed and the other half answering that this is not an option in their system. This possibly indicates that workers feel that they have opportunities to choose different alternatives and that perhaps there are informal routes of supporting families that workers can access (see Križ & Skivenes, 2012). As for providing help with housing, the findings show that the samples from Austria and Norway are split in half, with one-half saying that they would help with housing and the other half saying that is not an option in their system. These results suggest that workers enjoy some amount of discretion in choosing how to proceed. It might also point to a gap between welfare state provisions and child welfare system provisions. For the rest of the country samples, a majority of workers indicated that they would find a place to live for the family.

When we asked workers whether they would encourage parents to return to their home country, we saw significant country differences. In descending order, respondents in Spain (36%), Italy (28%), Estonia (27%), Norway (22%), and England (15%) would be more inclined to suggest that parents should return to their country of origin. We do not have a plausible explanation for this difference because these countries involve very different migration histories and represent all three types of child welfare systems and welfare states. They also rank very differently (high, medium, and low) on the latest child welfare index (UNICEF, 2013).

Undocumented migrants are a sensitive and difficult issue to deal with for states. In terms of child welfare, this becomes a particularly relevant issue when it involves children in families where family members, including children themselves, are undocumented. These children live in a situation in which they are much more dependent on their parents' actions and decisions than other children. Children who live in detention centers or in fear of being detained and deported and who experience uncertainty about their and their family's future grow up in an environment that is not conducive to their development and well-being (see, e.g., Abrego and Gonzales, 2010; Gonzales and Chavez, 2012; Sigona and Hughes, 2012). The previous chapters indicate that in these situations children's individual rights seem to be cast aside. We see this for example in Norway with the group of young children who were born in Norway or have spent most of their life in Norway but still face a constant risk of being deported. Even though the child welfare system has a responsibility for all children who are at risk in a country, the system seems to remain distant when it concerns undocumented and asylum-seeking children.

The workers surveyed all have some experience working with migrant children and their families and know the challenges and problems the child welfare system and the services users face. From the literature on street-level bureaucracy (Evans and Harris, 2004; Lipsky, 1980), we know that frontline workers matter not only because they implement welfare policies but also because they define a system's goals and services. To explore issues around undocumented migrant children, we presented child welfare workers with a very simple scenario about an undocumented child who does not attend school. We asked whether this child would be the responsibility of the child welfare system in their country. The findings show that most workers (75%) think that an undocumented child who does not attend school is the child welfare system's responsibility. However, there are country differences: Canada, Finland, and the United States scored significantly lower than the rest of the countries, saying that an undocumented child who is not attending school is not the child welfare system's responsibility. Finland exhibited the lowest level and also stands out because half of the sample responded with "I don't know" if an undocumented child who does not attend school is the responsibility of the child welfare system. In Canada, about 20% answered that they do not know. Overall, 13% of respondents expressed not knowing their area of responsibility when it comes to an undocumented child not attending school. We believe that this relatively high proportion of workers calls for further examination in the future. The fact that 25% of survey respondents did not consider undocumented children who are not attending school the child welfare system's responsibility indicates that this group of children may fall through the cracks of welfare states when it comes to educational access and social mobility.

In summary, the survey results demonstrate that there are variations within countries. Workers are split in their suggested decisions about how to proceed and their views on what services they can or should provide. In some countries there is a considerable number of workers who are uncertain about the policies and regulations around migrant children—a finding that we find worrying. Seen in a positive light, this is a problem that could be solved with appropriate information and training. We could not detect any systematic differences in the survey responses that correspond to different types of child welfare systems, welfare state models, or degree of child well-being index (on the dimensions established by UNICEF). Cross-country differences and similarities did not follow these dimensions. This may be due to the survey questions, but it may also be due to the fact that the issues we surveyed involved migrant children and families—a population that the child welfare and welfare state taxonomies and UNICEF indices do not specifically address.

PERSPECTIVES

Child Welfare Systems and Migrant Children's Well-Being and Rights

There is a dearth of scholarship on the relationship between welfare state types and types of child welfare systems (Pösö, Skivenes, and Hestbæk, 2013), even though the connection between these two systems often seems to be taken for granted. For example, on the one hand, the social democratic welfare states, with generous and universal welfare services, a high degree of decommodification and, perhaps, most importantly, a high degree of solidarity between individuals in society (in the sense of perceived responsibility of social inclusion for all), seem to offer family services systems with low thresholds for providing services and welfare state services (Pösö et al., 2013). In these systems, only a fine line demarcates where welfare state services end and child welfare services begin. On the other hand, the liberal welfare states rely on the family and private (market) providers of services that individuals in these societies can purchase (if they can afford them), with little collective responsibility for all individuals in society. In countries embracing this welfare state regime, we see that child welfare systems intervene primarily when there is a high risk and danger for the child. Clearly, these two types of welfare states and child welfare systems expect (and accept) differences in vulnerable children's living conditions and possibilities for development, education, and prosperity. We are particularly interested in this difference in perspectives because it may reflect a certain conceptualization of children and their rights. The differences in perspective also have different implications for migrant children and their families. Thus we would expect to see differences in migrant children's well-being and rights between countries based on the system differences.

The most recent UNICEF report measuring children's well-being, which we presented in chapter 1 in this book, does partially support this hypothesis if we use children's standard of well-being in a country as an accurate measurement of difference (UNICEF, 2013). Three of the four family service child welfare systems within social democratic welfare states—Finland, Norway, and the Netherlands—are ranked high on the child well-being list. On the bottom of the ranking we see the countries with child protection child welfare systems within liberal welfare states. Here two countries,[1] the United States and Estonia, score low on children's well-being standards. However, Canada and the United Kingdom, also two countries with child protection–oriented child welfare systems in liberal welfare regimes, are ranked in the middle category of children's well-being group, above Austria and Spain, whereas Italy is in the lowest well-being group. These rankings reveal that welfare state and child welfare system typologies themselves are not sufficient indicators for understanding the developments in children's well-being in different countries (see also Gilbert et al., 2011). We suspect that these differences may stem from differences in child-focused orientations and perspectives, an emerging orientation that Gilbert et al. call "child focus." The UNICEF child well-being ranking resonates with the preliminary findings that were pointed out by Gilbert et al.: Finland, Norway, and the Netherlands evidenced a strong child orientation, and England and Canada showed a clear focus on children's needs for protection.

How can this book, which is focused on migrant children, contribute conceptually to our understanding of the relationship between welfare states and child welfare systems when it comes to ethnic and national background, diversity, and childhood? While there are overlaps in the situation of vulnerable migrant and nonmigrant children who come into contact with child welfare systems, such as the likelihood of poverty as indicated in chapter 1, there are also significant differences related to a range of factors, including ethnic minority background, legal status, and migration experience. Can we see a pattern in the orientations toward migrant children in countries with child welfare systems with different orientations toward children?

Indeed, we did detect a pattern emerging in all child welfare systems concerning the needs and rights of migrant children: they have not been fully met by any system. The overall message from the 11 countries involved in this book is that all child welfare systems have some weaknesses and blind spots in meeting the needs of vulnerable groups of migrant children. This is true for countries with expansive services for children and families and high levels of recognition of children's rights, as well as for countries with more limited welfare services; it is also true for countries that have a long history of working with migrant families, as well as for those without such a long history. We saw, for example, that children's (or parents') legal migration status may trump children's needs and rights in decisions concerning a child in need of protection. Further, immigration services tend to have an adult-centered approach that excludes children and their particular needs from relevant public support. The chapters in this book have also demonstrated that all the child welfare systems provide protective measures to migrant children at immediate risk, but they might fail to provide preventive and supportive services to children who are undocumented. We claim that child welfare systems are at their strongest in protecting children and providing services to settled migrant communities—families and children who are documented and recognized by nation-state legislation and bureaucracy. However, the countries under study lack the ethos, policy, and practice to effectively work with migrant children and families who do not meet those criteria. This is a major problem as those groups of children may be in an extremely vulnerable position because they or their parents are undocumented.

Child welfare systems have not fully recognized that children may be exposed to different vulnerabilities in the migration process from those of adults. Rather, children tend to be treated as family members whose interests and rights are considered the same as that of the "family," especially parents. The tendency to address children in such an adult-centered way is strong also in migration policy and research in general (Dobson, 2009; White, Ní Laoire, Tyrrel, and Carpena-Mendez, 2011; Gardner, 2012). Most children migrate with their families, and therefore their family membership is important in terms of the country to which they migrate. However, child welfare systems also interact with children who migrate on their own without any parental care or existing family ties in the new country. Children are also left behind in countries of origin when their adult carers migrate (Parreñas, 2005). Children's migration routes, practices, and experiences may, in fact, significantly differ from those of their parents (White et al., 2011).

It is a challenge for child welfare systems to recognize children's specific experiences in migration (as opposed to their family members) and the variation in experiences of migrating children—for example, they may or may not have lived in war zones or grown up in refugee camps before migrating. It seems even more difficult and yet imperative to develop policy and practice that take these variations and specific experiences into account. It is of course far from straightforward to determine how state policy and child welfare practice should recognize the particular position of migrant children. Recent research suggests that migrant children tend to be treated as vulnerable and as needing (adult) protection, an approach that denies their agency and subjectivity (White et al., 2011).

This may be a special dilemma for child welfare systems as their ethics, policy and practice are motivated by the vulnerabilities of children: child welfare systems are built on the notion that children are in need of protection by the adult society. It is not easy to actualize a rights-based and agency-based type of child protection practice. How, then, can systems recognize the agency of migrant children who have interests and rights on their own, that is, independently of their parents' legal status, or children who are seeking asylum on their own or who are the victims of human trafficking? The country chapters in this book suggest that there are numerous challenges that child welfare systems need to resolve in the future: only a few of them report on child-focused child welfare practices with migrant children.

Toward Global Child Protection

We suggest that a conceptual framework involving the idea of "global child protection" needs to be developed for child protection policy, practice, and research that expands on the present child welfare systems' responses to migrant children and families. The term "global child protection" builds on the messages from the country chapters in this book that highlight that, first, there is a need to address migrant children as agents: migrant children's rights and specific needs should be recognized in their interactions with child welfare systems. Second, there is a need to address child protection as a global issue in which nation-states recognize their responsibilities and duties beyond the nation-state territory, citizens, and inhabitants. Thus this notion builds on the 1989 United Nations Conventions on the Rights of the Child, which, as stated in the introduction chapter of this book, provides a globally recognized normative structure for child welfare. With this concept of global child protection, we suggest that there is a need for recognition of migrant children in policy and practice at both the national level (through a country's laws and policies) and the supra-national level.

Such a global view on child protection recognizes that child welfare systems are as equally interrelated with "the world" as any other social and human systems, and this interrelatedness should be acknowledged (Therborn, 2011). Migration and its diverse impacts have fundamentally changed the agenda for nation-states' child protection systems, and the changes are likely to be even more drastic in the future. It is not only people migrating to another country but the very existence of transnational families (Heymann, Flores-Macias, Hayes, Kennedy, Lahaie, and Earle, 2009; Menjivar and Abrego, 2009; Suarez-Oroczo, 2011) that have challenged existing child welfare systems. The acknowledgment of migrant children's rights requires child welfare systems to consider children regardless of migration status.

Our suggestion for global child protection is built on three main principles:

(1) Children's rights should be recognized in every situation in which the state interacts with migrant children. The legal status of migrant children or their right to remain in the country should not diminish their right for protection (Bhabha, 2009). In other words, the right for protection should overrule any citizenship rule or other types of status related to individual nation-states. Children's agency should be recognized and supported by the child protection policy and practice, even (and especially) when they are in a situation that makes them vulnerable.

(2) Global child protection should recognize the three groups of children related to migration: children who migrate with their families and live in the new country (regardless of their legal status), children who migrate on their own and live in the new country (regardless of their legal status), and children who stay behind in their country of ori-gin while their parents (or other caregiving adults) have migrated. Migrant children who were at risk of harm in their country of origin and leave their country's territory may still be in need of protection and support even after leaving behind the situation that put them at risk in their country of origin.

(3) Children's vulnerability related specifically to migration may have particular characteristics that need attention from child protection policy and practice. The notions of ethnicity and multiculturalism cover, in terms of theory and practice, some of the vulnerabilities; however, children's vulnerability related to migration goes beyond such a framework and requires a more nuanced and comprehen-sive approach, including transnational cultural competency and an understanding of processes of discrimination targeting migrant chil-dren and families in particular. Professional training and research

need to focus on problems encountered by migrant children in the migration process and to produce relevant knowledge and practice recommendations.

To conclude, the global tasks suggested here require that child welfare systems reconsider their tasks and responsibilities in ways that correspond to migrant children's realities and needs, especially those of vulnerable migrant children. The historical roots of modern child welfare systems, which represent an organized institutional response to neglected and abused children, were radically innovative (Lindsey, 2004). It is high time we recultivated those innovative roots to meet the needs of vulnerable migrant children.

NOTE

1   Australia is not included because it did not provide sufficient data to the UNICEF report.

REFERENCES

Abrego, Leisy J., & Gonzales, R. (2010). Blocked paths, uncertain futures: The postsecondary education and labor market prospects of undocumented youth. *Journal of Education for Students Placed at Risk*, 15(1), 144–157.

Barn, R. (1993). *Black Children in the Public Care System*. London: Batsford.

———. (2007). "Race," ethnicity and child welfare: A fine balancing act, critical commentary. *British Journal of Social Work*, 37(8), 1425–1434.

Barn, R., Sinclair, R., & Ferdinand, D. (1997). *Acting on Principle: An Examination of Race and Ethnicity in Social Services Provision to Children and Families*. London: British Agencies for Adoption & Fostering.

Bhabha, J. (2009). Arendt's children: Do today's migrant children have a right to have rights? *Human Rights Quarterly*, 31(2), 410–451.

Chand, A. (2005). Do you speak English? Language barriers in child protection social work with minority ethnic families. *British Journal of Social Work*, 35, 807–321.

Dobson, M. (2009). Unpacking children in migration research. *Children's Geographies*, 3(7), 355–360.

Esping-Andersen, G. (1990). *The Three Worlds of Welfare Capitalism*. London: Polity Press.

Gilbert, N., Parton, N., & Skivenes, M., eds. (2011). *Child Protection Systems: International Trends and Emerging Orientations*. New York: Oxford University Press.

Global Initiative to End All Corporal Punishment of Children. (2012). *Ending Legalised Violence Against Children: Global Report 2012*. Geneva: Global Initiative to End All Corporal Punishment of Children. Retrieved August 6, 2014, from http://www.endcorporalpunishment.org/pages/pdfs/reports/GlobalReport2012.pdf.

Gonzales, Roberto G., & Chavez, Leo R. (2012). "Awakening to a nightmare:" Abjectivity and illegality in the lives of undocumented 1.5 generation Latino immigrants in the United States. *Current Anthropology*, 53(3), 255–281.

Heymann, J., Flores-Macias, F., Hayes, J.A., Kennedy, M., Lahaie, C., & Earle, A. (2009). The impact of migration on the well-being of transnational families: New data from sending communities in Mexico. *Community, Work & Family*, 12(1), 91–103.

Humphreys, C., Atkar, S., & Baldwin, N. (1999). Discrimination in child protection work: Recurring themes in work with Asian families. *Child and Family Social Work*, 4, 283–291.

Ife, J. (2001). *Human Rights and Social Work: Towards Rights-Based Practice*. Cambridge: Cambridge University Press.

Križ, K., & Skivenes, M. (2010). Lost in translation: How child welfare workers in Norway and England experience language difficulties when working with minority ethnic families. *British Journal of Social Work*, 40, 1353–1367.

———. (2012). How child welfare workers perceive their work with undocumented immigrant families: An explorative study of challenges and coping strategies. *Children and Youth Services Review*, 34, 790–797.

Lindsey, D. (2004). *The Welfare of Children*. New York: Oxford University Press.

Lipsky, M. (1980). *Street-Level Bureaucracy: Dilemmas of the Individual in Public Services*. New York: Russell Sage.

Menjivar, C., & Abrego, L. (2009). Parents and children across borders: Legal instability and intergenerational relations in Guatemalan and Salvadoran families. In N. Foner (Ed.), *Across Generations: Immigrant Families in America*, 160–189. New York: New York University Press.

Parreñas, R. (2005). *Children of Global Migration*. Stanford: Stanford University Press.

Pösö, T., Skivenes, M., & Hestbæk, A.-D. (2013). Child protection systems within the Danish, Finnish and Norwegian welfare states—Time for a child centric approach? *European Journal of Social Work*, 1, 1–16.

Sigona, N., & Hughes, V. (2012). *No Way Out, No Way In: Irregular Migrant Children and Families in the UK*. Oxford: Centre on Migration, Policy and Society.

Skytte, M. (2002). *Anbringelse av etniske minoritetsbørn* (Out of Home Placements of Ethnic Minority Children). Lund: Lunds Universitet.

Suarez-Orozco, C., Bang, H.J., & Kim, H.Y. (2011). I felt like my heart was staying behind: Psychological implications of family separations and reunifications for immigrant youth. *Journal of Adolescent Research*, 26(2), 222–257.

Therborn, G. (2011). *The World—A Beginner's Guide*. Cambridge: Polity Press.

UNICEF. (2009). *Children in Immigrant Families in Eight Affluent Countries: Their Family, National and International Context*. Florence: UNICEF. Retrieved April 22, 2013, from http://www.globalmigrationgroup.org/uploads/gmg-topics/children/2.A_Children_in_immigrant_families_in_eight_affluent_countries_UNICEF_IRC.pdf.

———. (2013). *Child Well-Being in Rich Countries: A Comparative Overview*. Florence: UNICEF. Retrieved on December 17, 2013, from http://www.unicef-irc.org/publications/pdf/rc11_eng.pdf.

Vericker, T., Kuehn, D., & Capps, R. (2007). *Title IV-E Funding: Funded Foster Care Placements by Child Generation and Ethnicity. Findings from Texas*. Urban Institute Child Welfare Research Program Brief 3. Washington, DC: Urban Institute.

White, A., Ni Laoire, C., Tyrrel, N., & Carpena-Mendez, F. (2011). Children's roles in transnational migration. *Journal of Ethnic and Migration Studies*, 8(37), 1159–1170.

Williamson, J.G. (2006). Global migration. *Finance and Development*, 43 (3). Retrieved August 18, 2012, from http://www.imf.org/external/pubs/ft/fandd/2006/09/williams.htm.

APPENDIX—SURVEY METHOD OVERVIEW

The survey examines the experiences that frontline child welfare workers have when working with migrant children and families. It also provides background information about the workers. We asked the same questions in all countries and presented workers with two vignettes. The survey was developed in English and was then translated back and forth to make sure we had the correct translation for the non-English-speaking countries. Detailed information about the practical steps in the data collection process can be found at http://www.hib.no/avd_ahs/fou/book_project.asp.

A total of 845 child welfare workers, from nine countries, contributed to the data collection in our survey. However, the number of participants answering the survey in each country varied, as shown in Table A.1. This is an important matter to keep in mind when reading the findings we present in the book.

Table A.1. Overview of countries and number of participants who answered the survey

Country	Number of participants
Norway	168
Estonia	22
Canada	33
USA	103
Italy	90
England	72
Austria	193
Spain	87
Finland	76

The first vignette that workers in nine countries were presented with is about a newborn baby:

CASE 1 Imagine that you as a child welfare worker are responsible for the following case

The child welfare agency is contacted by a hospital concerning a young mother and father with a newborn baby. The baby is healthy and the mother is recovering well after the birth. The parents speak limited English. Their housing condition is poor and lacks basic amenities. They left their home country because they could not find any work there and moved to England eight months ago to find a job. They have not been successful in finding work here either and live in extreme poverty. They do not have access to running warm water, and the parents look undernourished. The parents are desperate because they cannot see any future in their home country, but they do not find any ways to cope in this country, either.

Based on this case, we asked workers to assess the level of risk on a 5-point scale ranging from "no risk" to "very high risk," and thereafter we asked them to identify which factors in the case were decisive for their assessment. Furthermore we asked what they would do in the case, using closed answers from "do nothing" to "removal of the baby." We also asked a few knowledge and attitude questions based on the case.

The second vignette is about a 10-year-old girl who is beaten by her parents. For this case we tested whether there is any impact of parents' relation to the labor market (unemployed or employed) and welfare services.

CASE 2 Imagine again that you as a child welfare worker are responsible for the following case

A health nurse reported the case of a 10-year-old girl to the child welfare authorities who was apparently mistreated by her parents. The girl has marks on her arms and back. In an interview with the child welfare authorities, the girl reported being beaten by her parents. The parents are immigrants and came to England five years ago. *Both parents are employed and work long hours.* They do not think they mistreat their daughter and say they have to discipline her because she is lazy and does not do her chores. They also find her disrespectful of their family traditions.

We also asked about risk level in relation to this case and what workers would suggest should be done. A randomized half of the sample received the version of Case 2 as it was outlined above, and the rest of the sample were given an identical case, in which the sentence in italics was substituted with the following sentence: "Both parents are unemployed and receive financial support through welfare services."

INDEX